MAMMOGRAPHIC INTERPRETATION

MAMMOGRAPHIC INTERPRETATION

A Practical Approach

Second Edition

Marc J. Homer, M.D.

Professor of Radiology
Tufts University School of Medicine
Chief, Mammography Section
Senior Radiologist
New England Medical Center Hospitals
Boston, Massachusetts

Foreword by

Edward A. Sickles, M.D.

McGraw-Hill
HEALTH PROFESSIONS DIVISION

New York   St. Louis   San Francisco   Auckland Bogotá
Caracas   Lisbon London   Madrid   Mexico City   Milan
Montreal   New Delhi   San Juan   Singapore   Sydney   Tokyo   Toronto

McGraw-Hill

A Division of The **McGraw·Hill** Companies

MAMMOGRAPHIC INTERPRETATION
A Practical Approach, Second Edition

1 2 3 4 5 6 7 8 9 0 KGPKGP 9 8 7 6

ISBN 0-07-029720-7

This book was set in Century Schoolbook by York Graphic Services, Inc.
The editors were James T. Morgan and Steven Melvin;
the production supervisor was Richard Ruzycka;
the cover and text were designed by Marsha Cohen/Parallelogram;
the index was prepared by Jerry Ralya.
Quebecor/Kingsport was printer and binder.

This book is printed on acid-free paper.

Cataloguing-in-publication data is on file for this title at the Library of Congress.

To my wife, Diane, and my sons, Ross and Seth. I have tried my best to minimize the impact this project had on family time.

CONTENTS

Marc Homer has earned a nationwide reputation as an expert *teacher* of mammography interpretation, in no small part due to the very successful postgraduate breast imaging course he conducts both at his own New England Medical Center Hospitals and elsewhere around the country. More than most teachers, he has a keen ability to understand his students' insecurities and to overcome them by offering the practical solutions he has devised to solve his own imaging problems. Rather than using the language of statistics and literature citations to support a specific approach, he often chooses the more familiar language of common sense. Some of his most effective teaching comes by providing realistic analogies between common mammographic situations and those faced in general radiology practice. If, as he argues, it is unnecessary in reporting a normal chest x-ray examination to add that cancer cannot be excluded, why then must one incorporate such a disclaimer into the normal mammography report?

True to Dr. Homer's style of teaching, this book is intensely personal, directly focusing on the day-to-day needs of the working radiologist. It is a faithful translation into print of his postgraduate mammography course, both with respect to written material and illustrations. It is *not* a scholarly text book, nor is it intended to be. Rather, it is designed to be an "easy read," a guide to achieving peace of mind in interpreting mammograms, even if some of the message may be unconventional in format and content.

The radiologist inexperienced with mammography is likely to integrate many of Dr. Homer's teachings into his or her own practice, deriving maximum benefit from the book. Subspecialist mammographers, who already have devised their own successful strategies of interpretation, also will profit from exposure to the Homer ideology if only to gain a better understanding of the multiplicity of approaches with which mammographic problems can be solved. Radiologists who already have completed Dr. Homer's postgraduate course will find that the book reinforces now familiar concepts; those in the process of taking the course will find it a superb companion.

Edward A. Sickles, M.D.

PREFACE TO THE SECOND EDITION

This book is based on the course in mammographic interpretation that I have been giving in Boston since 1981 and this second edition reflects the evolutionary changes in that course. The preface to the first edition of this book describes the background and objectives of both the course and this text. References in every chapter have been updated. New concepts in interpretation such as the "tattoo sign" for the recognition of dermal calcifications, and new concepts regarding technique, such as the proper way to place a metallic marker on an area of focal concern, have been added.

Three new chapters appear in this second edition. The first is devoted to breast implants. The imaging of breast implants, and the recognition of associated abnormalities such as rupture, have assumed a great deal of importance in the last several years. At Tufts-New England Medical Center, we do not image a large number of patients with breast implants (fortunately!) so our experience in this area is limited. Kathleen M. Harris, M.D., has written a chapter about breast implants for this second edition. In it she draws upon her experience from her practice at Magee Breast Center in Pittsburgh.

The ancillary role of ultrasound as a complement to mammography for the detection of breast cancer continues to increase in importance. New advances in technology allow the radiologist to better identify and evaluate normal and abnormal processes in the breast. In addition, the field of interventional breast ultrasound has exploded within the past several years. Its use in aspiration, core biopsy, and needle localization has been clearly established. Frederick J. Doherty, M.D., who is the head of the ultrasound section at Tufts-New England Medical Center and gives the ultrasound lecture in the course, has authored the new ultrasound chapter. Aspects of both diagnosis and intervention are presented.

Delay of diagnosis of cancer is one of the most serious malpractice claims that can be brought against a physician. Within the last several years, breast cancer has become the most frequent cancer where a delay of diagnosis is alleged. As the utilization of mammography increases, inevitably the number of radiologists who become involved in lawsuits dealing with delay of diagnosis of breast cancer increases. All radiologists involved in the field of breast imaging should be aware of the medicolegal issues which involve many aspects of breast cancer diagnosis and intervention. I have written the final chapter of this edition to address malpractice issues regarding mammography. The chapter defines the extent of the problem, identifies common areas of malpractice exposure, and offers suggestions of how to minimize these exposures.

Finally additional test cases have been added to the second portion of the book. They have been selected to present challenges in interpretation or management. I am grateful to Dr. Harris for submitting cases about breast implants to supplement my own material.

In writing this second edition, it became apparent to me that the principles of mammographic interpretation that I use and teach have remained the same since my first course in 1981. This is as it should be because the goal of every teacher is to give students principles which have withstood the test of time. The concepts of interpretation in this text meet this goal. I hope that the material in this second edition either reinforces principles of interpretation the reader already uses, or introduces new ones to be considered and tested in clinical practice.

PREFACE TO THE FIRST EDITION

This book is based upon the course in mammographic interpretation that I have been giving since 1981. It is divided into two sections. The first section presents and illustrates the principles used in mammographic interpretation, reviews the signs of malignant and benign breast disease, and covers other topics, including the mammography report, male breast disease, mammography of breast conservation therapy, and percutaneous needle localization of nonpalpable breast lesions. The second section consists of test cases, which illustrate how the principles of mammographic interpretation are used.

The material in this book should prove helpful to all radiologists who interpret mammograms regardless of their level of training. Those with less experience will be presented with a logical pragmatic approach to mammographic interpretation. Those with more experience will appreciate the material on a different level, since they will recognize that the principles and cases address recurrent problems that they confront in daily practice. The test cases should also prove especially useful for radiology residents preparing for their boards in diagnostic radiology.

Since the approach in this book places a great deal of emphasis on the interaction between the radiologist and the referring clinician, physicians who order mammographic examinations of their patients should also find the material helpful in their practice. To provide optimal patient care, such specialists as gynecologists, surgeons, internists, and family practitioners must be knowledgeable about the role of mammography in the detection of breast cancer.

In the older days (pre-1980), very few radiologists willingly became involved with mammography as a result of an interest developed and nurtured during their residency training. My interest in mammography began rather abruptly when I was told by my future chairman Dr. Robert E. Paul, Jr., that when I joined the staff of the Department of Radiology of New England Medical Center Hospitals (NEMCH), the primary teaching hospital of Tufts University School of Medicine, my responsibilities would include interpreting the one or two mammograms done daily. Dr. Paul was unperturbed by my immediate confession that I had never been systematically trained how to read a mammogram and had never, in fact, read a mammogram in my life. I remember confessing to a total and complete ignorance regarding this diagnostic radiology examination. He appreciated my honesty and advised me to use the next few months before the start of my job to read about mammography. He further assured me that he would be understanding and felt certain that after a few months of actually reading mammograms and taking courses, I would feel more comfortable about this examination. I accepted the position and for the next months voraciously devoured mammographic texts, motivated by a real terror that soon I alone would be assuming total responsibility for interpreting the Department's mammograms.

Thus my professional experience with actually interpreting mammograms can be dated precisely to when I began my job at NEMCH, on July 1, 1977. I started this assignment feeling confident, since the wisdom of others was fresh in my mind from recent months of intense reading. I understood the differences between benign and malignant breast masses, and I felt that I could distinguish between benign and malignant breast microcalcifications. I had read all the literature pertaining to the increasingly important technique of preoperative percutaneous needle localization for nonpalpable breast lesions. However, my confidence was quickly shattered by the realization that the more experience in mammographic interpretation I accumulated, the less I understood. What I felt certain was benign more often than not turned out to be malignant, and vice versa. My frustrations mounted daily.

However, throughout this ordeal I was very fortunate to have had the support and encouragement of my chairman. In addition, I had the support of the surgeons who biopsied the lesions that I localized. My surgical colleagues who deserve thanks for their understanding and patience include Drs. Douglas J. Marchant, Thomas J. Smith, George W. Mitchell, Jr., Harry H. Miller, and Decio M. Rangel. None of the correlation between my needle localizations, gross pathology, and the definitive histology could have been accomplished without the assistance of the many pathologists who patiently sliced each specimen and waited for me to perform repeat specimen radiography of the tissue sections so that precise analysis was possible. I could never have learned anything without this accurate correlation. I owe thanks to Dr. Homa Safaii, whose expertise in breast pathology was so important in many of my projects. I am also indebted to my oncology colleagues Drs. Nicholas J. Robert and Steven W. Papish and my radiation therapy colleagues Drs. Rupert Schmidt-Ullrich and David E. Wazer for teaching me about the treatment of breast cancer. My very special thanks go to Patricia M. Izzo, senior mammography technologist at NEMCH, who has worked with me from the beginning.

After my first year, I confided to my chairman that despite his prediction, I still did not feel comfortable with mammographic interpretation. But of one thing I was pretty certain: I saw more breast cancers in that one year than all of the colon, kidney, pancreas, and stomach cancers that I saw during the entire three years of my residency in diagnostic radiology. I recognized not only that this disease was as common as the literature stated (1 in 13 in those days), but also that its occurrence in women below the age of 40 was not a rarity. It was these realizations that fueled my desire to understand mammography, because it was the only test available that enabled early detection of what was obviously a common disease.

It is a unique experience for a physician to learn about an examination with absolutely no preconceived biases from past teachers. Since no one taught me about mammography during my residency years, I was able to approach it as a blank slate, believing only what my own experience proved to me to be true.

In the spring of 1981, I offered my first teaching course in mammographic interpretation at NEMCH.

This course could never have been offered without the administrative support and encouragement of Ed Cohen. Although there were only five registrants, I taught the course anyway. Their enthusiastic comments and suggestions encouraged me to offer it again, and since then hundreds of radiologists have trained with me. Their feedback by phone and letter has been gratifying. Through this feedback I realized that the effort put into the course was appreciated because its contents, principles, and practical approach have helped radiologists to recognize the limitations of mammography, define their role on the team of physicians who care for patients with breast cancer, and provide practical help in mammographic interpretation and breast ultrasound, resulting in better patient care. This text is an outgrowth of the course, I am grateful to Drs. Rick Doherty and Bob Zamenhof for their participation in this course. My final thanks go to Judy Dean, who maintained a reasonable sense of humor as she was typing this text.

My course is the result of a sincere desire to teach what I have painfully learned on my own. Its goal is to help others get off to a better start interpreting mammograms by avoiding common mistakes and pitfalls. Judging by the feedback of my colleagues who have trained with me, this goal has often been achieved. If this text helps realize the same goal, then the time that I have devoted to it was well spent.

MAMMOGRAPHIC INTERPRETATION

OBJECTIVES AND THOUGHTS

OBJECTIVES _____

At the outset it might be helpful to clearly define what this teaching text is not meant to be as well as what it is meant to be. It is not meant to be an encyclopedic compilation of every disease that can involve the breast, nor is it meant to be a radiographic collection of breast pathology. It is not intended to present a multidisciplinary approach to every abnormal disease state of the breast. Finally, it is not meant to review every modality that can be used to image the breast. Excellent texts covering this material already exist, and duplication is unnecessary.

The first portion of this text presents a logical approach to aid in the interpretation of mammographic findings. Also, the ancillary role of ultrasound as it relates to the interpretation of mammographic findings will be included. Ultrasound has proved to be invaluable for aiding in the analysis of certain mammographic problems and should be viewed as a necessary adjunct to mammographic interpretation.

The emphasis in this text is placed upon practicality and patient care. While a rare disease may fleetingly capture one's interest, and while radiographs with dramatic findings can arouse any lethargic reader, most who practice radiology will never see rare diseases or uncommon radiographic findings. The material covered in this text is meant to be extremely practical and clinically oriented. Everyday problems in mammographic interpretation will be presented, and a rational approach for management options will be proposed. Thus the exclusion from this teaching text of rare breast diseases and unusual infrequent mammographic findings is deliberate. Readers who hope to find within these pages an illustration of hemangiosarcoma of the breast will be sorely disappointed.

The second portion of this text consists of test cases. Cases were chosen not because they represent unusual entities but because they highlight recurrent diagnostic problems faced in the daily practice of mammography. In many instances, the teaching points relate more to patient management than to the mammographic findings.

THE CLINICAL SETTING OF ONE'S MAMMOGRAPHIC PRACTICE _____

It is quite understandable that many of the perceptions that one has about the practice of mammography come from one's personal experience. Naturally, this experience may vary widely and differ significantly because of the difference in practice settings. The radiologist who works at an academic center and has referrals exclusively from breast surgeons will undoubtedly be able to manage patients and dictate reports much differently than will a radiologist who receives referrals primarily from family practitioners. Both of these radiologists will function differently from those who screen self-referred women. The radiologist who has the permission of colleagues to perform needle cytology immediately upon the discovery of a breast abnormality certainly will have an approach that differs from that of a radiologist who does not have this option.

What works in one clinical setting may be absolutely unsuitable and unacceptable for a different clinical setting, but not necessarily because a particular approach is wrong. I have always found it helpful when listening to colleagues explain how they manage patients to inquire about their particular practice setting. If this setting is quite different from mine, then I can understand why some of their approaches may not work for me.

The patients I see at New England Medical Center Hospitals (NEMCH) are a mix of second opinion cases with referrals directly from breast surgeons and patients who are referred from physicians for routine screening examinations. Some of these patients, in fact, are referred from non-M.D. health care providers. It is my policy not to accept self-referred patients.

INSTITUTING CHANGE

Over the years, radiologists who have returned to their clinical setting from my course have frequently expressed a real sense of frustration about being unable to modify practices regarding mammography. This problem is important enough to consider at this time. Only a naive person will believe that modifying a current practice will be speedy and painless. In my experience, as well as in the experience of others, such change is often painful and slow. Interestingly, not only is there resistance from our colleagues in other disciplines, but there is often a resistance from our partners who do not want to quickly change their long-standing practices. This resistance is understandable, since one is naturally reluctant to change old practices unless there is a real perception of a need for change.

I would like the reader to know that if there are some new perceptions that come from this text that lead to the desire to change or modify current practice, one should not be surprised if resistance is encountered. My only advice is not to let this frustration lead to the abandonment of the desire to change. The resistance to change can be attributed to many reasons that can vary widely from ego to economics. I advise you to be patient. In my own situation, it took 4 to 5 years before many of the concepts presented in this text were eventually accepted (sometimes only grudgingly, at best) by all of my clinicians and pathologists.

MAMMOGRAPHY AS A DIAGNOSTIC X-RAY EXAMINATION

For reasons that will be explained in the next chapter, many radiologists believe that mammography is so different from other diagnostic radiologic examinations that there is a much higher level of anxiety associated

with it. I would disagree. If radiologists would approach a mammographic problem with the same standards and insights that they use when approaching other diagnostic radiologic examinations, I believe that some of the apparent differences between mammography and other examinations would disappear. One of the techniques that I use in my course, and which will be used throughout this text, will be to draw analogies between mammographic situations and more familiar situations in general diagnostic radiology. I believe that this helps put problems into a more familiar context, which makes them much easier to relate to and deal with.

For example, many radiologists express real concern about the inability to quantitate certain things on the mammogram. I am unable to give anyone a measurement as to how much subareolar asymmetry is allowed between the right breast and left breast. I am unable to define how large a microcalcification is. I am also unable to give a measurement for deciding when localized skin thickening becomes generalized skin thickening. Why should this uncertainty be viewed any differently than other uncertainties we constantly live with in other areas of diagnostic radiology? I would be willing to wager that the reader has had the occasion to look at a chest radiograph where the hilar areas appear somewhat prominent. Scrutiny of the paratracheal stripe, the mediastinum, and the azygos node region reveals them to be normal in size. The lateral chest x-ray similarly is quite normal. When the history states "preoperative chest x-ray for dental extraction in a 23-year-old male," the report probably will come out with a conclusion of "normal chest x-ray." This same chest x-ray with a different history stating "rule out lymphoma" will generate a different report that would probably question the possibility of hilar prominence and would recommend a CT.

We are guided by the clinical context when we interpret other diagnostic x-rays, and similarly, this weighs into the equation when reading a mammogram. As a general diagnostic radiologist, I have learned to live with the fact that I cannot rely on an absolute measurement for the volume of a hilus or a scientific way to radiographically differentiate between a large area of atelectasis and a pneumonia. We recognize that we cannot adequately interpret a radiograph in the absence of appropriate clinical information. The uncertainties in mammography are not unique.

VIEWING ANOTHER APPROACH

Concepts presented in this text have evolved from my experience over the years based upon close clinical, radiographic, surgical, and pathologic correlation. I am fully cognizant of the fact that there are different ways to approach and analyze mammographic problems. This is not an earth-shattering insight, since physicians know that there are probably few medical areas where there is only one correct course of action. In fact, there are often excellent physicians who strongly disagree about aspects of diagnosis or disease management. Mammography is no different, and I want to state unequivocally now that I never mean to imply that a particular approach presented here is necessarily more acceptable than others.

Some of the approaches within this text may be at variance with the teachings of others. One should not be surprised if there are significant differences between concepts in this text and one's current practices. Hopefully, the concepts in this text will be intuitively correct to those readers who have experience in mammographic interpretation. Whenever anyone teaches, I always would encourage the listener to be skeptical and have an attitude that says "prove it to me." In my teaching course I challenge radiologists to be skeptical but open-minded. I offer the same challenge to the readers of this text.

WHY MAMMOGRAPHY IS PERCEIVED TO BE "DIFFERENT"

Many radiologists perceive mammography to be different from other diagnostic radiographic examinations. This perception is probably a cause for the heightened level of anxiety some radiologists have about the examination. While there are certain aspects of mammography that make it appear to be a more formidable challenge when compared with other radiographic examinations, in reality most of these aspects are not unique to mammography. When these aspects are defined, put into perspective, and fully understood, one might be able to approach mammography with a less frightened and more positive attitude. Conquering the beast requires knowledge of its strengths and weaknesses.

FALSE-NEGATIVE RATE

Imagine you were asked to perform an upper GI series on a patient with a known 3-cm pre-pyloric ulcer on the lesser curvature of the stomach documented by endoscopy. It is a reasonable expectation that a competent radiologist should not have too much difficulty in finding the ulcer, taking films to document its existence, and defining its features. I would be willing to wager that if there were a 10-percent failure rate in being able to find this 3-cm ulcer, there would be a perpetually high level of anxiety regarding the upper GI series. Every radiologist interpreting mammograms will experience (unfortunately more than once) a situation in which the mammogram shows no variation

from normal despite the fact that the clinician, the patient, and even the radiologist are able to palpate a definite mass. The false-negative rate for mammography is estimated to be approximately 5 to 15 percent.[1-3] In a reported consecutive series of 70 patients with palpable breast carcinoma, I did not detect malignancy in five cases, or 7 percent. In a retrospective review of these five cases, one cancer could have been identified because of the presence of subtle architectural distortion, but in the other four cases I still could not recognize any direct or indirect sign of malignancy.[4] Table 2-1 lists the major causes of the false-negative mammogram. These causes include some that are avoidable, some that can be minimized, and some that are unavoidable.

Imaging the Region of Interest

In the situation in which the patient knows where a suspected mass is located, one should strive to image

TABLE 2-1 _____
REASONS FOR THE FALSE-NEGATIVE MAMMOGRAM

1. Failure to image the region of interest
2. Obscuration of the mass by overlying breast tissue
3. Poor image quality
4. Errors of perception
5. Breast cancer indistinguishable from "normal" breast tissue

the area on the mammogram. The responsibility to do this rests squarely upon the shoulders of both the technologist and the radiologist. Sometimes ancillary views are required to image certain areas of the breast, such as far medially (Fig. 2-1), far laterally (Fig. 2-2), in the axillary region,[5] or deep near the chest wall[6] (Fig. 2-3). Tricks, including using a coat hanger, have been helpful in imaging a palpable mass.[7]

Occasionally, the area of the suspected palpable abnormality is impossible to image despite special maneuvers. This will be particularly true when the patient has some skeletal deformity preventing optimal positioning, when the patient is uncooperative (such as a mentally retarded patient who cannot sit still during the exposure), or when the woman has such painful breasts that she cannot tolerate optimal compression. When the area under question cannot be imaged, the radiology report should contain this information so that the clinician clearly understands that the region of concern is off the film and cannot be analyzed and that the mammogram, therefore, provides no information about the abnormality. In my practice, if there is a palpable area, the technologist will place a metallic marker on the area and obtain a view in true lateral projection

as well as a compression magnification view in craniocaudal (CC) projection.

Sometimes the questioned palpable breast mass is unable to be imaged on the mammogram because it is, in fact, not in the breast. Rib lesions and soft tissue masses adjacent to the breast on occasion may be mistakenly thought to be within the breast. In this situation the radiology report should transmit this information to the clinician by stating that the palpable mass is not imaged on the mammogram because it is not contained in breast parenchyma.

Another pitfall is mistaking a mammographic abnormality for the palpable abnormality. If a woman presents with a palpable mass in the breast and the radiologist detects an abnormality in the area, the question must always be asked: Does the palpable finding correspond to the mammographic finding? If there is any doubt, the question usually can be simply resolved by placing a metallic marker over the palpable abnormality and obtaining another film. To automatically assume that a mammographic abnormality and a palpable abnormality are the same thing can be dangerous (Fig. 2-4).

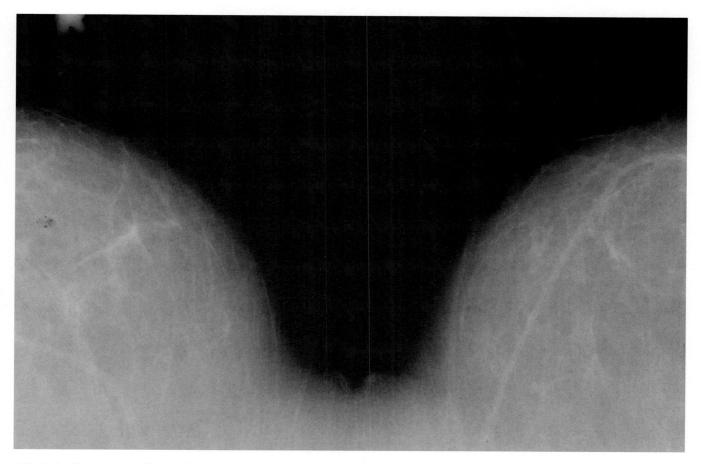

FIG. 2-1 *The most medial portion of each breast can be imaged on this single cleavage view.*

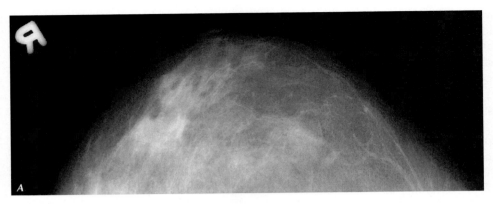

FIG. 2-2 **A.** *Mammogram was performed to evaluate a palpable mass in the right upper outer quadrant. CC view shows no abnormality.*

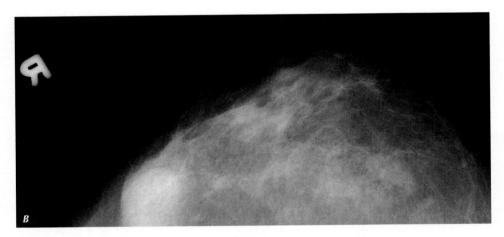

FIG. 2-2 *(Continued)* **B.** *On this CC view with the patient rotated medially, the 3-cm mass is easily seen. Histology revealed a benign fibroadenoma.*

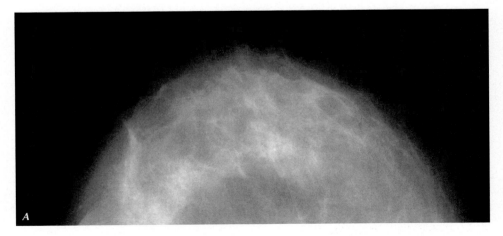

FIG. 2-3 **A.** *Mammogram was performed to evaluate a 2-cm palpable mass in the right breast, close to the chest wall in the 12 o'clock position. CC view is unremarkable.*

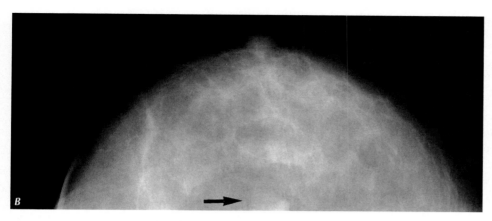

FIG. 2-3 *(Continued)* **B.** *Modified CC projection using wedge-shaped sponge demonstrates the mass (arrow) at the chest wall. Histology revealed a benign fibroadenoma.*

Overlying Breast Tissue

Usually the routine number of views taken of each breast is two. These are the CC view and an oblique (OBL) projection. When these views do not optimally project a palpable mass away from normal dense breast parenchyma or fibrosis to allow it to be recognized, ancillary views may be required to discern the mass. However, sometimes the breast is so dense that no view will succeed in separating a mass from the other tissue density to allow its recognition.

Poor Images

Poor images may be caused by technical factors, including overpenetration, underpenetration, poor positioning, and suboptimal compression. Technologists

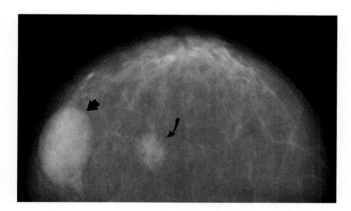

FIG. 2-4 *This 65-year-old woman had a mammogram for a palpable mass in the right breast. After reviewing the mammogram with the clinician it became clear that the mass with the sharp borders (straight arrow) was the palpable abnormality, while the mass with irregular borders (curved arrow) was nonpalpable. The large mass proved to be a benign fibroadenoma, and the smaller one was an invasive ductal carcinoma.*

performing mammography should know how to quality control the images. This is particularly important in a practice setting where the radiologist is not available to review every examination before the patient leaves. Obviously, a balance must exist between the reluctance to repeat additional views of the breast and the desire to be certain that the examination is diagnostically acceptable. This is no different than with other radiographic examinations.

Another area related to poor images that deserves attention is poor processing. Considerable information is lost by using processors that are not optimized for mammography or that are not maintained properly. Film companies are most eager to assist the interested radiologist in evaluating, optimizing, and correcting processor problems. A final area causing inadequate images is poor equipment. As with all radiographic equipment, periodic quality control by an experienced person must be performed regularly.[8] The Mammography Quality Standards Act of 1992 established a national standard for quality assurance.

Errors of Perception

Radiologists commit errors of two kinds: not perceiving the abnormality and misinterpreting the significance of the abnormality. While education will decrease the incidence of misinterpretation of findings, errors of perception are more difficult to overcome. The signs of breast cancer, especially early breast cancer, may be extremely subtle. Radiologists should not read mammograms when they are fatigued or rushed. There are very few "emergency" mammograms demanding a stat reading. At the end of the day when one's level of fatigue is the greatest, perhaps one can read the routine preoperative chest x-rays or the bone films from the emergency room, but one should not read the mammograms. While errors of perception can never be totally eliminated, they must be minimized as much as possible.

Tumors Indistinguishable from Breast Tissue

Some breast carcinomas do not make a mass and do not make tumor calcifications. Instead they infiltrate in a fashion that makes the malignancy indistinguishable from normal breast parenchyma. Invasive lobular carcinoma typically infiltrates in this fashion.[9] This is an uncontrollable false-negative and indeed a frightening one. This means that despite optimal technique, a conscientious technologist, good patient cooperation, and expert mammographic interpretation, there are some breast carcinomas that will defy detection by mammography even though they are large enough to be clinically palpable. This is a reality of mammography that radiologists must recognize and accept or they should not be involved with the examination.

DEPENDENCE UPON THE TECHNOLOGIST

There are imaging modalities that are totally dependent upon the expertise of the one performing the examination. Mammography, ultrasound, and GI fluoroscopy are some examinations that share this characteristic. One cannot help but be concerned when one compares a recently performed mammogram with a previous study and sees a difference in the amount of breast tissue imaged without any change in the patient's weight. One cannot automatically assume that the fault lies with the technologist. Possibly during one study the patient had such severe breast pain that no technologist could have compressed or pulled harder to image more breast tissue. This dependence upon the person performing the examination is a real limitation, but if we have learned to accept it for other diagnostic radiographic examinations, we can certainly live with it for mammography. One obvious caveat is that when the examination is judged to be inadequate, the radiologist should not hesitate to recommend a repeat examination.

THE "NORMAL" APPEARANCE OF THE BREAST

If each of us took a pencil and paper and drew a normal kidney, colon, stomach, or pancreas, I suspect that our pictures would look similar. If this exercise were applied to the breast, probably dissimilarity would be the rule. There is no normal appearance of the breast that can be memorized. The breast varies in appearance over the years, changing from the normally dense breast in the younger woman to a more fat-replaced breast in the older woman. It has a different appearance during pregnancy and in the postpartum period. The breast is like a fingerprint; each one is unique. Often the best that we can do on an initial mammogram is to decide whether the breast appearance falls outside of our acceptable "normal" range of appearance. This is a highly subjective determination that evolves as our experience increases. It cannot be easily taught to others. Certainly a more reliable way to recognize an abnormality is by comparing the current mammogram with a prior examination to assess any interval change. The most subtle signs of breast carcinoma can sometimes only be detected in this way (Fig. 2-5).

Though the inability to recognize the appearance of a "normal" breast is rightfully a concern for those interpreting mammograms, we live with similar uncertainty in other areas of diagnostic imaging: How wide is the superior mediastinum allowed to be? How prominent are gastric rugae allowed to be? When do the interstitial markings in the lung become abnormally prominent? Absolute measurements in radiology are usually less reliable than one's experience. The abdominal film provides an appropriate analogy. The gas pattern of the bowel is constantly changing, and a normal appearance defies memorization. The best we can do is determine whether a gas pattern fits within our "normal" acceptable range based upon our experience. So while our inability to draw a normal breast is real, this inability is not confined to this organ. There are few absolute measurements that can be applied to help interpret the breast, and similar limitations exist with other organs.

EXPERIENCE OF THE CLINICIAN

Few clinicians have developed experience during their training to help them understand the significance of mammographic findings. While no clinician should have a problem deciding what to do with the patient with a nonpalpable stellate mass interpreted by the radiologist as being highly suspicious for malignancy, what does that clinician do when the radiologist reports that the patient has an asymmetric density? In fact, because most clinicians have had no previous training about how to manage the nonpalpable mammographic abnormality, they must be guided by the ra-

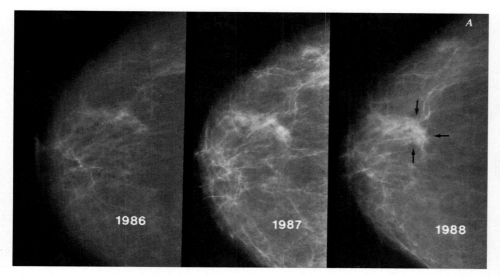

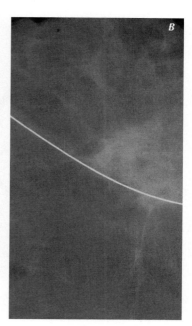

FIG. 2-5 *A. The enlarging nonpalpable carcinoma (arrows) is easily perceived when comparing CC views of the same breast over time. B. Specimen radiograph confirms excision of what proved to be a stellate invasive ductal carcinoma.*

diologist when such findings are discovered. This is especially important in the asymptomatic patient.

Such guidance is less crucial in other areas of radiology. For example, when a patient comes in with a cough and a fever and the radiologist detects an infiltrate, the clinician understands the significance of the findings and will treat the patient for pneumonia. Clinicians are familiar with the standard practice from their training. In fact, regardless of whether the radiologist describes the parenchymal process as alveolar, interstitial, air space disease, and so on, the significance of the findings and of their appropriate management should be clear to the knowledgeable clinician. I submit that a report stating "There is a cluster of four microcalcifications in the right upper outer quadrant without an associated mass density. Recommend clinical correlation," can leave the most astute clinician adrift without guidance.

Even when a new technology comes on the scene and the clinician is totally unfamiliar with it, once one understands the findings, experience directs the appropriate management. For example, a clinician may never understand the difference between a T1- and T2-weighted image of a vertebral body, but when the conclusion is that there is a destructive lesion of the bone, this anatomic information and its implications are familiar to the clinician and the workup will proceed in the usual fashion.

REFERENCES

1. Baker LH. The breast cancer detection demonstration project: five year summary report. CA **32**:194–225, 1982.
2. Linver MN, Paster SB, Rosenberg RD, et al. Improvement in mammography interpretation skills in a community radiology practice after dedicated teaching courses: 2 year medical audit of 38,633 cases. Radiology **184**:39–43, 1992.
3. Linver MN, Osuch JR, Brenner RJ, et al. The mammography audit: a primer for the mammography quality standards act. AJR **165**:19–25, 1995.
4. Homer MJ. Analysis of patients undergoing breast biopsy: the role of mammography. JAMA **243**:677–679, 1980.
5. Goodrich WA. The Cleopatra view in xeromammography: a semi-reclining position for the tail of the breast. Radiology **128**:811–812, 1978.
6. Bassett LW, Axelrod S. A modification of the craniocaudal view in mammography. Radiology **132**:222–224, 1979.
7. Logan WW, Janus J. Use of special mammographic views to maximize radiographic information. Radiol Clin North Am **25**:953–959, 1981.
8. Zamenhof RG, Homer MJ. Mammography: evaluation of equipment and guidelines for quality assurance. Appl Radiol **13**:51–54, 1984.
9. Krecke KN, Gisvold JJ. Invasive lobular carcinoma of the breast: mammographic findings and extent of disease at diagnosis in 184 patients. AJR **161**:957–960, 1993.

Chapter 3

THE TECHNOLOGIST'S RESPONSIBILITIES

The four necessary components for obtaining high-quality mammography are a motivated and competent technologist, a cooperative patient, good equipment, and a knowledgeable radiologist. Of the four components, the motivated and competent technologist is the key because without her the importance of the other three is greatly decreased. The wise radiologist has learned early that an invaluable asset to the practice is an interested, reliable, enthusiastic technologist. The extra pair of eyes and ears that a technologist can provide may often avoid potential problems that can arise. Nowhere is this more true than with mammography, especially when the examination is performed without a radiologist on site. However, it is unfair to place increased responsibility upon our technologists without formally training them about what we expect from them and without clearly defining their responsibilities. Ideally we should try to transmit some of our enthusiasm about mammography to our technologists. I have tried to channel mine into three paths: selection, motivation, and education.

CHOOSING A TECHNOLOGIST

There is general agreement that male technologists, if at all possible, should not perform mammography. There is probably no other area in diagnostic imaging where such bias exists, but mammography is such a highly charged, anxiety-provoking examination that having a female perform it is preferred. However, it is equally important to realize that not all female technologists should be made to perform mammography.

There is a certain patience, compassion, and sensitivity that the technologist doing mammography needs in order to make the patient feel as comfortable as possible. I do not think that these qualities can easily be taught, and I recognize that some technologists clearly do not possess these traits. Some practices may be small and must require all female technologists to rotate through mammography. However, if one has the luxury of a large pool of female technologists, I think that the ideal is to select those who would like to do the procedure.

When I first started at NEMCH, the technologist who "lost the choose" did mammography for the day. Over the course of weeks it was painfully clear that the quality of the examination varied from excellent to embarrassing. With the permission of the chief technologist, I held a meeting with the entire group of female technologists. I told them that I recognized that some of them were not happy doing mammograms for many reasons, ranging from personal emotions about breast cancer to the difficulty of knowing just how vigorously to compress the breast. I proposed that I wanted only technologists interested in doing the examination to do it and that I would personally educate them about breast disease in general and mammography in particular. They would be assuming additional significant responsibilities other than just producing the images, since the radiologist might not always be there for immediate supervision. By a show of hands the interested technologists declared themselves, and in one moment not only did I identify a cadre of motivated technologists, but I also gained gratitude from the other technologists who no longer had to suffer doing the examination.

MALPRACTICE

Most malpractice lawyers will tell you that the patients who are more prone to sue are those who are angry with their physicians, not necessarily because of negligent care but because of their *perception* that the physician was too busy to spend time explaining things, was rude, or was just not friendly enough. In other words, a key factor in whether the patient initiates a lawsuit is the rapport between the physician and the patient. With mammography, the patient often spends most or all of her time with the technologist and not the radiologist. Any displeasure generated by the patient-technologist interaction can be transferred to the radiologist, even though the radiologist had nothing at all to do with it. The technologist should view herself as an extension of the radiologist. The radiologist is directly responsible for her actions.

We cannot overemphasize to our technologists that the patient often perceives the radiologist and technologist, the mammography team, as a single entity.[1] I have instructed my technologists to notify me immediately when they believe that a patient may be upset at something so that I can learn of the specifics of the event while the facts are still fresh. Even if I can't rectify them, I have often avoided difficulty by immediately calling the referring physician, alerting him or her to the potential problem (whether real or perceived), and when appropriate, offering either explanation or apology over the telephone. Not only are my clinical colleagues grateful to be forewarned, but on occasion, when the patient does complain, the clinician is prepared and able to deal with the complaint.

DETAILED RESPONSIBILITIES

My technologists' responsibilities cover several broad areas, and these will now be covered in sequence.

The Patient History Form

The technologist takes a brief but directed history from every patient. One of the first facts asked is the patient's age, since the rule at NEMCH is that mammograms are not performed on women 29 years of age or younger unless approved by a radiologist. Data exist showing that there are very few valid indications for mammography in women below the 30 to 35 age group.[2–4] While we do not encourage routine screening on women 30 to 35 years of age, we allow it because of the many cancers we have found in this age group. If there is no appropriate indication for performing the examination in the younger women, the mammogram will not be done. The radiologist speaks to the patient to explain why the examination is not going to be performed and telephones the referring clinician's office.

Next the technologist reviews the history form that every patient is required to complete prior to the performance of the mammographic examination. The order of information on the form parallels the standard sequence used by our clinical colleagues; specifically, chief complaint, history of present illness, past medical history, family history, and physical findings. The patient is required to answer whether the examination is routine. If it is not, she is requested to describe her breast problem.

Past medical history includes questions about prior breast surgery, including biopsies and aspirations. There is a question regarding the use of hormones, such as estrogen, which might be the explanation for increasing parenchymal density within the breast (Fig. 3-1), or the development of cysts.[5,6] The patient is asked whether she has breast fed within the past 3 months, because this may cause the development of new asymmetric densities. The patient is asked whether she has had a weight change of more than 10 lb within the past year. This information is requested because a significant weight change may explain a change in breast size (Fig. 3-2), increased density within the breast (decreased fat due to weight loss), or decreased density within the breast (deposition of fat due to weight gain). If the patient notes on the form that she has had a weight change of more than 10 lb within the past year,

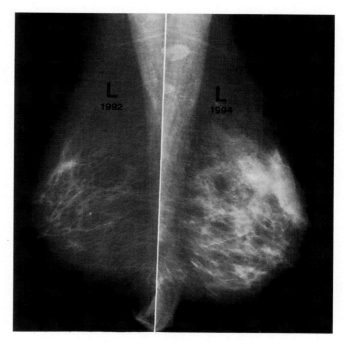

FIG. 3-1 *The development of increased parenchymal density in the left breast is caused by hormonal replacement which the patient began taking in 1992.*

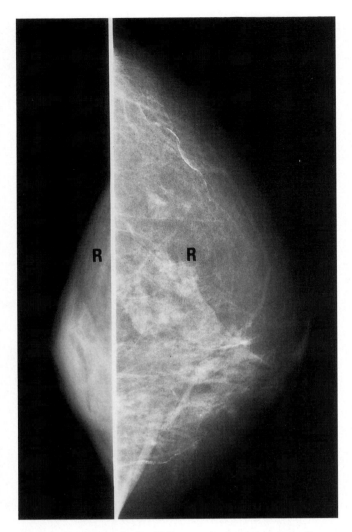

FIG. 3-2 *The dramatic difference in breast size on these CC views of the right breast was caused by a weight gain of 120 pounds.*

the technologist, in the privacy of the mammography suite, asks the patient whether there was weight gain or loss and how much. The question about weight change has been purposefully crafted in a neutral way to avoid any potential embarrassment to the patient, so, hopefully, she will answer the question honestly. There is also a question about past trauma to the breast, because this might be an explanation for mammographic findings that could mimic changes of malignancy. The final question about past medical history asks whether the patient has had a child, and, if so, her age at first birth. The age at first birth is important to obtain because the risk is increased for women who were 30 years of age or older at the time of birth of their first child.[7]

The section on family history requires the patient to indicate whether there is any breast cancer in the immediate family, including mother, sister, and grandmother, and, if so, the age at diagnosis. Both maternal and paternal sides contribute to risk.[8] A mammography questionnaire that asks about the presence of a family history of breast cancer without requesting the age at diagnosis does not obtain the most accurate picture of the patient's true risk. The development of premenopausal breast cancer in a family member is a much more important risk factor than the development of postmenopausal breast cancer in the same relative.

The final portion of the patient history form deals with physical findings. These may or may not be related to the reason the patient is having the mammogram. The technologist notes all pertinent physical findings on the diagrammatic representation of the breasts that is present on every form.

Depending on the breast facility, the patient history forms may be either brief or extensive and detailed. Since these forms take time for the patient to complete and for the technologist to review, I believe that the radiologist should be certain that the form does not contain any extraneous material. The form should be as concise as possible to avoid needless wasting of time on the part of both the patient and the technologist. One rule that I have is that if a question is important enough to be asked on the history form, it is important enough to be answered. My technologists are taught that since I have limited my patient history form to those questions that I believe are absolutely necessary, there must be a response to every question. There will be more about this principle in an upcoming chapter that deals with malpractice issues.

Visual Inspection of the Breast

The technologist then visually inspects the breasts and knows to meticulously mark things on the diagram. A diagram only showing the breast in frontal projection (Fig. 3-3) cannot adequately portray the dimension of depth. How can the technologist accurately mark the location of a palpable mass, at the 6 o'clock position of the breast near the chest wall, on a diagram of the breast in frontal projection? I believe that an appropriate diagram must allow the technologist to indicate not only distance of an abnormality from the nipple, but also its relationship to the chest wall (Fig. 3-4). Biopsy scars, skin lesions such as moles or keloids, and anything unusual appearing on the breast are carefully drawn on the diagram. Often one breast may be larger than the other. The technologist should note this so that the radiologist will realize when a discrepancy in breast size depicted on the mammogram reflects actual anatomic disparity between the breasts rather than inadequate compression. The nipples are carefully observed, and if there is any asymmetry between them, the patient is questioned as to whether she has noticed

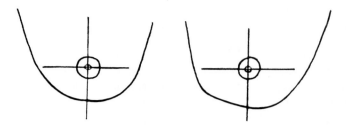

FIG. 3-3 *This diagram in frontal projection does not allow the technologist to accurately note the depth of a palpable lesion.*

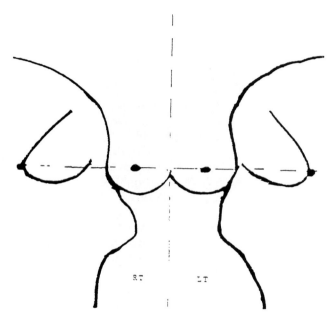

FIG. 3-4 *This type of diagram permits accurate depiction of the location of a palpable mass.*

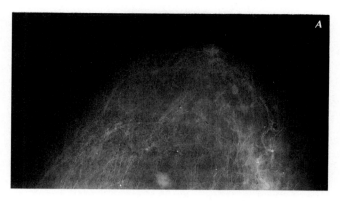

FIG. 3-5 **A.** *CC view from a screening mammogram shows what appears to be a poorly defined mass near the chest wall.*

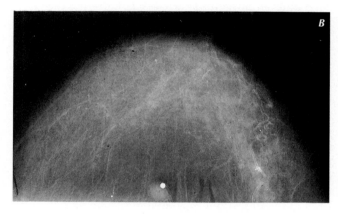

FIG. 3-5 (Continued) **B.** *When the undersurface of the breast was examined, a sebaceous cyst was obvious in the inframammary region. A metallic marker placed on the skin lesion proved that it was the suspected breast mass seen on the initial examination.*

the difference, and, if so, for how long she has been aware of it.

Pendulous breasts cannot be visually inspected without touching them. In particular, the most common errors made are forgetting to lift up the breast to carefully examine the undersurface (Fig. 3-5), and failure to separate the breasts to carefully examine their medial aspects, especially areas close to the chest wall.

My technologists have been taught that anything that projects either over or on the breast should be noted, because it may be significant or because its omission may confuse mammographic interpretation. Noting tattoos on the skin is an obvious example, but other examples include powder retained in moles, which can appear as a cluster of microcalcifications (Fig. 3-6), and subcutaneous calcifications such as those seen in dermatomyositis (Fig. 3-7), which may be

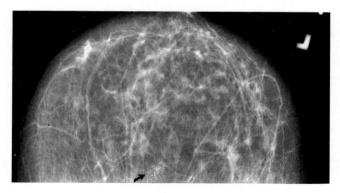

FIG. 3-6 *This patient was referred for localization and excision of a geographic cluster of microcalcifications (arrow) deep at the chest wall. On inspection of the breast, it proved to be a skin mole containing powder on the undersurface of the breast.*

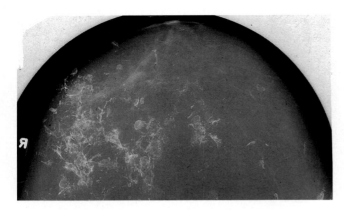

FIG. 3-7 *This patient has dermatomyositis. None of these calcifications are within breast tissue.*

mistaken for parenchymal calcifications and even subcutaneous emphysema (Fig. 3-8*A*, *B*, and *C*) of the chest wall.

Breast Palpation

At NEMCH the woman does not receive a complete breast palpation as part of the mammography examination, but the technologist may perform a breast palpation to correlate with the patient's problems. If the patient has described a mass, the technologist palpates the area. She does this because she must make the decision whether the area is going to be successfully imaged on our routine views. Sometimes the mass is not even in the breast but is related to the rib or is in close proximity to the breast, such as a fibroma in adjacent skin. It is crucial to note this because if that is the case, the radiologist should dictate into the report that the area of the palpable mass is not imaged on the mammogram at all and may not be related to the breast. In any event, management must be based upon clinical grounds. If the woman complains of skin thickening or dimpling the technologist determines whether this is real and palpable, because if it is detected by palpation, it should be possible to reproduce it on the mammogram. A special obliquity may be required to image skin thickening or dimpling in tangent.

Compression

The success of mammography is directly related to the degree of compression that can be applied. The technologist explains to each patient the necessity for vigorous compression. It is helpful to have an illustrative case on display so that the woman can see for herself how compression can make a breast mass more easily perceived. This will help her realize its importance.

I believe that the next step that we perform is the key to why we have been successful in virtually elimi-

nating the letters we used to receive from angry patients complaining of painful breasts from too much compression.

There is an interaction that takes place between the patient and the technologist to "titrate" the amount of compression that the patient is able to tolerate. The patient is an active participant in this decision. I disagree with those who require the technologist to arbitrarily decide how much to compress a breast without the patient's involvement in the process. We tell the patient that to make the examination as good as possible, the compression should be as uncomfortable as the patient can tolerate but should not be painful. However, what is perceived as pain by one person may not be

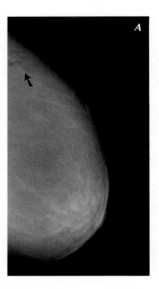

FIG. 3-8 A. *LAT view shows unusual lucencies (arrow) in the upper portion of the breast.*

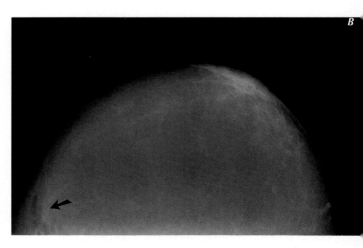

FIG. 3-8 *(Continued)* **B.** *CC view demonstrates the lucencies again in the medial portion of the breast (arrow).*

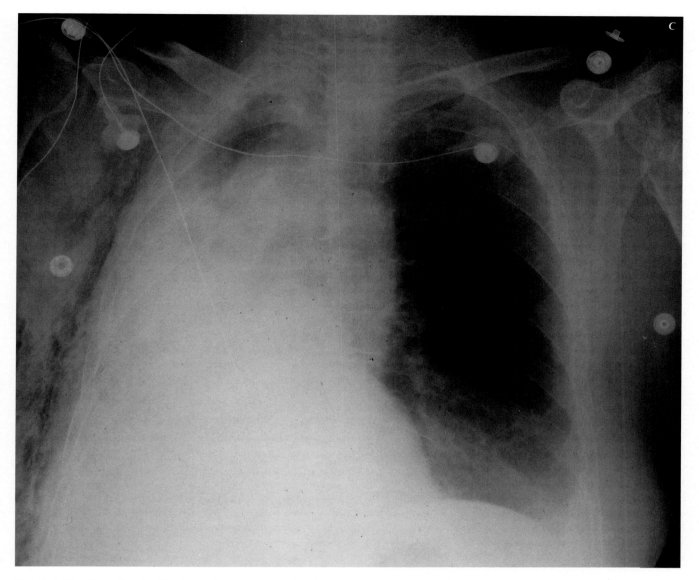

FIG. 3-8 *(Continued)* **C.** *The lucencies represented subcutaneous emphysema involving the entire right side of the chest wall.*

perceived as pain by another, and therefore only the patient herself can be the judge of this. The technologist tells the patient that she is going to lower the compression device so that it is as uncomfortable as the patient can bear, but if it is painful, the patient must let the technologist know so that the compression can be released slightly. The patient is then told that the compression will last only for seconds and will be completely released after the mammogram is obtained.[9]

On occasion one of my clinicians will phone stating that a patient has complained of painful compression. I explain to the clinician that it is not our policy to have the technologist arbitrarily decide how much compression to apply, and I ask the clinician to call the patient back to ask if indeed an interaction took place between the patient and the technologist in order to determine how much compression to apply. I instruct the clinician to tell the patient that if the examination was truly painful, then she pushed herself as much as she could and allowed us to get as good a mammogram as possible on her, but to tell the patient the next time not to be so heroic. I request feedback so that I can know whether this interaction had indeed taken place. Thus far, the return calls from my clinicians almost always confirm that this interaction had indeed taken place, and the patient usually admits that though she did experience pain, this was because she allowed the technologist to apply too much compression.

Quality Control

As with all other radiographic examinations, the technologist views her mammogram films for things such as motion, position, technique, and film-screen contact. Assuming that the breasts are the same size anatomically, the amount of breast imaged on each side should be the same. If the breasts appear greatly different in size from a previous examination (either larger or smaller), the technologist should go back and inquire whether the patient has experienced a significant weight change since the previous examination, which might explain it.

The technologist strives to get the nipple in tangent on all views but knows that it is almost impossible to image inferiorly placed nipples in tangent on the CC view. In this situation, if the nipple is caught in tangent on the LAT or OBL view, the technologist need not automatically obtain a spot compression film of the nipple in tangent. Unless the patient has a specific nipple or periareolar problem, I do not find that this extra view adds much to the examination, and therefore I do not require my technologist to obtain it routinely.

Technologists who perform mammography are required to take continuing medical education courses to maintain their level of skill. As a result, there is a better understanding and appreciation for those components that are necessary for the production of mammograms of diagnostic image quality.[10] In addition to technical factors such as exposure and contrast, proper positioning is necessary for optimal images.[11] Various parameters are being established to allow both the technologist and radiologist to recognize whether a breast is properly positioned.[12] For example, on the OBL view, ideally the pectoral muscle should extend down to the level of the nipple. One of the most basic judgments is whether an adequate amount of breast tissue is visualized on the CC view relative to the OBL view. The posterior nipple line (Fig. 3-9) is defined as an oblique line drawn perpendicular to the pectoral muscle, extending from the nipple to the muscle or the edge of the film (whichever comes first). The length of this line should be no longer than 1 cm more than the length of a line drawn on the CC view from the nipple to the pectoral muscle or the edge of the film, whichever comes first (Fig. 3-10). If there is more than a 1-cm difference, it should be possible to image deeper tissue on the CC projection.

Extra Views

In many practices, the radiologist is not always on site to check every film before the patient leaves. This is the situation at NEMCH. I have given my technologists the option of obtaining ancillary views if they deem it

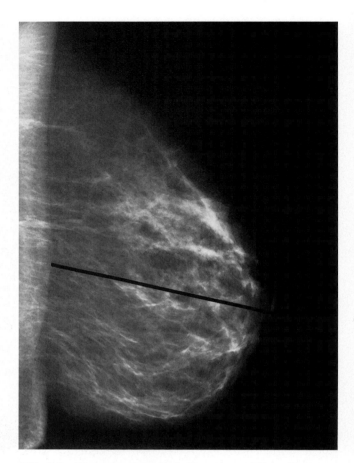

FIG. 3-9 *The posterior nipple line is an oblique line extending from the nipple to the pectoral muscle or the edge of the film, whichever comes first. It is drawn perpendicular to the pectoral muscle.*

necessary, but they must note on the form why the views were obtained.

A mammogram will image only a portion of the skin in tangent. For example, on the CC view only the skin on the 3 o'clock–9 o'clock axis is caught in tangent. Similarly, on the true LAT view, only the skin on the 12 o'clock–6 o'clock axis is caught in tangent. If the patient has a breast biopsy scar in the upper outer quadrant, one can easily understand why it might not be imaged on the mammogram even though it is palpable and even visually obvious. My technologists are instructed that if the patient has a definite thickening or dimpling of the skin that is not seen on the standard mammographic views, they may go back and obtain a tangential view of the area.

While I do not hold my technologists responsible for scrutinizing the mammogram for microcalcifications, I do encourage them to judge whether there are gross asymmetric densities present. If a radiologist is not available for review of the films and the technolo-

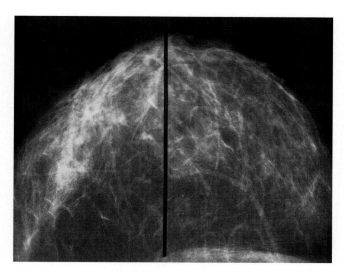

FIG. 3-10 *The depth of breast tissue imaged on the CC view is measured by a line drawn from the nipple to the pectoral muscle or the edge of the film, whichever comes first.*

gist perceives one or more asymmetric densities, she may obtain a third view. My preference for analyzing asymmetric densities is to have CC, LAT, and OBL views. If more information is required the patient is scheduled to return for additional views to be performed under the supervision of a radiologist. When the patient states that she feels a lump, it is my current practice to have the technologist place a metallic marker over the focal area, after the standard OBL and CC views are obtained, and perform two additional views in true lateral and coned compression magnification CC projections. These added views with a metallic marker are only performed if the patient can locate the area of focal concern for the technologist. Regardless of whether I or my technologist can feel anything palpable at the site, as long as the patient alleges that there is a palpable abnormality, it is my job to adequately image the area.

My purpose for the metallic marker in this setting is to positively identify the site of focal concern (usually a palpable lump) on the view being obtained. The proper technique for placement of the marker is often misunderstood by both the technologist and the radiologist. The position of the marker does not necessarily correspond to the location at which the lump is most easily palpable. The marker is correctly positioned when it superimposes directly over the area of focal concern on the projection being obtained. To accomplish this, the hand placing the marker approaches the breast in a path parallel to the central ray of the x-ray beam for the view being obtained and the marker is placed directly upon the focal area of concern. For a CC view, the hand placing the marker is moving in a

vertical direction paralleling the central ray of the CC view (Fig. 3-11). For a true LAT projection, the hand holding the metallic marker is moving in a horizontal direction (Fig. 3-12). The marker often has to be repositioned on different views to correspond to the shifting location of the focal area in different projections (Fig. 3-13). The radiologist can easily determine whether this maneuver is being performed, because if the technologist is merely placing the marker on the location where a lump is most easily palpable, it is being done incorrectly.[13]

In addition to our four standard views, the technologist will always try to obtain a magnification view of the lumpectomy site for all breast cancer patients being treated with breast conservation therapy. If at all possible, the magnification view is obtained in the same projection every time in order to allow easier comparison between examinations.

Shared responsibility is a real concept in my practice. Whenever my technologists add an extra view, it is their responsibility to write down on their form why they did it so that I can understand its purpose. It is my responsibility to let them know whether I would have done the same thing and to tell them my final interpretation. I find that I rarely disagree with my technologists.

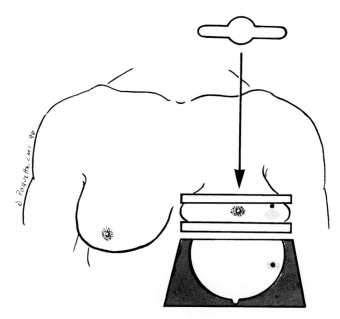

FIG. 3-11 *On this CC view, the marker is placed so that it superimposes over a palpable mass. (Reprinted by permission of the publisher from Homer MJ: Proper placement of a metallic marker on an area of focal concern within the breast. AJR 167:390–391, 1996.)*

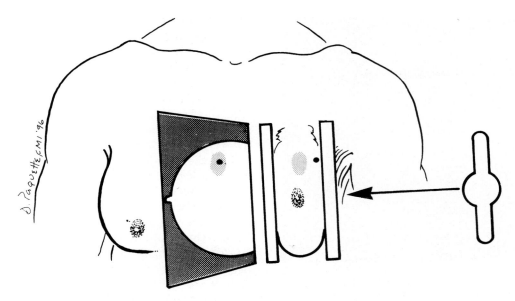

FIG. 3-12 *The marker has been repositioned for this lateromedial view and again is positioned so that it superimposes over a palpable mass. (Reprinted by permission of the publisher from Homer MJ: Proper placement of a metallic marker on an area of focal concern within the breast. AJR **167:**390–391, 1996.)*

Trouble or Difficulty during the Examination

As stated previously, my technologists are instructed to alert me to any problem that they may have encountered with the patient. The problem may vary from a patient who is angry because her examination was performed later than the appointment time, a patient complaining about painful compression, or a patient with a neurological disorder who cannot hold still during the exposure. These problems are all to be written on the technologist's form. In this way there is documentation for the future should the incident have to be recalled. When necessary I will telephone the referring clinician about the problem.

FEEDBACK

It has been my experience that technologists appreciate feedback from the radiologist so that they can understand what is expected of them in order to provide high-quality films. Radiologists must always remember that this feedback should not just be limited to the negative kind. My technologists know that when they have done something that I consider to be very good, I will seek them out and congratulate them for a job well done. They also understand that when they have done something that I consider to be wrong or sloppy, my intent in speaking with them is not to humiliate them but to try to explain how dependent I am upon them and

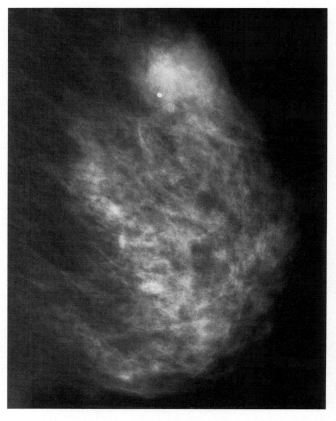

FIG. 3-13 A. *This woman presented for evaluation of a palpable lump in the 12 o'clock position of the left breast. The technologist placed a metallic marker over the lump and obtained a LAT view. The marker superimposes over a noncalcified mass with irregular margins.*

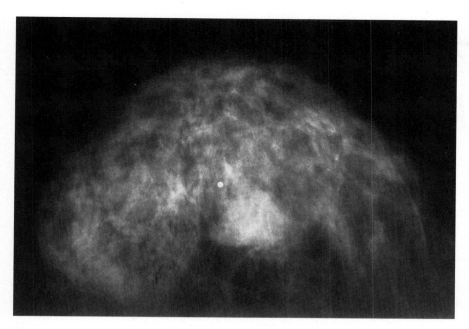

FIG. 3-13 *(Continued)* ***B.*** *The marker was then repositioned to project over the mass in a CC projection and this view was obtained. It is superimposed over the edge of a noncalcified mass with irregular margins. Histology revealed an invasive ductal carcinoma.*

to educate them as to what they did incorrectly in order to try to help them prevent this from happening again in the future.

REFERENCES

1. Fox SA, Klos DS, Worthen NJ, et al. Improving the adherence of urban women to mammography guidelines: strategies for radiologists. Radiology **174**:203–206, 1990.
2. Harris VJ, Jackson VP. Indications for breast imaging in women under age 35 years. Radiology **172**:445–448, 1989.
3. Homer MJ. Mammography in young asymptomatic women: a survey of current practice. Breast Dis **1**:59–63, 1988.
4. Williams SM, Kaplan PA, Petersen JC, et al. Mammography in women under age 30: is there clinical benefit? Radiology **161**:49–51, 1986.
5. Cyrlak D, Wong CH. Mammographic changes in postmenopausal women undergoing hormonal replacement therapy. AJR **161**:1177–1183, 1993.
6. Laya MB, Gallagher JC, Schreiman JS, et al. Effect of postmenopausal hormonal replacement on mammographic density and parenchymal pattern. Radiology **196**:433–437, 1995.
7. Seidman H, Stellman SD, Mushinski MH. A different perspective on breast cancer risk factors: Some implications of the nonattributable risk. CA Cancer Clin **32**:301–313, 1982.
8. King MC, Rowell S, Love SM. Inherited breast and ovarian cancer: what are the risks? What are the choices? JAMA **269**:1975–1980, 1993.
9. Eklund GW. Mammographic compression: science or art? Radiology **181**:339–341, 1991.
10. Eklund GW, Cardenosa G, Parsons W. Assessing adequacy of mammographic image quality. Radiology **190**:297–307, 1994.
11. Eklund GW, Cardenosa G. The art of mammographic positioning. Radiol Clin North Am **30**:21–53, 1992.
12. Bassett LW, Hirbawi IA, DeBruhl N, et al. Mammographic positioning: evaluation from the view box. Radiology **188**:803–806, 1993.
13. Homer MJ. Proper placement of a metallic marker on an area of focal concern within the breast. AJR **167**:390–391, 1996.).

GENERAL PRINCIPLES

RED FLAG APPROACH _____

In general, I use mammography to detect a solitary geographic area of the breast different from all other areas in the ipsilateral and contralateral breast. The challenges of mammography are to find the area, determine that it is indeed a solitary geographic abnormality, judge whether it can possibly be a normal variation, and, if it cannot be a normal variation, formulate appropriate recommendation options. The radiologist's job is not primarily to differentiate benign from malignant. In fact, there is someone whose job it is to differentiate benign from malignant—the pathologist.

Although the rules differentiating benign from malignant processes in the breast based upon mammographic appearance are valid in large numbers of patients, these rules are less helpful for the specific case on the view box. *The emphasis of using mammography to define an area with a different appearance from other areas in the breast rather than using it to differentiate benign from malignant may be the single most important concept in this text.* If one can accept this concept, then the mammographic examination takes on a completely different challenge and relieves the radiologist from the primary responsibility of differentiating benign from malignant. This responsibility is difficult at best and often fraught with danger.

THE PRINCIPLE OF MULTIPLICITY AND BILATERALITY _____

When there are bilateral abnormalities all of similar appearance possessing features that have a high probability of being benign, then the choice of follow-up rather than biopsy is appropriate. It is an extremely reassuring mammographic finding to see bilateral abnor-

malities. However, if there are masses in one breast and none in the other (Fig. 4-1) or multiple clusters of microcalcifications in one breast but none in the other (Fig. 4-2), in other words, when there is multiplicity without bilaterality, it is more disturbing because the other breast should be undergoing the same influences to produce the same changes. In a case of multiplicity without bilaterality, one should at least consider the option of a biopsy of one or perhaps two of the unilateral abnormalities.

THE PRINCIPLE OF BIOPSY _____

For solitary lesions that have a high probability of being benign, the management options are either biopsy to definitively establish the nature of the process or follow-up. At NEMCH, biopsy of a lesion that has a high probability of being benign will be considered if afterward the surgeon can say to the woman, "You have had the biopsy, the area is benign as we thought it most probably would be, and now you go back into the normal category." As a general rule, we will not biopsy one of multiple bilateral abnormalities all with the same appearance and each having a high probability of being benign, because though one or even two might be excised and prove to be benign, one cannot guarantee that the other abnormalities are of similar pathology, so the patient still must undergo follow-up.

THE CONCEPT OF GEOGRAPHIC ABNORMALITY _____

The concept of geographic abnormality defies measurement. Four or five microcalcifications in a tight cluster are a geographic abnormality just as microcalcifications located in only one quadrant are a geographic abnormality (Fig. 4-3). In both situations, the radiologist can define an area of the breast that differs from other areas in the ipsilateral or contralateral breast. Even unilateral microcalcifications in an entire breast are a geographic abnormality because the other half of the organ (the contralateral breast) is uninvolved. Obviously, the longer an occult malignancy remains undiscovered, the larger the geographic area it will involve. One should beware of a false sense of security when analyzing a large geographic area of microcalcifications and assuming that it must be benign because nothing is palpable and the patient is asymptomatic. If it is geographic, then it is worrisome. The concept of geographic abnormality will appear again in Chap. 6.

One important exception to this relates to ducts. In the asymptomatic patient with a normal breast palpation, a solitary enlarged duct is a focal geographic abnormality that requires excision or follow-up. However, in the case of unilateral subareolar dilated ducts coupled with a normal breast palpation, no nipple discharge, and a normal appearing nipple, I advise follow-up rather than excision even though this is in essence a geographic abnormality. The reason is that to have diffuse carcinoma in multiple subareolar ducts in an asymptomatic patient without a palpable abnor-

mality is highly improbable, and resection of the entire ductal system in one breast is extensive surgery for a mammographic finding that has a very low probability of being malignant. Management of enlarged ducts will be discussed in Chap. 6.

THE ROLE OF ULTRASOUND IN AIDING MAMMOGRAPHIC INTERPRETATION

At NEMCH, the primary use of ultrasound is to differentiate a simple cyst from a solid mass in the breast. The kidney provides a good analogy to how breast ultrasound is used. When a renal mass undergoes ultrasound evaluation, it is either a simple cyst or "something else." When it is "something else," the differential diagnosis includes both benign and malignant entities. In either case, further investigation is usually required. Similarly, in the breast a mass is proved by ultrasound to be either a simple cyst or "something else." If it falls into the latter category, it requires further investigation to establish its nature. At NEMCH, all ultrasound is tar-

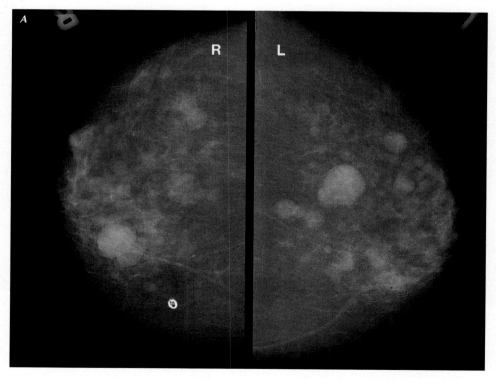

FIG. 4-1 A. *CC views of each breast demonstrate multiple bilateral noncalcified masses. This is an example of multiplicity and bilaterality. Since there was no dominant mass by palpation, this patient was placed into follow-up to assess stability of the masses.*

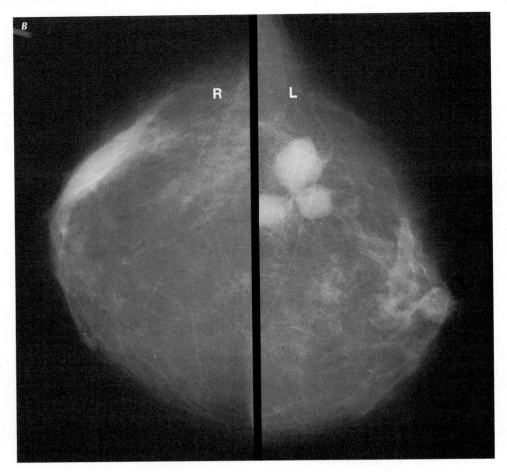

FIG. 4-1 *(Continued)* **B.** *CC views of each breast demonstrate multiple noncalcified masses in the left breast. This is an example of multiplicity without bilaterality. Biopsy revealed multicentric invasive ductal carcinoma.*

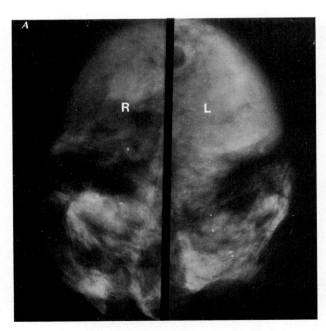

FIG. 4-2 **A.** *This woman has had bilateral breast reductions. CC views of each breast demonstrate bilateral microcalcifications. This is an example of multiplicity and bilaterality. Since there was no palpable abnormality, this patient was placed into follow-up to assess stability of the microcalcifications.*

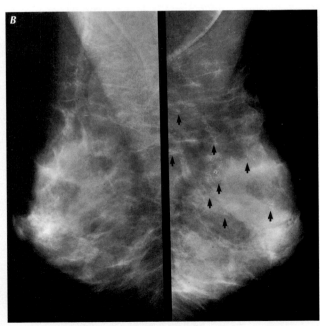

FIG. 4-2 *(Continued)* **B.** *OBL views from a routine screening mammogram reveal numerous clusters of microcalcifications in the right breast (arrows). There are no microcalcifications on the left side. This is an example of multiplicity without bilaterality. Biopsy revealed multicentric foci of intraductal and invasive ductal carcinoma.*

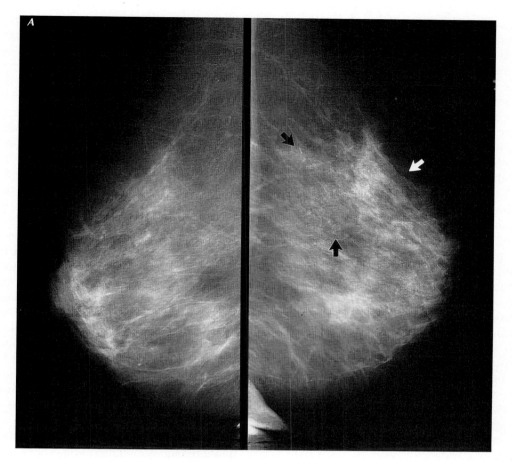

FIG. 4-3 **A.** *This screening mammogram demonstrates a large geographic area of punctate microcalcifications occupying the upper half of the right breast (arrows).*

geted to define a specific mammographic abnormality. We do not use ultrasound to image a dense breast or a breast with multiple masses.

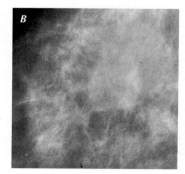

FIG. 4-3 *(Continued)* **B.** *Magnification view shows the microcalcifications to better advantage. Biopsy revealed extensive intraductal and invasive ductal carcinoma.*

THE PHILOSOPHY OF FOLLOW-UP

Often a decision is made not to biopsy a solitary nonpalpable abnormality with a mammographic appearance that has a high probability of being benign.[1] When this is done, the patient is placed into a follow-up protocol to be certain that the abnormality remains stable in appearance. This protocol can also be used in situations in which there are multiple bilateral abnormalities that have a high probability of being benign, such as asymmetric densities, microcalcifications, or masses. To use the follow-up protocol correctly, one should have a clear understanding of what is being accomplished by the examination. It is to document stability of mammographic finding or findings that have a high probability, based upon appearance, of being benign. Therefore, if there is a change over time, whether in shape, number (such as the number of microcalcifications in a cluster), or size, then the lesion is not stable and the initial decision to follow the mammographic abnormality must be reevaluated. Some changes reinforce the decision to follow. For example, if over time microcalcifications become macrocalcifications, this change to a "more benign" appearance is good.

The recommendation for a follow-up is not the same as recommending future mammography (even annually), according to suggested mammographic guidelines for screening. Recommendations for screening may not be followed by either the clinician or the patient if one or the other does not adhere to the guidelines. The follow-up protocol is altogether different because the radiologist is recommending it for a specific reason, and if the clinician chooses to ignore this recommendation, then the responsibility rests with the clinician. Distinction between a follow-up protocol and the recommendation of annual mammography according to screening guidelines is an important one to realize. When the patient is put into a follow-up, she has been pulled out of the routine screening pool because of mammographic findings.

The protocol that I use for follow-up is based upon a national survey that I reported several years ago.[2] The information from this survey is summarized in Tables 4-1 and 4-2. This survey cannot substitute for a prospective study to determine a "correct" sequence for follow-up, but such a study has not been done. The survey represents the practice of experienced mammographers. When something has not yet been established by the scientific method, the next best thing is at least to be certain that one's practice is consistent with the prevailing standard of care.

There are three parts to a follow-up protocol: the time of the initial follow-up examination, the interval between follow-up examinations, and the total length of time required to allow the radiologist to conclude that when an abnormality is stable there is no need for further follow-up to assess interval change. Based upon the results of the survey, most radiologists trigger the initial study within 3 to 6 months and continue to follow the abnormality for at least 2 to 3 years. What was not determined from the survey was the interval for follow-up between the initial study and the final study.

My particular follow-up protocol calls for the initial examination to be performed within 6 months, although on occasion I have recommended that the first follow-up examination be performed as soon as 3 months after the initial study. If the lesion is stable at the 6-month period, then I recommend additional examinations to provide a total follow-up of $2\frac{1}{2}$ to 3 years from the time of the initial mammogram. If the abnormality has remained unchanged for this length of time, I recommend future mammography as per usual clinical indications. In other words, I am not requiring any future mammography for follow-up. If future mammograms are ordered, it is because the clinician desires it. Breast cancers that have not changed for $2\frac{1}{2}$ to 3 years on good quality mammographic studies are very unusual. If a radiologist wants to carry out the follow-up for a period longer than 3 years, that is certainly acceptable, but it is not my usual practice to do this.

Not all lesions qualify for mammographic follow-up. As a general principle, no mammographic finding should be considered for follow-up unless it has a highly probable benign appearance based upon traditional mammographic criteria. Therefore, the mammographic stability for $2\frac{1}{2}$ to 3 years of a breast lesion that would never have qualified for follow-up does not guarantee that the lesion is benign.

Some colleagues have told me that they prefer to trigger the interval follow-up examinations every 6 months. This is an altogether reasonable option. It is not even always necessary to obtain full set mammography (two views of each breast) on someone in a follow-up protocol. If bilateral abnormalities are not being evaluated, then perhaps only the ipsilateral breast need be imaged. If the mammographic finding in question can be adequately analyzed for change on a single view, then the examination can even be limited to one view. If the mammographic abnormality disappears during the follow-up protocol, then obviously the protocol can be terminated. In other words, when one triggers a follow-up protocol, one is not necessarily committed to the entire $2\frac{1}{2}$ to 3 years if findings change, nor is one committed to a full set examination each time. The protocol should be modified as required. Common sense dictates that if a new abnormality develops during a follow-up protocol, it must be evaluated separately and it may require immediate biopsy even though the other abnormalities remain stable.

I have been told by colleagues that some clinicians are upset when mammographic follow-up is recommended. These clinicians expect radiologists to report

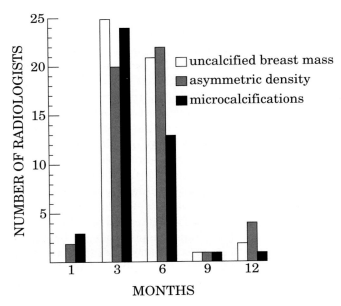

TABLE 4-1

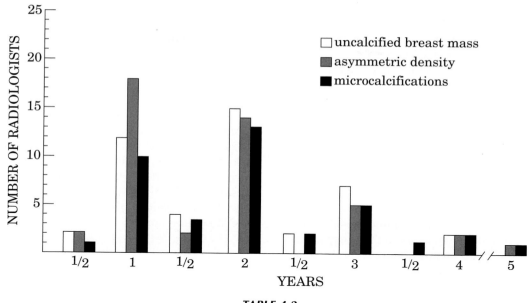

TABLE 4-2

that the mammogram is normal or that biopsy is necessary. However, in many cases mammography cannot do this. Certainly there is anxiety in a mammographic follow-up, but it is no different from the anxiety generated in a clinical follow-up. If my clinicians were only allowed to choose between calling an area in the breast normal or recommending biopsy based upon palpation, then I could understand why I should be held to the same standards and not be able to offer the option of recommending follow-up. However, it is quite common for a woman to come in with a thickening or for the clinician to feel an area of the breast and explain to the woman that though it is not definite enough to demand a biopsy at this time, he or she would like to reexamine it again in several weeks or months. Since clinical follow-up is an accepted recommendation in breast disease management, I see no reason for a radiologist to be prohibited from recommending a mammographic follow-up for the many indeterminate lesions that are visualized on the mammogram. Follow-up of the lesion with a high probability of being benign is an acceptable management option, and its efficacy has been validated by others.[3–6]

VIEWING THE MAMMOGRAM

Ideally, mammograms should be interpreted in a quiet place free from the usual distractions of a busy radiology department. Needless to say, this ideal is not often realized. Though someone with perfect vision may feel that using a magnifying glass is unnecessary, I believe that a magnifying glass aids in appreciating very subtle abnormalities and forces one to slow down when scanning the image. I do not interpret mammograms without a magnifying glass in hand.

While many radiologists routinely mount the LAT or OBL views back to back, they place the CC views side by side on the view box to correspond to the anatomic position in which the films were taken. Comparison of the right breast to the left breast is done for evaluation of symmetry. The symmetry demanded of breast tissue on the LAT and OBL views must also be present on the CC projection. Perceptual psychologists have proven that the eye can more easily perceive asymmetric densities when patterns are scanned in a mirror-image fashion rather than side by side. I evaluate mammograms in a mirror-image fashion with both the LAT, OBL, *and* CC views mounted back to back. Some radiologists mount the right mammogram on the right and the left one on the left. Others prefer to view the mammograms as if they are facing the patient. I am more concerned about evaluating symmetry and do not have a rule as to which side of the image pair I mount on the right and which on the left. This explains why in this text the right breast is not always on the right side of an image pair.

Viewing the mammogram is a two-step procedure. First, one sits back and evaluates the general contour of the breast, the size of the breast, and scans for asymmetric density. A discrepancy in breast size demands an explanation. Most commonly, this is caused by poor positioning. However, it is not unusual for one breast to be considerably larger than the other. When this is the case, obviously the larger breast should appear larger on all views. If it does not, the radiologist cannot accept the explanation of a difference in breast size. In my practice, when the technologist judges that there is great difference in breast size, she must note this on the history form for documentation.

The next step in interpretation is coming up close to the mammogram to examine the skin and the nipple region. Depending on the penetration of the film, this might require a bright light. Then, with a magnifying glass in hand, each area of the breast is carefully examined for the presence of microcalcifications. If one immediately proceeds to this last step (close inspection of the mammogram with a magnifying glass), then asymmetric breast densities and contour abnormalities can be easily overlooked.

Even when there are prior mammograms available for comparison, my first step is always to compare the right breast to the left breast on the current examination. Then I compare this examination to a previous one, evaluating the right breast over time and then the left breast over time. If one only compares the right breast on the current study to the right breast on an earlier study, a slowly evolving asymmetric density may be overlooked. Since an asymmetric density can only be perceived as asymmetric because it is not present on the contralateral side, I feel that it is necessary to compare the right side to the left side.

I have no firm rule as to which previous mammogram I select for comparison. One might think that the earliest mammogram should always be selected because any interval change can best be appreciated when comparing the earliest examination to the current examination. While theoretically this might be true, often the difference in technique over the years is so great as we change film-screen combinations, begin using grids, and purchase newer units with smaller focal spots, that comparison with the earliest examination may prove to be extremely difficult. A more recent examination could be more suitable for comparison. Similarly, it may be unwise to always select the immediately previous examination for comparison. While

the technique may be more similar, making the comparison easier to accomplish, an enlarging neodensity might not be appreciated. The analogy to interpreting chest radiographs on the intensive care unit (ICU) board should make this last point clear. Sometimes an evolving pneumonia is difficult to recognize if one only compares the current chest radiograph to the most recent previous examination. The pneumonia is often more easily perceived when one pulls out examinations done several days earlier. Just as there is no set rule which chest radiograph to use for comparison, there is no absolute rule with mammography. Suffice to say that the comparison need not be limited to either the immediately previous mammogram or the earliest mammogram.

REFERENCES

1. Brenner RJ, Sickles EA. Acceptability of periodic follow-up as an alternative to biopsy for mammographically detected lesions interpreted as probably benign. Radiology **171**:645–646, 1989.
2. Homer MJ. Nonpalpable mammographic abnormalities: timing the follow-up studies. AJR **136**:923–926, 1981.
3. Adler DD, Helvie MA, Ikeda DM. Nonpalpable, probably benign breast lesions: follow-up strategies after initial detection on mammography. AJR **155**:1195–1201, 1990.
4. Sickles EA. Periodic mammographic follow-up of probably benign lesions: results in 3,184 consecutive cases. Radiology **179**:463–468, 1991.
5. Helvie MA, Pennes DR, Rebner M, Adler DD. Mammographic follow-up of low suspicion lesions: compliance rate and diagnostic yield. Radiology **178**:155–158, 1991.
6. Varas X, Leborgne F, Leborgne JH. Nonpalpable, probably benign lesions: role of follow-up mammography. Radiology **184**:409–414, 1992.

THE MAMMOGRAPHY REPORT

The creation of a radiology report is an idiosyncratic and subjective exercise. While one radiologist can dictate a normal chest radiograph in two sentences, another requires three paragraphs to reach the identical conclusion for the same chest radiograph. Though the goals of this chapter are to crystallize problems with the mammography report and propose solutions, it is not my intent to suggest that my specific verbiage or form is the only correct way to solve the problem. I hope to stimulate readers to consider problems, anticipate difficulties, and create solutions that are appropriate for their unique practice setting. Examples of the more commonly used reports at NEMCH are listed in Table 5-1.

The mammography report, like all other radiograph reports, is a legal document. Not only will the referring clinician be looking at this communication, but others, including nonphysicians, may eventually be reading it. The report is the vehicle for transmitting information to the referring clinician, and in most cases it is the only proof that the radiologist has of his or her interpretation. One of my key principles is that whatever form a mammography report takes, the information it conveys must be able to be clearly understood not only by the referring clinician but also by a judge, an expert witness, a tribunal, or a jury of one's peers.

There is an aspect of mammography that makes it unique, and it would be wise for the mammography report to reflect this. Most clinicians have had little training in mammography. In other areas of radiology, even when the report is not carefully constructed, the clinician usually understands its meaning, can relate it to the patient's symptoms, and will draw upon his or her own experience to manage the patient appropriately. For example, if a patient comes in with a cough and fever and there is an infiltrate in the left lower lobe, it is usually inconsequential how the radiologist describes the process. When the finding of a pulmonary abnormality is communicated to the clinician, he or she understands that in all likelihood it represents a pneumonia and will treat the patient accordingly. Furthermore, the clinician knows that if the infiltrate does not go away or if the patient's symptoms do not improve, either the wrong antibiotic was given or other causes must be considered, such as an obstructing endobronchial lesion causing a distal pneumonia, pulmonary infarction, or alveolar cell carcinoma. However, if the radiologist simply describes the finding of a moderately well-defined noncalcified density in the left upper outer quadrant, the clinician may not fully understand the implications of the finding, nor might the clinician have any experience in knowing what the next appropriate step is. When subtle findings of early breast cancer are discovered on a routine mammogram, especially in the asymptomatic patient, I believe it is necessary for the report to clearly relate to the clinician the finding, its implications, and recommendations.

PRINCIPLES OF REPORTING _____

My clinicians are primarily interested in knowing three things from my mammography report: Is the mammogram normal? If it is not normal, must a biopsy be done now? If it is not normal but biopsy is not indicated at this time, what must be done? The basic reports listed in Table 5-1 are used in more than 90 percent of my mammography case load. They are brief and can be easily computerized.

TABLE 5-1
MAMMOGRAPHY REPORTS

1. THE NORMAL REPORT

IMPRESSION: I see no dominant mass or suspicious calcifications.

The false-negative rate of mammography is approximately 10%. Management of a palpable abnormality must be based upon clinical grounds.

2. THE NORMAL-DENSE REPORT

IMPRESSION: The breasts are dense, limiting the sensitivity of the examination. A mass could easily be hidden.

I see no dominant mass or suspicious calcifications.

The false-negative rate of mammography is approximately 10%. Management of a palpable abnormality must be based upon clinical grounds.

3. THE MUST BIOPSY REPORT

IMPRESSION: There is a *(description)* in the *(location)* quadrant. These are characteristics highly suggestive of cancer.

I recommend biopsy to rule out breast cancer.

4. THE MULTIPLICITY REPORT

IMPRESSION: There are multiple   (masses) (asymmetric densities) (microcalcifications)

No one area appears more suspicious to merit biopsy at this time. I recommend a repeat examination within   months to assess the stability of these areas.

The false-negative rate of mammography is approximately 10%. Management of a palpable abnormality must be based upon clinical grounds.

5. THE NEUTRAL REPORT

IMPRESSION: There is a *(description)* in the *(location)* quadrant. This has a high probability of being benign. It can be localized prior to biopsy to establish histology. If biopsy is deferred, I recommend a follow-up examination within 6 months to assess its stability.

The false-negative rate of mammography is approximately 10%. Management of a palpable abnormality must be based upon clinical grounds.

There are basic concepts that I follow in mammographic reporting that are not unique to mammography. The first is consistency. If the radiologist believes that a certain finding requires follow-up, then the recommendation for follow-up should be standardized. It is understandably confusing to our clinicians when one report recommends a 3-month follow-up while another recommends an 8-month follow-up for the same abnormality. Next, the mammography report should be concise and to the point. Traditionally, a radiology report consists of a body and an impression.[1] The reality is that often our busy clinicians do not read the body of the report as carefully as we want them to. Some do not even read the body of the report at all. Without judging whether this practice is correct (it is obviously not correct), the reality we must recognize is that it is important to be concise. Therefore, it is my practice that all important information regarding my findings is contained within the impression.

I believe that the radiologist should be directive in the mammography report. If a radiologist simply recommends a follow-up examination, does that mean a follow-up in 1 month, 3 months, or 1 year? The radiologist should make the directive clear. If the clinician chooses to ignore a clear directive, then that is his or her decision. Radiologists are expected to make recommendations in other radiology reports, and there is no reason why a mammography report should be different.

THE DISCLAIMER

Many radiologists include what is popularly known as a "disclaimer" in their reports. The reason is that one of the most common scenarios for malpractice concerning breast cancer is the clinician who feels a lump but ignores the finding because the mammogram is interpreted as normal. I can see nothing inherently wrong in using a disclaimer, but the disclaimer should be appropriate. The disclaimer is not needed for the intelligent health care provider but serves to protect the radiologist from the ignorant clinician who is not knowledgeable about the limitations of mammography and the meaning of a normal report. Appropriate material in the disclaimer can include information such as the false-negative rate of mammography or a statement about the management of a palpable mass. I use a disclaimer because I do not want to depend upon my lawyer to convince a jury that it should be common knowledge that a normal mammogram report should not delay the biopsy of a palpable mass. My specific verbiage is, "The false-negative rate of mammography is approximately 10 percent. Management of a palpable abnormality must be based upon clinical grounds."

CLINICAL HISTORY

Clinical history is extremely important for correct performance and interpretation of the mammogram. I believe that the radiologist is a consultant.[2] I do not view the radiology requisition as a demand for me to perform a procedure but rather as a consultation request from a colleague to help solve a specific clinical problem. The requisition suggests an imaging procedure to accomplish this and in the majority of cases the suggestion is correct. However, if the examination proposed is inappropriate, then I believe it is my responsibility not only to the clinician but also to the patient not to perform the examination. In the role of a consultant, it is customary that appropriate clinical history be provided. I cannot imagine a clinician requesting a pulmonary consultation for his or her patient and telling the consultant, "I am not going to let you know anything about the patient because I want your findings to be unbiased." The consultant needs to know the reason for the consultation and to have the patient's chart available for review. To be effective, the radiologist also requires such information.[3] The battle to persuade our colleagues to provide us with pertinent information must be fought.

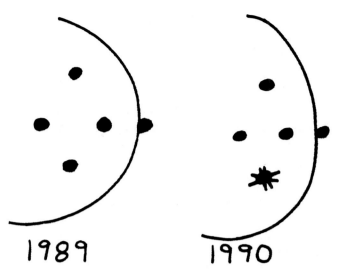

FIG. 5-1 *Routine screening mammogram in 1989 is interpreted as normal. Routine screening mammogram a year later demonstrates a nonpalpable stellate mass.*

SPECIFIC REPORTS

The Normal Report

The nightmare of every radiologist is illustrated in Fig. 5-1. The 1989 mammogram appears normal. There are four rather similarly appearing densities in the breast. In 1990, unequivocally the density in the lower part of the breast now has characteristics of a stellate mass. A biopsy reveals an invasive ductal carcinoma. The radiologist is sued for failure to diagnose the cancer in 1989. The plaintiff's lawyer shows the radiologist the stellate mass present in 1990 and asks whether it is a cancer. The answer is yes because that is the truth. If the radiologist answers no, the lawyer will show the pathology slides proving that it is a cancer. He or she then points to the 1989 mammogram and asks, "Doctor, is this area the same area that you just identified as malignant in 1990?" The radiologist had better answer yes because in this case that is the truth. If he or she answers no, the expert witness will state that the round area present in 1989 does indeed correspond to what is now known to be a cancer in 1990. Actually, the lawyer did not even require an expert witness because anyone in the jury can plainly see the fact. The lawyer now reads the impression from the 1989 report stating "normal mammogram." He or she is finished questioning. It is likely that the jury will be quite impressed because anyone can see that the cancer in 1990 was clearly present in 1989. Of course, you and I know that in 1989 the cancer had no telltale signs of malignancy. However, now the radiologist's lawyer must convince the jury that the normal impression in 1989 was correct.

Let us imagine that I am sued in a case like this. My lawyer would ask, "Dr. Homer, let me read you your report in 1989. It says:

> I see no dominant mass or suspicious calcifications.
> The false-negative rate of mammography is approximately 10 percent. Management of a palpable abnormality must be based upon clinical grounds.

What does that mean?" Now I have the opportunity to explain the limitations of mammography. Every mammogram is unique just as a fingerprint is unique. I cannot tell what normal is just as I cannot tell what a normal fingerprint is. The best thing I can hope to do with a mammogram is to determine whether it is in the realm of acceptable variation. In 1989 I saw no dominant mass. In 1989 I saw no suspicious calcifications. While it is true that the round density in the lower half of the breast in 1989 turned out to be a cancer that developed characteristic features in 1990, I could not diagnose it a year earlier because it did not vary from other areas in the breast. My report also includes a disclaimer. Finally, I would be certain to emphasize that the density in the lower half of the breast was not only impossible to diagnose by mammography in 1989 but it was not diagnosed by palpation either.

Once, during a deposition, I was asked by a lawyer what I meant by the word *dominant*. I explained that when I used the word I meant that there was nothing about any of the masses that made it dominant by radiographic criteria. A mass could be dominant by one of a number of features, including size, shape, margins, and the presence of microcalcifications. No feature of the mass dominated the mammogram to allow me to recognize it to be different from other areas in the breast.

In summary, my "normal" mammography report consists of a single sentence plus my standard disclaimer. The word "normal" does not appear in my mammography report because I am uncomfortable using it in the context of the mammographic examination.[4] The appearance of a normal breast changes with age and can vary from a totally dense breast in the younger woman to a fat-replaced breast over time.

The Normal-Dense Report

The sensitivity of mammography is very high in the fat-replaced breast and much lower in the dense breast. This is important information to communicate to the clinician so that the sensitivity of the examination in this type of patient is understood.[5] My clinicians certainly want to know this. Therefore, I have a separate report for the *normal-dense* breast:

> The breasts are dense, limiting the sensitivity of the examination. A mass could easily be hidden. I see no dominant mass or suspicious calcifications.
> The false-negative rate of mammography is approximately 10 percent. Management of a palpable abnormality must be based upon clinical grounds.

In other words, the components of this report are my "normal" report and a statement to alert the clinician that the sensitivity of the mammographic examination is decreased in the patient with dense breasts.

The Must Biopsy Report

When there is an abnormality on the mammogram that has a high probability of being a cancer, I generate what I call a *must biopsy* report. This is a firm report, and I use it when a prompt biopsy is necessary. There is no equivocation. For example, a typical report for a stellate mass would be as follows:

> There is a 1.5-cm stellate mass in the right upper outer quadrant. These are characteristics highly suggestive of carcinoma.
> I recommend biopsy to rule out breast cancer.

Since this report forces action, I use it only on occasions when a mammographic lesion must be excised as soon as possible.

The Multiplicity Report

One of the dilemmas facing mammographers is how to word a report when there are multiple abnormalities, all of a rather similar benign appearance. These abnormalities could be masses, asymmetric densities, or calcifications. I have a report that simply states:

> | | (masses) |
> |---|---|
> | There are multiple | (asymmetric densities) |
> | | (microcalcifications) |
>
> No one area appears more suspicious to merit biopsy at this time.
> I recommend a repeat examination within ___ months to assess the stability of these areas.

This is then followed by my disclaimer. The specific follow-up protocol I use (triggering the first follow-up within 6 months and continuing the follow-up for a minimum of $2\frac{1}{2}$ to 3 years) has been detailed previously. In cases with multiple abnormalities it is not my usual practice to describe or measure each abnormality. I can understand why radiologists are accustomed to generating a descriptive report of multiple abnormalities, but since my recommendation and management are the same in all situations of multiplicity and bilaterality, my clinicians do not desire or require a long descriptive report. Some radiologists have told me that the reason they generate lengthy descriptive reports is that should the mammogram be lost, at least they have a description of the previous abnormalities to decide whether there has been an interval change that merits biopsy. In my experience with cases of multiplicity, a report cannot be descriptive enough to allow this judgment to be made. But I reemphasize that certainly it is the prerogative of the individual radiologist as to how descriptive to be.

In this *multiplicity* report, the follow-up directive is not optional. It is a clear recommendation, and if it is disregarded by the clinician, he or she assumes responsibility for the consequences. It is not the same as recommending annual mammography according to screening guidelines.

The Neutral Report

One recurring situation is handling a mammographic finding that has a very low probability of representing carcinoma. What kind of report should be generated for a mammographic finding that has less than a 5 percent chance of representing cancer? In this situation, I am uncomfortable being the one to choose between biopsy or follow-up. What might be considered to be the appropriate choice for a healthy 45-year-old woman could be inappropriate for a frail, 80-year-old woman. What might be appropriate for a 40-year-old woman with no risk factors might be inappropriate for a 40-year-old woman who already has had a contralateral mastectomy. In these cases I generate what I call a *neutral* report. For example, if a solitary geographic cluster of four microcalcifications unassociated with a mass is present, the report reads as follows:

> There is a cluster of four microcalcifications in the right upper outer quadrant. This has a high probability of being benign. The area can be localized prior to biopsy to establish histology. If biopsy is deferred, I recommend a follow-up examination within 6 months to assess its stability.

Notice that the words *malignant, cancer, mandatory,* and *must* do not appear in this report. The purpose of this neutral report is to give the clinician flexibility to determine the optimal management for a

mammographic abnormality with a very low chance of representing carcinoma. Circumstances best known to the clinician and not the radiologist may determine the appropriate course of management for a particular patient. My neutral report fulfills the obligation I have as a radiologist. I make the radiographic finding, convey to the clinician the sense of its probability of being either benign or malignant, and then make a recommendation. My recommendation is neutral in the sense that the abnormality under discussion can be either subject to biopsy or followed, since in my judgment both of these are appropriate management courses. Notice, however, that the one option my neutral report does not allow is for the clinician to ignore the finding.

Some of my radiology colleagues have said that no matter how they might word a neutral report, the surgeons tell them that they are forced to biopsy something once anything is found on the mammogram. This is nonsense. As long as the report is not worded in a way to force biopsy, there is absolutely no reason that a surgeon should feel any more compelled to subject to biopsy something described on the mammogram than he or she is compelled to subject to biopsy every thickening or nodularity in a breast that he or she decides requires follow-up. I believe that the surgeon who tells his or her radiologist that the detection of any mammographic abnormality automatically leaves him or her no option to use clinical judgment whether to subject it to biopsy or follow it is abrogating his or her responsibility as a physician. If the clinician's response is that the current legal environment forces him or her to subject to biopsy anything and everything that the radiologist describes, then that clinician is no longer *practicing* medicine. Being cognizant of the legal realities of our society does not justify allowing lawyers to determine patient management. In such a situation, I would agree with the radiologist that there is absolutely no verbiage that can be used in a mammography report to help this type of physician.

PUTTING MAMMOGRAPHIC GUIDELINES IN THE MAMMOGRAPHY REPORT

I do not believe that putting guidelines for mammographic utilization in the mammography report, whether those of the ACS or those of any other organization, is appropriate. Guidelines are only suggestions and may change. For instance, the ACS guidelines regarding mammography were different before 1980, were updated in 1983, and were modified again in 1989. If you put guidelines in your mammography report and they change in several years, are you going to retrieve your reports in order to make corrections? Imagine the predicament that a clinician might be in if he or she chooses not to order annual mammography on a woman younger than 50 years of age and she develops a breast cancer. The plaintiff's lawyer will show the mammogram report and say, "You did not follow the clear recommendation given by your consultant radiologist, which was to obtain annual mammograms, and therefore the delay in diagnosis of the woman's breast cancer was directly attributable to your refusal to follow these recommendations." I do not want to be responsible for placing my clinicians in this situation.

Some radiologists tell me that their reason for putting guidelines in the report is educational. I, too, think that education is important. If you want to educate your clinicians, there are other, more appropriate ways to do this such as putting guidelines of mammographic utilization inserts on a separate piece of paper accompanying the mammography report. When the clinician gets the report, he or she will see the guidelines you recommend without them being incorporated into the body of the report.

THE TECHNOLOGIST'S DIAGRAM

Although many may not consider the diagram and data sheet that our mammography technologists fill out relevant to the body of the report, I do. My technologist must carefully fill out a diagram of the breast, noting visible scars, dermatologic conditions, location of masses, and so on. She must ask the patient to describe symptoms. The information that the technologist receives can be an important complement to the mammography report and can be used as evidence in court. As discussed previously, diagrams should not consist of a single frontal projection but should include both a frontal and a lateral projection of each breast in order to document the precise location of a palpable abnormality. I would encourage every radiologist to instruct the technologist to meticulously fill in the information so it can serve as a check upon the information that the clinician provides. In addition, the technologist should be required to put down an answer on the data sheet for *every* question. For example, if the question states, "Previous biopsy?" rather than leave it blank, the technologist should fill it in with the word *no*. This documents the fact that the patient has been asked the question and that the technologist has recorded an answer. Other specifics of the technologist's role have been detailed in Chap. 3.

GETTING THE REPORT TO THE CLINICIAN

The million-dollar question is, "What is the radiologist's responsibility in getting the mammography report, or any radiology report for that matter, to the clinician?" Probably, the 100 percent foolproof solution is to have every radiology report sent by registered mail. I suspect that few of us do this. I think it would be prudent for radiologists to meet with their own legal counsels in order to understand the specific rules that apply to their hospitals, communities, and states.

Some radiologists tell me that in addition to the report, they rely upon a telephone call to get information to the clinician. The telephone call is good but may not be sufficient. First of all, what is your proof that the telephone call was made and what is your proof of the content of the telephone call? If you do not speak directly to the clinician, how do you know if the secretary or nurse delivered the message correctly? I also make telephone calls, but in addition to stating in my mammography report that a telephone call was made and the name of the person who received the telephone call, I keep a running log book that contains the name of the patient, and who received the call. This log is my proof that I made a reasonable attempt to get the message to the clinician. I have been told by lawyers that this log is strong evidence in the radiologist's favor. Ask your own lawyer about this.

Radiologists have told me that their clinicians do not allow them to be directive in their reports, so instead, they describe the finding and recommend clinical correlation. They use the telephone call to tell the surgeon of the exact findings. Recommending clinical correlation for a nonpalpable mammographic abnormality is insufficient. Imagine the following sequence of events. An asymptomatic woman has a routine screening mammogram and an irregular mass is identified. The radiologist correctly recognizes this as a lesion with a high probability of being carcinoma and immediately telephones the clinician with this information. However, the report only recommends clinical correlation. Such a report does not convey any sense of the high probability that this lesion represents carcinoma. Assume that for some reason the biopsy was not performed. Perhaps the surgeon decided that because his or her repeat breast palpation was normal, the radiologist was incorrectly interpreting an insignificant region on the mammogram and does not perform a biopsy. In court, your report shows that you recommended clinical correlation. The clinician says that indeed he or she followed your recommendation and performed clinical correlation. He or she produces office records, which show that the patient was called back a week later, palpated, and no abnormality was noted. While you are squirming in your seat knowing that the stellate mass about which you telephoned should have been immediately excised, the clinician simply states that he or she followed your recommendation. You really should have generated a *must biopsy* report. I do not believe that you are off the hook by recommending clinical correlation without being more directive. I would encourage you to describe this theoretical situation to your lawyer and listen to his or her response.[6]

USE OF THE WORD DYSPLASIA

In Chap. 8 there is a detailed discussion about why I believe that dysplasia cannot be diagnosed on the mammogram. At this time, it is sufficient to state that *dysplasia* is a term regarding cells and that the mammogram does not image cells. The diagnosis of dysplasia can only be made by the pathologist and not the radiologist.[7] My concern for the radiologist's inappropriate use of the word *dysplasia* is more practical than philosophical. When the pathologist diagnoses dysplasia from biopsy tissue, this carries a significant prognosis for the patient. Some pathologists believe that forms of very severe dysplasia with marked atypia are premalignant conditions. Some surgeons might even consider prophylactic mastectomy for severe dysplasia when the woman has other high-risk factors, such as a mother and sister with premenopausal breast cancer. The radiologist who uses the term *dysplasia* is not using it correctly and I am certain does not mean to convey the same implications as does the pathologist. In order to minimize confusion, radiologists should try as often as possible to use descriptive terms compatible with the pathologist's terms.[8]

REFERENCES

1. Friedman PJ. Radiologic reporting: structure. AJR **140**:171–172, 1980.
2. Homer MJ. A radiologist's point of view. JAMA **246**:2581–2582, 1981.
3. Berbaum KS, EL-Khoury GY, Franken EA, et al. Impact of clinical history on fracture detection with radiography. Radiology **168**:507–511, 1988.
4. Homer MJ. The mammography report. AJR **142**:643–644, 1984.
5. Hall FM. Mammographic reporting. Radiology **136**:258, 1980.
6. Berlin L. To telephone or not to telephone: how high is the standard? AJR **159**:1335–1339, 1992.
7. Page DL, Winfield AC. The dense mammogram. AJR **147**:487–489, 1986.
8. Friedman PJ. Radiologic reporting: the description of alveolar filling. AJR **141**:617–618, 1983.

LOCALIZING SIGNS OF BREAST CANCER

Radiologists are constantly trying to identify signs that will allow reliable differentiation between benign and malignant processes. The history of radiology is replete with examples showing that the initial enthusiasm for signs believed to accomplish this differentiation disappeared after experience proved that they were not reliable enough. Many of us have spent a great deal of time during residency being taught to recognize the difference between benign and malignant calcifications in a renal mass. We now know that the overlap is too great to confidently use it to differentiate between benign and malignant renal calcifications. Similarly, many of us were taught how to differentiate benign from malignant periosteal new bone formation. We now accept that while the appearance of periosteal reaction reflects aggressiveness, it cannot reliably differentiate benign from malignant. There are numerous other examples where radiographic signs have proved too unreliable for differentiating the benign from the malignant, such as with gastric ulcers, lung masses, and lytic bone lesions. Mammography is no different. While signs used to differentiate benign breast disease from malignant breast disease generally prove adequate in large groups of cases, lack of reliability lessens their value in determining patient management in the individual case. Every sign of malignant disease can be found in benign breast disease and vice versa.

The signs of malignancy in the breast have traditionally been divided into direct, or primary, signs reflecting the cancer itself and indirect, or secondary, signs evoked by the cancer. Since the ultimate question from a mammographic point of view is whether to biopsy, I prefer to divide the signs of breast cancer into localizing and nonlocalizing signs. A localizing sign of cancer means that when the radiologist identifies the sign on two views, the location of the suspected breast cancer is known. A nonlocalizing sign of breast cancer means that even if a breast cancer is causing the sign, its location is still not known and, therefore, biopsy is not an option. Table 6-1 lists the localizing signs of breast cancer. Each is discussed in sequence. For the purposes of this discussion, the assumption always is that the mammographic abnormality is nonpalpable unless stated otherwise. When a mammographic abnormality is palpable, the additional information from clinical findings is of crucial importance in determining patient management and becomes a primary consideration in each individual case.

LOCALIZING SIGNS

Mass

When a nonpalpable stellate mass is identified on the mammogram in an asymptomatic woman and there is no causal explanation for this finding such as prior biopsy, trauma, or infection, then there should be little difficulty in recognizing this as a worrisome sign of

TABLE 6-1
LOCALIZING SIGNS OF BREAST CANCER

1. Mass
2. Microcalcification
3. Asymmetric density
4. Neodensity
5. Architectural distortion
6. Enlarged duct

malignancy, which usually demands prompt biopsy. While benign entities such as focal sclerosing adenosis and radial scar may have stellate margins, biopsy is almost always necessary to exclude the presence of cancer. Stellate projections of cancer may represent either actual tumor infiltration into the breast tissue or non-tumor areas of desmoplastic fibrosis. These projections explain why often a breast cancer palpates larger than it appears by mammography.

What about the moderately well-circumscribed breast mass? Moderately well-circumscribed carcinomas include medullary carcinoma, intracystic carcinoma, colloid carcinoma, and on occasion "run-of-the-mill" ductal carcinoma (Fig. 6-1). The presence of a halo sign is not an absolute indication that the lesion is benign.[1] In fact, the halo sign has been shown to represent a Mach band reflecting an optical illusion rather than an anatomic sign indicating absence of infiltration of tissue adjacent to a mass.[2] Conversely, benign entities such as fibroadenoma and cystic masses may have poorly defined margins (Fig. 6-2). Often their margins, even when well-defined, cannot be evaluated adequately because of overlap from adjacent breast tissue or fibrosis. If sharply marginated masses may be malignant and masses with poorly defined borders may be benign, possibly too much time is spent analyzing borders. Perhaps reliance upon the sharpness of the border of a breast mass as a sign differentiating benign from malignant is less important than many believe it to be.

When there is a moderately well-circumscribed mass in the breast, an important determination is whether it is solitary or not. If there are other masses present in both breasts, all with similar features (multiplicity and bilaterality), then placing the patient in a

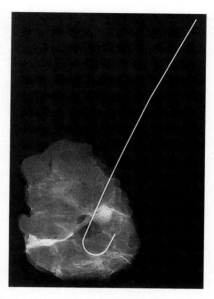

FIG. 6-1 *(Continued)* **B.** *Specimen radiograph of a well-circumscribed 7-mm invasive ductal carcinoma.*

follow-up protocol is more reasonable than random excision of one of the many mammographic masses.[3] Excising one of the masses and proving it to be benign does not prove that the other masses are benign nor does it eliminate the need for placing the patient into a follow-up protocol. If the masses are unilateral (multiplicity without bilaterality), then some consideration must still be given to performing a biopsy because the lack of bilaterality somewhat decreases the probability of the masses being benign. There are no reliable rules that can apply to this situation, and each case must be evaluated on an individual basis.

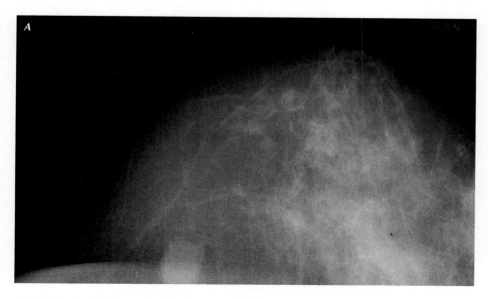

FIG. 6-1 **A.** *CC view of well-circumscribed invasive ductal carcinoma.*

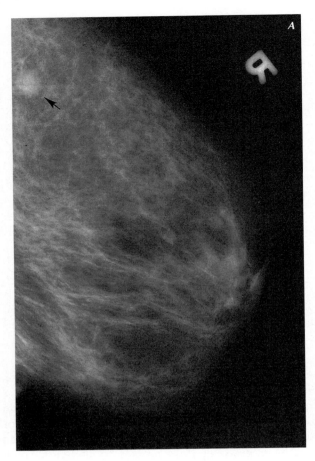

FIG. 6-2 A. *LAT view of a benign fibroadenoma with irregular margins.*

If there are no other masses in the breast—in other words, if the mass is a solitary dominant geographic abnormality—then biopsy becomes a much more acceptable option and the next determination should be whether there is any chance that the mammographic mass represents a cyst. If there is any possibility that it could be a cyst, an ultrasound examination should be performed to make this differentiation. As a general rule, any moderately well-circumscribed noncalcified mass should undergo ultrasound examination if it could be a cyst. If the mass contains calcium, the probability of it being a simple cyst becomes much less likely and ultrasound may be bypassed. An exception is when the mass has a form of benign punctate calcium. This is easily recognized because discrete calcium particles layer at the bottom of the mass which in reality is a macrocyst.[4] This layering phenomenon is demonstrated on a horizontal beam projection (Fig. 6-3). If this sign is present, then the benign nature of the mass may be assumed. My practice then is to place the patient in the standard follow-up protocol to confirm stability after ultrasound shows the mass to be a cyst.

There is an exception to the principle that a nonpalpable dominant solitary geographic mass with sharply marginated borders should undergo ultrasound to rule out a simple cyst prior to establishing its histology by obtaining tissue. In general the parameter of size in predicting the benign or malignant nature of any sharply defined noncalcified mass is not very reliable.[5] A very common finding in the breast is the small sharply circumscribed mass with no internal microcalcifica-

FIG. 6-2 (Continued) B. *Specimen radiograph of a different patient showing a poorly defined benign fibroadenoma.*

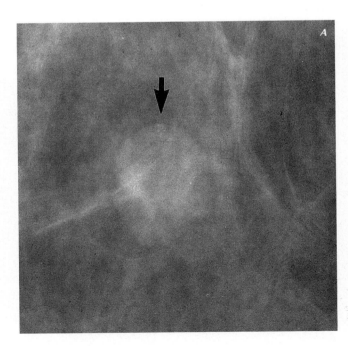

FIG. 6-3 A. *Vertical beam (CC view) of a macrocyst containing punctate calcifications.*

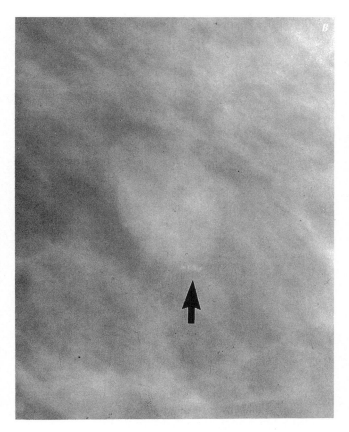

FIG. 6-3 *(Continued)* **B.** *Horizontal beam projection (LAT view) demonstrates layering of the punctate calcifications at the bottom of the benign cyst.*

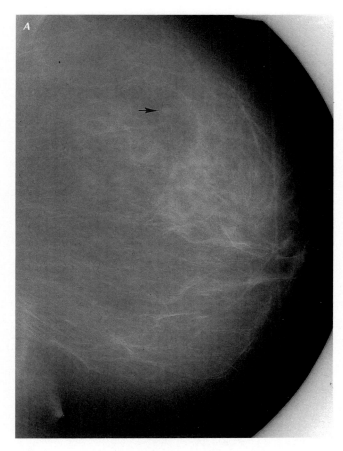

FIG. 6-4 **A.** *LAT view of sharply marginated noncalcified 5-mm mass.*

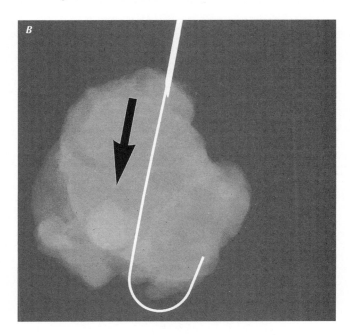

FIG. 6-4 *(Continued)* **B.** *Specimen radiograph from a different patient showing a well-defined noncalcified 6-mm mass. Although follow-up was recommended, the patient opted for excision. Histology revealed a benign fibroadenoma.*

tions. These masses measure no larger than 1 to 1.5 cm in greatest diametrer, and most are usually smaller (Fig. 6-4). It is my practice that a very sharply defined noncalcified nonpalpable mass measuring less than 1.5 cm in greatest diameter, is placed into follow-up. Often these masses are multiple and are commonly found in elderly patients. While these masses should not be ignored because occasionally they will indeed represent an early carcinoma (Fig. 6-5), they are so common a finding in the breast that excising them all would lead to an unacceptably high number of false-positive biopsies. The differential diagnosis of such masses includes fibroadenoma, intramammary lymph node, benign focus of fibrocystic change, small benign simple cyst, and rarely carcinoma.[6] When these masses are very small (below 0.5 cm in greatest diameter) I usually do not recommend ultrasound for these mammographic lesions that have a high probability of being benign for three reasons. First, they are usually so small that often they cannot be identified by ultrasound. Second, even if they are identified by ultrasound, they are usually too small for the examination to conclusively demonstrate a benign simple cyst (anechoic mass with sharp margins and good through transmission). Therefore, ultrasound does not allow

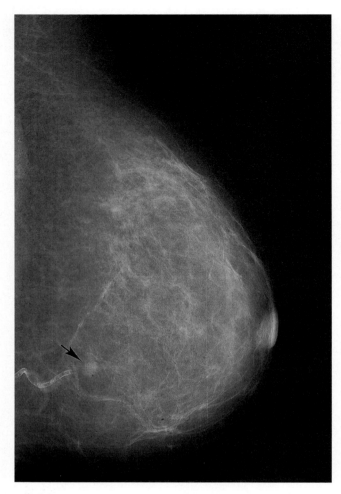

FIG. 6-5 *LAT view showing a sharply marginated noncalcified 5-mm mass. It was excised because it was not present on a previous examination. Histology revealed an invasive ductal carcinoma.*

the ultrasonographer to unequivocally make the diagnosis of a simple cyst and stop the workup from proceeding further. Their small size usually makes aspiration impossible. Finally, since these masses are most often solid (statistically the mass represents either a fibroadenoma, intramammary lymph node, or a type of benign fibrocystic change), the ultrasound study will, in fact, demonstrate echoes. This would make it even more difficult for a surgeon to opt for follow-up rather than biopsy

It must be emphasized that the mammographic characteristics of the small mass, as described above, must be strictly fulfilled in order to qualify as the lesion under discussion. Magnification mammography often will prove helpful in demonstrating these features. If the mass does not fulfill the strict criteria, then although it is still a mammographic abnormality with a high probability of being benign, the degree of confidence in its benign nature is decreased. The presence of a notch (hilus) and/or fat within the center of these

small sharply marginated masses are additional mammographic features that strongly support the specific diagnosis of an intramammary lymph node (Fig. 6-6).[7] Certainly in these cases every attempt should be made to discourage a biopsy from being performed.

Conventional wisdom holds that a mass of high density is more likely to be malignant than a low-density mass. In my experience, the smaller the breast cancer, the less tissue volume it has and the more likely it is to be isodense or even of lower density when compared to areas of fibrotic breast parenchyma. This is becoming increasingly more common as mammography allows the detection of very small cancers. It is for this reason that density analysis of masses is not a reliable feature in differentiating benign from malignant. In addition, density analysis is a subjective determination that has been shown to have considerable interobserver disagreement.[8]

MICROCALCIFICATIONS

Microcalcifications may be the only mammographic sign of breast cancer. As a general rule, microcalcifications with irregular, pleomorphic, branching, and rod shapes without polarity (not oriented toward the nipple) have a higher probability of being associated with malignant disease, while those with round or oval shapes and more uniform size have a higher probability of being associated with benign disease. However, since there is such a great similarity between the appearance of benign microcalcification and that of malignant microcalcification, in the great majority of situations it is difficult to be absolutely certain of the nature of the process that is creating the microcalcifications.[9] When a radiologist identifies an area of microcalcification and the obvious benign etiologies such as dermal, vascular, and fat necrosis have been ruled out, I believe there are only two options: either put the patient in a follow-up protocol to be certain that the microcalcifications remain stable or establish their histology by obtaining tissue.

Rather than attempting to divide microcalcifications into benign and malignant, my approach is to divide them into those that are more likely to be benign and those that are more likely to be malignant. This is not a mere semantic distinction because the radiologist's role becomes one of judging whether the patient should have a tissue diagnosis immediately or should be placed in a follow-up rather than deciding whether the calcifications are benign (requiring no further action) or malignant. The finding of microcalcifications in the asymptomatic woman takes her out of the routine screening population and places her either into a follow-up or biopsy category. I do not believe there are any features of microcalcifications that can reliably

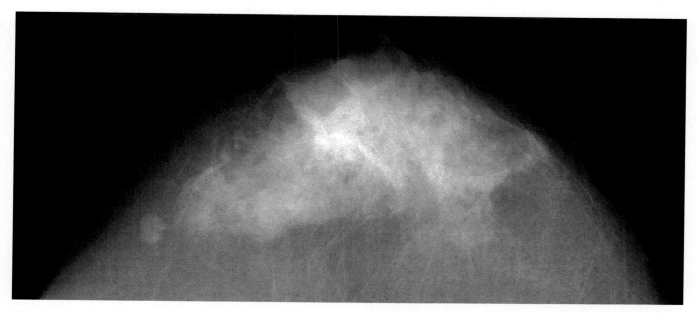

FIG. 6-6 *CC view showing a typical intramammary lymph node on the axillary side. Notice the sharp margins and central hilus.*

help distinguish benign from malignant except for a very few categories that have a virtually pathognomonic appearance. These benign calcifications are described later. Microcalcifications can be analyzed by size, shape, number, volume in which they are contained, and their association with density.

Size

The traditional teaching is that cancer is associated with microcalcification, while benign breast disease is associated with macrocalcification. If this is correct and we could agree upon a diameter at which *micro* becomes *macro*, much of the problem of differentiating benign from malignant would seem to be solved. How large is a microcalcification? My answer is that numbers will not help. To those who use a millimeter size to differentiate *micro* from *macro*, my "tongue-in-cheek" question is, How can you be certain that the cancer knows your measurement? While a reasonable arbitrary size for *micro* is often taken to be less than 0.5 mm,[10] anyone experienced in mammographic interpretation knows that tumor calcium may be larger.

Microcalcification can grow to macrocalcification over time. If a breast cancer is laying down calcium, initially the calcium is only visible microscopically and is too small to be resolved by mammography. As the process continues, the calcifications grow and eventually become large enough to be resolved by mammography. If the cancer remains undisturbed, calcium may continue to form and eventually *micro* can become *macro*. The well-known evolution of calcium development in a fibroadenoma is a good example of this

process. All fibroadenomas begin uncalcified. Then they develop histologic calcification and eventually small, mammographically visible microcalcification will be identified. When the calcification process continues uninterrupted, the calcium grows into the easily recognizable dense macrocalcification characteristic of the degenerating fibroadenoma. Therefore, I do not believe that making a distinction between *micro* and *macro* is as critical as many believe it to be. Cancers may even develop large areas of dense, popcornlike calcification if they are left alone long enough to permit the calcification process to continue undisturbed (Fig. 6-7).

Shape

The shape of microcalcification is considered by many to be the single most important feature in differentiating benign from malignant. Quite simply, the more round or oval and uniform the shape, the more likely the benign nature of the process, and the more irregular the shape, the more likely it is to be associated with malignancy. Extensive detailed analysis and description of malignant microcalcification exists.[11] Despite this, others believe that shape cannot reliably help to differentiate benign from malignant.[9] I have finally accepted the reality that after years of determined effort, I am still unable to confidently master differentiation between benign and malignant calcifications based upon shape. Round, oval, punctate calcium may be produced by malignancy (Fig. 6-8), and bizarre, pleomorphic branching calcium may be produced by benign processes (Fig. 6-9). I have also demonstrated that

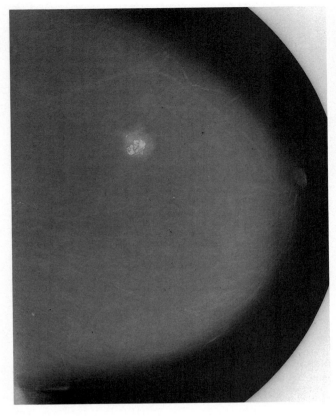

FIG. 6-7 *LAT view of a stellate invasive ductal carcinoma containing central popcornlike macrocalcification.*

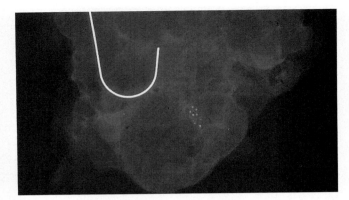

FIG. 6-8 *Specimen radiograph of an intraductal carcinoma containing punctate round microcalcifications.*

hundreds of other radiologists who have taken test cases of mine similarly cannot make this differentiation with more than 70 percent accuracy.[12] This percentage of accuracy is not good enough for determining a patient management decision.

Some place a great deal of emphasis on differentiating ductal calcification from lobular calcification by shape. The former has a rod-shaped appearance with branching linear forms, while the latter has a more regular rounded punctate appearance. The rationale for this discrimination is that since most breast cancer is ductal, recognition of this form of calcium is important

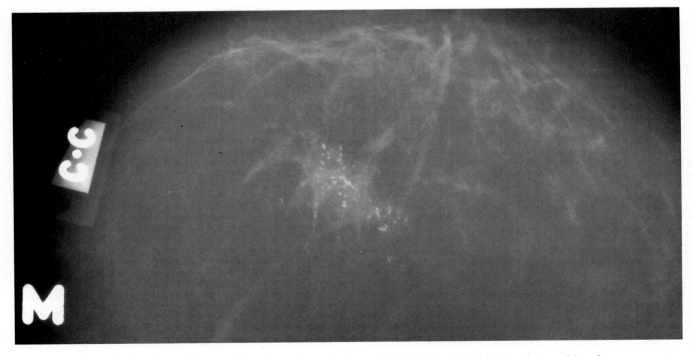

FIG. 6-9 *CC view reveals geographic area of pleomorphic microcalcifications with linear and branching forms. Excisional biopsy revealed benign fibrocystic changes.*

for diagnosis. The logic behind this should be carefully examined before accepting the premise. Ductal carcinoma may obstruct the egress of lobular contents, causing the development of "benign" lobular calcifications from the resultant stasis (Fig. 6-10). If the carcinoma itself remains noncalcified and its soft tissue component is too small to be detected as a mass by mammography, then the only clue to its presence will be the adjacent lobular calcification. The calcification, therefore, serves as a marker for cancer even though in reality it is truly benign lobular calcium. This phenomenon of mammographically visible calcium located in areas of benign breast parenchyma adjacent to the carcinoma, but not within the carcinoma, is well known.[13–15] Finally, pathologists have long recognized that not only can ductal carcinoma spread toward the nipple, but it can also migrate retrograde to involve the lobules (Fig. 6-11). This is called cancerization of the lobules.[16,17] Therefore, since lobular calcification may be caused by ductal carcinoma, differentiating between ductal and lobular calcifications has less value than many believe.

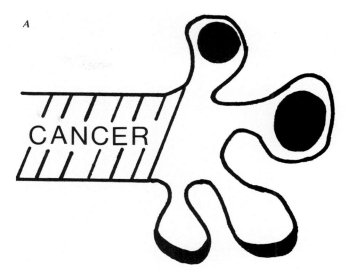

FIG. 6-10 A. *Diagram illustrating how an obstructing occult ductal carcinoma can cause lobular calcification of both punctate and milk-of-calcium forms.*

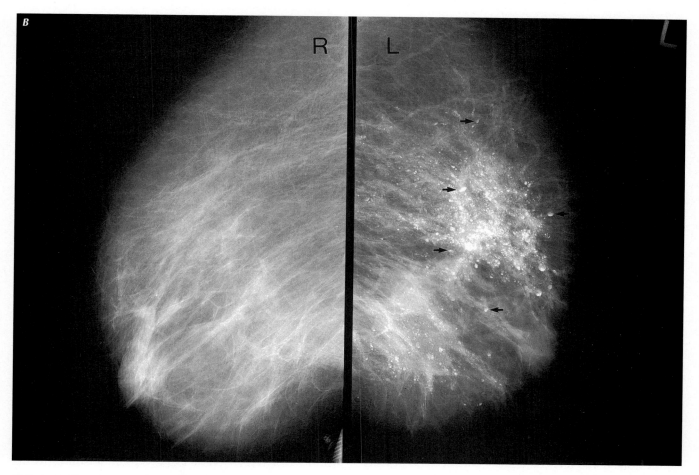

FIG. 6-10 *(Continued)* **B.** *OBL views from a routine screening mammogram. The right breast is normal. The left breast contains numerous benign-appearing macrocalcifications, milk of calcium (arrows), and microcalcifications. No discrete mass was evident by mammography or breast repalpation.*

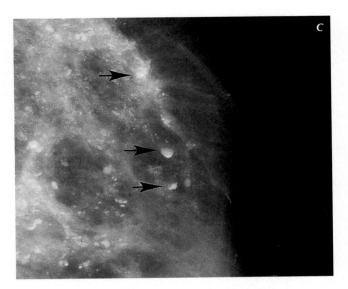

FIG. 6-10 *(Continued)* **C.** *Close-up LAT view shows definite milk-of-calcium levels. Histology revealed that the entire left breast was involved with intraductal and invasive ductal carcinoma. The tumor was blocking ducts, causing stasis and the development of benign calcium. (Courtesy of Phoebe A. Kaplan, M.D., Omaha, Nebraska.)*

Number

The number of microcalcifications has been used as an indicator of a benign lesion or a malignant one. Most would agree that a solitary cluster of microcalcifications should be excised, but the age-old question is, How many microcalcifications constitute a cluster? This question possibly may have more metaphysical interest than practical importance. My belief is that everyone has to pick an arbitrary number of how many microcalcifications make a cluster. My magic number is four, and your magic number may be five or six. In any event, we must all agree that the number generally be within this range rather than 10, 15, or 20. The reason that this is an arbitrary number is that if the mammogram can resolve 4, 5, or 6 microcalcifications, a magnification view of the area will probably demonstrate more microcalcifications, while specimen radiography will usually show even more than that! If you have any doubt about this, review your own specimen radiography of microcalcifications after you have counted how many microcalcifications appear to be present on the original mammogram. The number of microcalcifications visualized on the mammogram is almost always less than the number actually present within the tissue.

Once your arbitrary number is selected, biopsy can be considered an option if the cluster contains this number or more. If the number contained in the cluster is one less than your magic number, the calcium must not be viewed as insignificant, but the patient

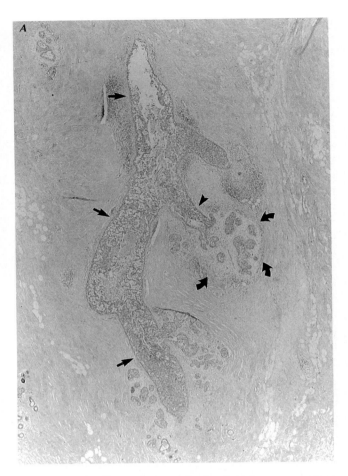

FIG. 6-11 **A.** *Photomicrograph of a duct in cross section (arrows) containing tumor. The tumor is spreading retrograde through an interlobular duct (arrowhead) to involve a lobular unit (curved arrows). Within the lobular unit are ductules filled with tumor. (Reprinted by permission of the publisher from Homer MJ, Safaii H: Cancerization of the Lobule: Implication regarding Analysis of Microcalcification Shape. Breast Disease 3:131–133, 1990. Copyright © 1990 by Elsevier Science Publishing Company, Inc.)*

should be placed into a follow-up protocol. Follow-up is necessary because while you may have decided how many calcifications constitute a cluster, you have no way of knowing whether the cancer agrees with you! For instance, if your number is 5, there is no guarantee that an area with 3 or 4 microcalcifications does not represent an early carcinoma, which, if left alone, will eventually develop more calcifications (Fig. 6-12).

Since my magic number is 4, usually a patient with a solitary focus of 2 or 3 microcalcifications is placed in my follow-up protocol. If I see 1 microcalcification, it is not my usual policy to recommend a follow-up protocol unless there is a special circumstance to the case. However, even putting a patient with a single calcification in follow-up is a practice that can be defended.[18]

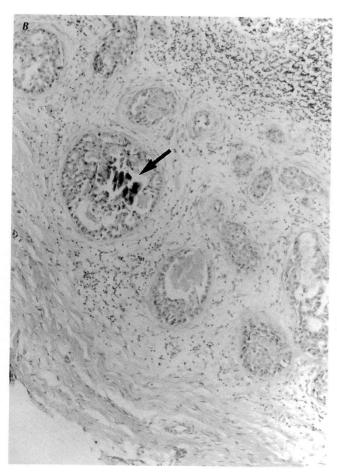

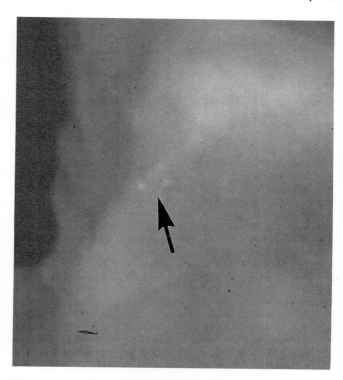

FIG. 6-12 *Magnification specimen radiograph showing an intraductal carcinoma presenting on the mammogram as four punctate microcalcifications.*

FIG. 6-11 *(Continued)* **B.** *Photomicrograph from an adjacent field shows a lobular unit containing ductules filled with tumor. The tumor contains microcalcifications (arrow). (Reprinted by permission of the publisher from Homer MJ, Safaii H: Cancerization of the Lobule: Implication regarding Analysis of Microcalcification Shape. Breast Disease 3:131–133, 1990. Copyright © 1990 by Elsevier Science Publishing Company, Inc.)*

There is one final situation in which a solitary geographic area of microcalcification containing less than your magic number may merit consideration for prompt biopsy. The development over time of more microcalcifications in the same area is important, even if the total number is still smaller than the magic number that you have arbitrarily chosen. For example, assume that your magic number is 5 and that on the present examination you detect an area of 4 microcalcifications. If on a previous examination there were only 2 microcalcifications in the area, and no other focus of calcium exists in either the ipsilateral or contralateral breast, biopsy should be considered even though your magic number of five has still not been reached. A magnification view may show even more calcium. At least the patient should be placed into a follow-up protocol. The increase in number of microcalcifications in a solitary geographic focus (Fig. 6-13) is a disturbing change.

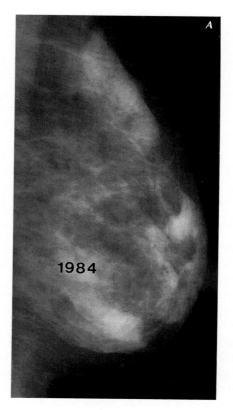

FIG. 6-13 **A.** *Normal LAT mammogram.*

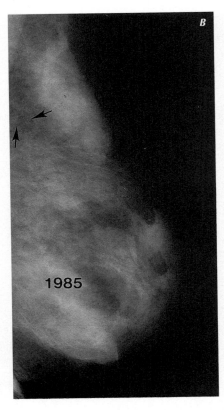

FIG. 6-13 (Continued) **B.** *The next year, two punctate microcalcifications have appeared.*

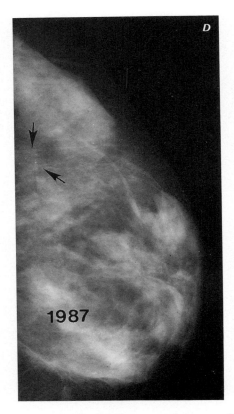

FIG. 6-13 (Continued) **D.** *Two years later, a solitary geographic cluster is evident.*

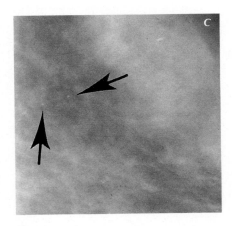

FIG. 6-13 (Continued) **C.** *Close-up view.*

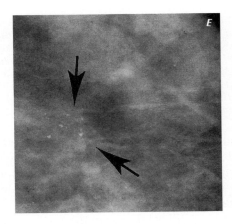

FIG. 6-13 (Continued) **E.** *Close-up; histology revealed intraductal carcinoma.*

Volume

The volume of what constitutes a significant grouping of microcalcifications has been proposed to be 1 cm³.[10] This is certainly an acceptable definition. In addition to volume, I also use the concept of *geographic abnormality*, but this concept defies quantification. A geographic abnormality in the case of microcalcifications, contained within a volume smaller than 1 cm³ (Fig. 6-14), within one half of the breast (Fig. 6-15), or throughout an entire breast (Fig. 6-16), all indicate that the process causing the calcium formation is only occurring in a defined region. In other words, it is a solitary geographic abnormality, and in all of these situations serious consideration should be given to establishing a tissue diagnosis.

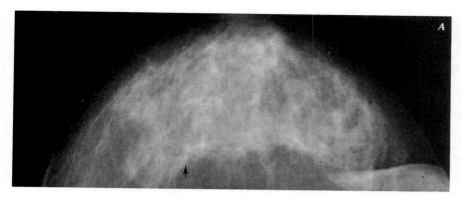

FIG. 6-14   A. *CC view of 2-mm geographic area of microcalcifications (arrow).*

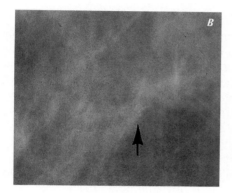

FIG. 6-14 *(Continued)*   **B.** *Close-up view. Histology revealed intraductal carcinoma.*

Association with Density

The association of microcalcifications with density seems to worry some radiologists, while the presence of the same microcalcifications with no density does not. I fail to understand the logic behind this. While I agree that the presence of a density with microcalcifications might convince the radiologist to recommend immediate biopsy rather than follow-up, I do not comprehend the rationale for considering a cluster of microcalcifications unassociated with density to be unimportant. Intraductal and microinvasive ductal carcinomas are early stages in the evolution of breast cancer, and often at this point in time the cancer may not have formed a large enough tissue volume to be perceived as a density on the mammogram. The presence of a density associated with microcalcifications in what proves to be a carcinoma increases the probability that the malignancy is already invasive. The absence of a density with microcalcifications should not by itself be used as the reason to declare a cluster of microcalcifications benign (Fig. 6-17).

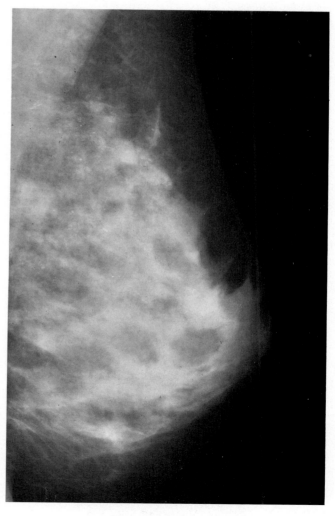

FIG. 6-15 *OBL view of the right breast demonstrates a process producing microcalcifications in the upper half of the breast. There was no palpable abnormality. Histology revealed predominantly intraductal carcinoma with a few areas of focal invasion.*

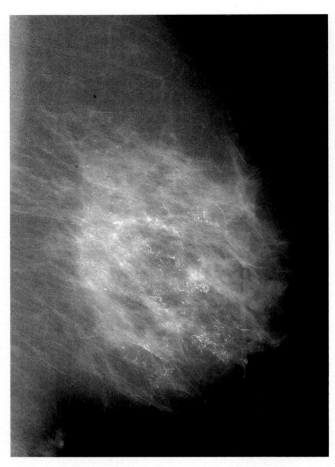

FIG. 6-16 *LAT view of left breast demonstrates involvement of almost the entire breast by a process producing microcalcifications. Histology revealed extensive intraductal and invasive ductal carcinoma.*

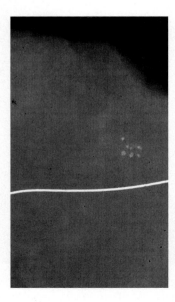

FIG. 6-17 *Specimen radiograph of a 3-mm geographic cluster of microcalcifications without an associated density. Histology revealed intraductal carcinoma.*

Virtually Pathognomonic Features of Benign Microcalcification

Although most features of microcalcifications cannot reliably differentiate a benign lesion from a malignant one, there are several types of microcalcifications with characteristics that are associated with benign or probably benign disease.

DERMAL CALCIUM

Dermal calcifications may appear to mimic a cluster of microcalcifications within breast tissue.[19,20] Since the breast is a flaccid organ that is easily compressed, dermal calcifications can appear to project deep within the breast on two views, even when the views are at 90-degree angles. In reality, however, they are not in breast parenchyma (Fig. 6-18).

There are clues to help recognize dermal calcifications (Table 6-2). Microcalcifications with lucent centers (Fig. 6-19), microcalcifications having polygonal shapes (Fig. 6-20), clustered microcalcifications that are located quite peripherally (even on one projection) (Fig. 6-21), calcifications that have a linear orientation (Fig. 6-22); and calcifications that maintain a fixed relationship to each other (Fig 6-23), should all raise the possibility of dermal calcification.

Since intramammary calcifications are located in compressible fibroglandular tissue and fat, they are not in a fixed position and can change their relationships to each other. In contradistinction, dermal calcifications have a fixed position within the dermal layer of the skin and the calcific particles maintain a constant relationship to each other. Similar to a tattoo which has a fixed pattern on the skin, dermal calcifications maintain a fixed relationship to each other when similar projections of mammograms are compared to each other, even if obtained at different times. This fixed relationship has been referred to as the tattoo sign.[21] When calcifications exhibit a tattoo sign, the radiologist should be alerted to the possibility of their dermal location. This observation can help avoid inadvertent needle localization and biopsy for dermal calcifications. In patients undergoing needle localization for microcalcifications without an associated mass, a helpful step prior to insertion of the needle, would be to compare the initial mammogram of the breast in the compression template with an earlier mammogram obtained in a similar projection. If the calcium particles show the tattoo sign by maintaining a fixed relationship to each other, their dermal location should be suspected and confirmed using standard methods.

A linear orientation is often seen with dermal calcium, since the calcium assumes this position when the skin is caught in tangent. Even when a single microcalcification in a cluster has a lucent center, the

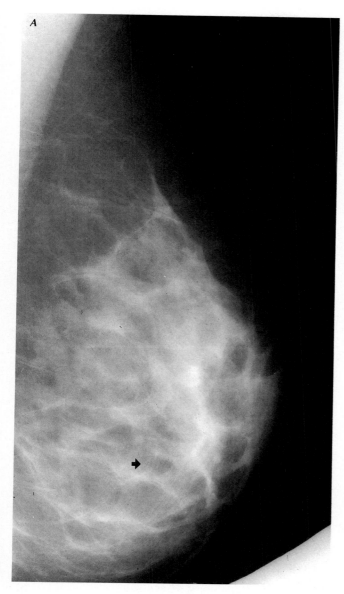

FIG. 6-18 **A.** *LAT view of 3-mm geographic cluster of microcalcifications.*

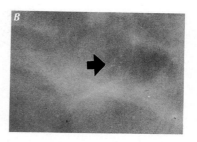

FIG. 6-18 *(Continued)* **B.** *Close-up view.*

possibility of the entire cluster being in the dermal layer should be considered. If there is a question of whether a microcalcification has a lucent center, a magnification mammogram may prove helpful for clarification (Fig. 6-24). It is important to remember that, unfortunately, dermal calcifications may possess none of these telltale clues. It must also be emphasized that the presence of a lucent center in a microcalcification is not a pathognomonic sign that the location of the cluster is dermal. If calcium is caught in tangent within the dermal layer on a routine view, then there is no need for further proof of its location (Fig. 6-25).

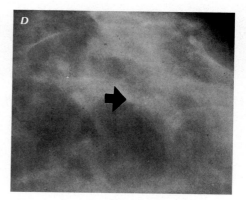

FIG. 6-18 *(Continued)* **D.** *Close-up view of the microcalcifications. These were proven to be dermal in location.*

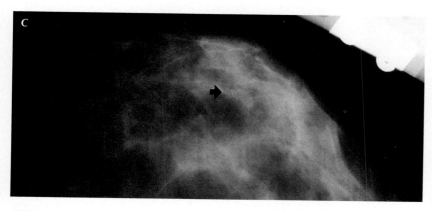

FIG. 6-18 *(Continued)* **C.** *CC view of the same cluster. On both this view and the LAT view it appears to project within breast parenchyma.*

TABLE 6-2 _____
CHARACTERISTICS OF DERMAL CALCIUM

1. Lucent center
2. Polygonal shape
3. Peripheral location
4. Linear orientation
5. Calcific particles maintain a fixed relationship to each other

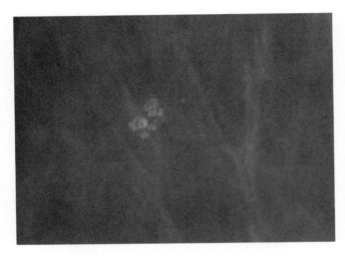

FIG. 6-19 *Notice the lucent centers in many of these dermal calcifications.*

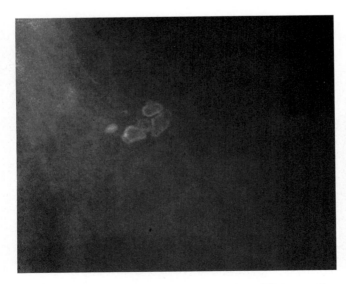

FIG. 6-20 *Notice the polygonal shapes in addition to the lucent centers of this dermal calcium cluster.*

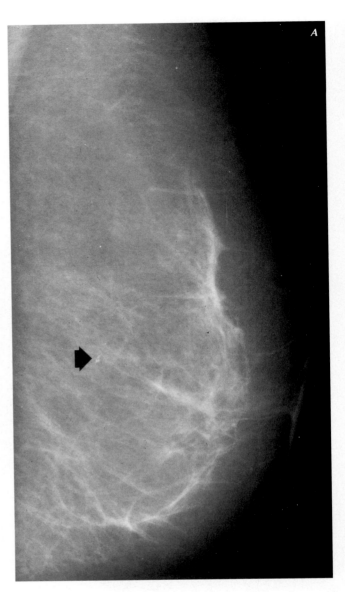

FIG. 6-21 **A.** *LAT view demonstrates a solitary cluster of microcalcifications (arrow) located 6 cm deep to the nipple.*

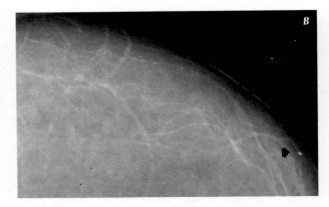

FIG. 6-21 *(Continued)* **B.** *CC view shows that the cluster (arrow) is very peripheral in location. This is the clue to its dermal location.*

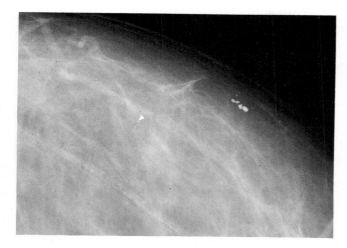

FIG. 6-22 *Notice the linear orientation of this dermal calcium as it comes close to being imaged in tangent.*

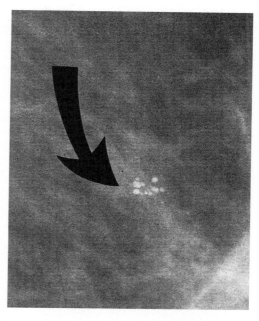

FIG. 6-23 *(Continued)* **B.** *Close-up view.*

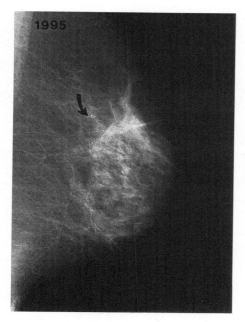

FIG. 6-23 **A.** *OBL view of the left breast revealed a solitary cluster of microcalcifications.*

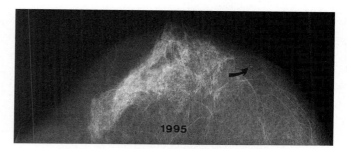

FIG. 6-23 *(Continued)* **C.** *CC view demonstrates the cluster.*

Proving the dermal location of a cluster of microcalcifications using a superficial marking technique is simple and can be performed by either the radiologist or technologist.[20] From the craniocaudal view, the posterior and medial or lateral distance between the cluster and the nipple is measured. If the lateral view shows that the cluster is in the upper half of the breast, a radiopaque marker is placed on the upper half of the breast at the measured point. Conversely, if according to the lateral view the cluster is in the lower half of the breast, then the measurements are made on the undersurface of the breast and the radiopaque marker is

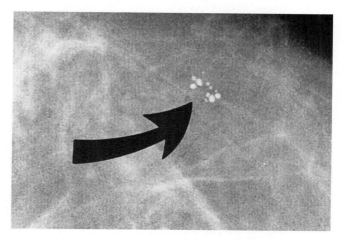

FIG. 6-23 *(Continued)* **D.** *Close-up view. Biopsy was recommended unless prior mammograms could be obtained for review.*

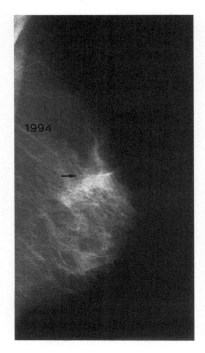

FIG. 6-23 *(Continued)* **E.** *OBL view 1 year earlier shows that the cluster was present.*

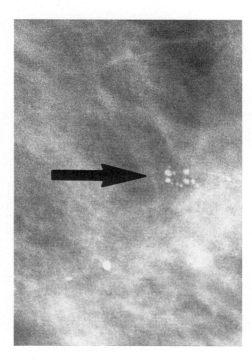

FIG. 6-23 *(Continued)* **F.** *Close-up view. Notice that the calcific particles have the same relationship to each other as on the OBL view of 1995.*

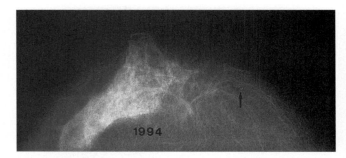

FIG. 6-23 *(Continued)* **G.** *CC view 1 year earlier also demonstrates the cluster of microcalcifications.*

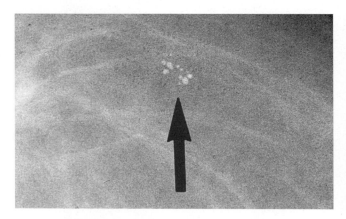

FIG. 6-23 *(Continued)* **H.** *Close-up view again demonstrates that the particles maintain a fixed relationship to each other. When this "tattoo sign" was recognized, the dermal location of the calcifications was suspected.*

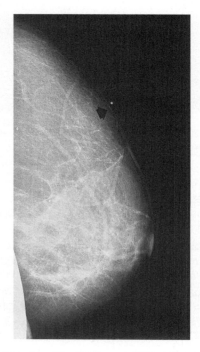

FIG. 6-23 *(Continued)* **I.** *Tangential view confirms the dermal location of the calcific particles. The needle localization was canceled.*

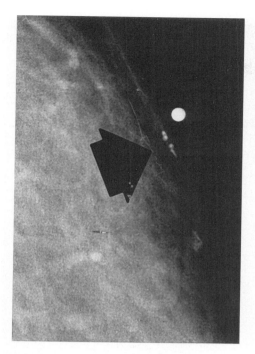

FIG. 6-23 *(Continued)* **J.** *Close-up view.*

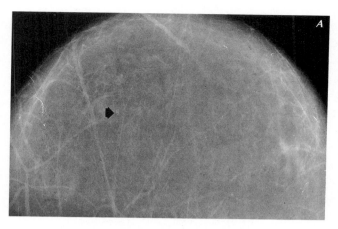

FIG. 6-25 **A.** *CC view demonstrates a solitary geographic cluster of calcium.*

4 mm or less of each other on any view (Fig. 6-26). A wider separation raises the possibility that the calcification may be very superficial but not necessarily within the dermal layer. This technique can also be performed using a standard coordinate-labeled localization template compression device.[22]

placed there. A craniocaudal view is then obtained in order to document that the marker is positioned directly over the cluster. If it is not, it must be repositioned until the final craniocaudal view shows that it is. Another view such as a lateral, an oblique, or a tangential projection is obtained to demonstrate the constant close relationship between the cluster and the superficial radiopaque skin marker. Maintenance of this relationship proves its dermal location. The marker and calcification should remain within approximately

FIG. 6-24 *On this magnification view, the dermal location of this cluster should be suspected, since one of the calcifications has a lucent center (arrow).*

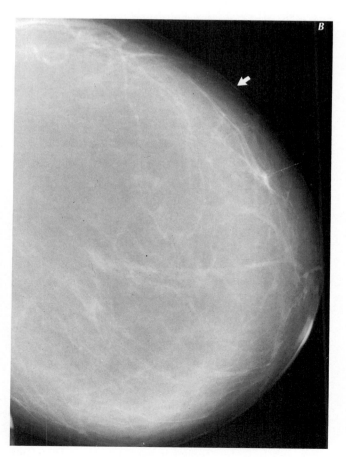

FIG. 6-25 *(Continued)* **B.** *On an OBL view the calcium is imaged tangentially in the dermal layer (arrow).*

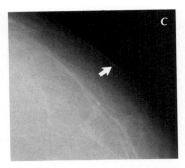

FIG. 6-25 *(Continued)* **C.** *Close-up view of a dermal location of calcium.*

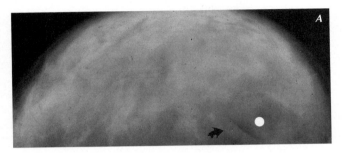

FIG. 6-26 **A.** *CC view demonstrates that the metallic marker is close to but not on the suspected dermal calcium. Repositioning of the marker is necessary.*

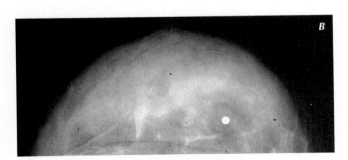

FIG. 6-26 *(Continued)* **B.** *CC view shows that the metallic marker is directly over the calcifications.*

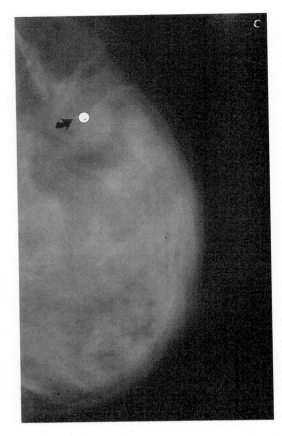

FIG. 6-26 *(Continued)* **C.** *LAT view demonstrates that the calcium does not separate from the metallic marker.*

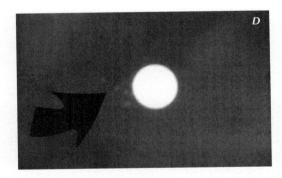

FIG. 6-26 *(Continued)* **D.** *Close-up view.*

Whenever I diagnose and confirm a cluster of dermal calcifications, I immediately discuss it with the patient. Since this entity is not well recognized by all radiologists, I am trying to avoid the possibility that at some future date the woman will have a mammogram elsewhere and that someone will recommend localization for the cluster of dermal calcifications. It is my practice to explain the entity to the woman as best as I can and have her repeat it back to me so that I am certain that she understands. I have her look at her breast in the area of the dermal calcium so that she can see that there is no visual skin abnormality. Sometimes it takes two or three explanations before I am convinced that she understands that there is nothing wrong with her breast, that this is a normal variation of no significance, and that this can potentially be misinterpreted for a significant abnormality. I tell her that in the future, if anyone wants to perform a biopsy of the area because of calcification, she must remember to tell her doctor that she has dermal calcification in the

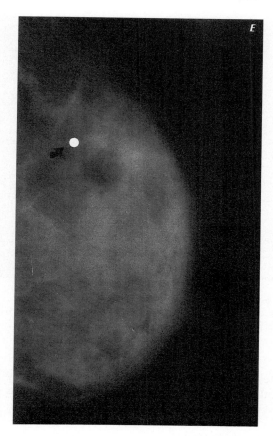

FIG. 6-26 *(Continued)* **E.** *OBL view demonstrates the inability to separate dermal calcium from the metallic marker.*

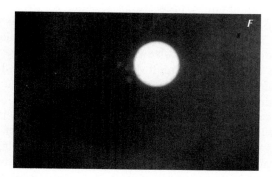

FIG. 6-26 *(Continued)* **F.** *Close-up view.*

area and ask if that could be the cause for concern. Another aid to help the woman remember this important finding is to hand her a written explanation or even a copy of the mammogram report and tell her to file it with other important papers she keeps at home. Not recognizing the dermal location of punctate microcalcification is a significant error because localization and excision will almost always fail. The reason is that it is not customary for the surgeon to include der-

mis in a breast biopsy. I have seen women unsuccessfully localized several times for failure to excise what proves to be dermal calcium.

RIM CALCIUM

Another calcium pattern which has a high association with a benign process is rim, or peripheral, calcium.[10] This type of calcification may surround all or part of the border of a mass (Fig. 6-27). The presence of rim calcium may be a reason to opt for follow-up rather than excision, since breast cancer typically does not contain this pattern.

MILK OF CALCIUM

Still another type of microcalcification that should be recognized as benign is milk of calcium.[23,24] This form of calcium settles at the bottom of microcysts and appears as smudgelike particles on vertical beam mammography and has flat or meniscus levels on the horizontal beam view (Fig. 6-28). It must be stressed that for an area of milk of calcium to be considered benign, all of the calcium present must adhere to the criterion of milk of calcium. If the lesion is mixed, containing both milk of calcium and punctate microcalcification, then it cannot be assumed that the lesion is benign[25] (Fig. 6-29). Milk of calcium may also present as a focal process[26] instead of the more usual diffuse form.

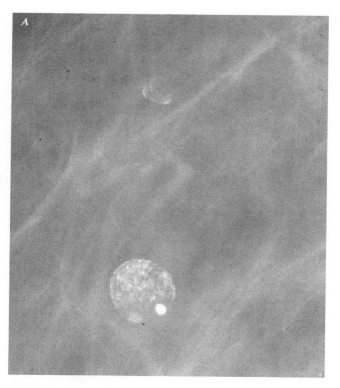

FIG. 6-27 **A.** *Notice the rim calcium around these masses. The patient was put into a follow-up protocol and because they remained unchanged, biopsy was avoided.*

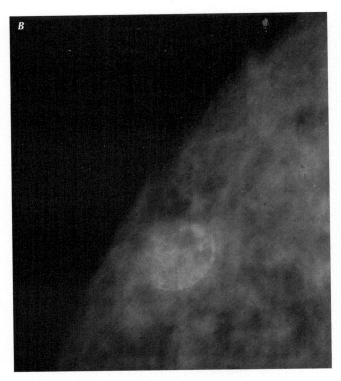

FIG. 6-27 (Continued) **B.** *Another example of rim calcium around a benign mass.*

DISAPPEARING CALCIFICATIONS

Intramammary calcifications can spontaneously disappear from the breast. This can occur with both macrocalcification and microcalcification. The mechanism responsible for this is unknown. Disappearance of breast calcification is more likely to reflect a benign

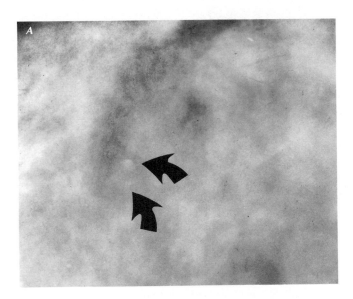

FIG. 6-28 **A.** *Close-up of CC view (vertical beam) showing milk of calcium as smudgelike particles.*

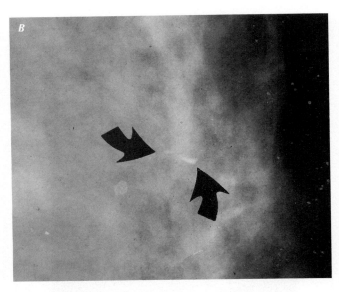

FIG. 6-28 (Continued) **B.** *Close-up of LAT view (horizontal beam) demonstrating the characteristic milk-of-calcium levels.*

process.[27] Unless a mass or new "malignant-type" microcalcifications develop at the site, biopsy is not indicated.

OTHER VARIATIONS

A variation of layering calcium previously described is that of punctate calcification that can layer at the bottom of a macrocyst.[4] As with milk of calcium, this characteristic appearance is also demonstrated on horizontal beam mammography.

A final type of benign calcium in the breast is vascular calcification, which has an appearance similar to vascular calcification elsewhere in the body. Early vascular calcification which does not have a typical appearance can be mistaken for parenchymal calcium and undergo needle localization.[28]

In summary, my magic number of microcalcifications in a cluster is 4. When I identify a cluster of 4 or more microcalcifications, I spend less time trying to characterize their appearance and more time determining whether they are confined to a geographic area. I spend most of my efforts carefully scrutinizing the remaining ipsilateral breast as well as the contralateral breast for the presence of other microcalcification foci. Magnification views of other areas of the breast often prove quite helpful in identifying additional foci, especially in the dense breast. If other foci are present bilaterally and all of the microcalcifications have a similar appearance, then one has proven that there are multiplicity and bilaterality so follow-up becomes a reasonable option. However, if there are other calcium foci but they are unilateral, a determination must be made as to whether to perform a biopsy because mul-

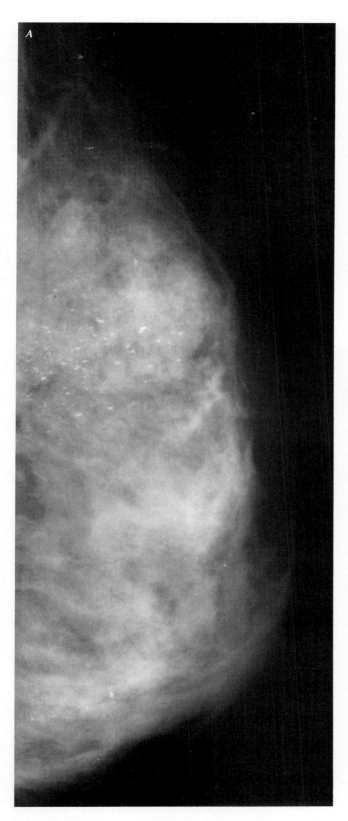

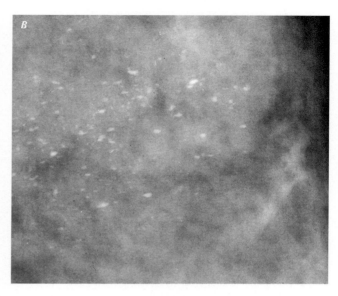

FIG. 6-29 (Continued) **B.** Close-up view.

FIG. 6-29 A. LAT view (horizontal beam) demonstrates a large geographic area containing both milk of calcium and numerous microcalcifications. The patient preferred biopsy rather than follow-up. Histology revealed fibrocystic changes with no evidence of malignancy.

tiplicity and unilaterality are definitely more disturbing than multiplicity and bilaterality. Analyzing microcalcification shape takes on more importance when one has to determine whether all foci of microcalcification are of similar appearance. For instance, if there are multiple foci of rounded, more uniform, punctate microcalcifications and there is one focus of branching, irregular microcalcifications, one must not interpret this as the pattern of multiplicity. The latter focus is different from the others and therefore becomes the dominant cluster. If there are no other areas of microcalcification in either the ipsilateral or contralateral breast, then one has proven that the cluster is a solitary dominant geographic abnormality and strong consideration should be given to establishing its histology.

Perhaps management of microcalcification would be easier if the radiologist interpreted its presence to indicate cellular activity rather than a benign or malignant lesion. I have resigned myself to my failure to reliably differentiate benign calcification from malignant calcification. I think I understand why I cannot master the differentiation and why I do not really feel too bad about it. First, by definition microcalcifications are so small that it will always be extremely difficult to confidently analyze their shapes, even with magnification. There necessarily will be a great deal of subjectivity in making this determination. For example, look at the crisply defined microcalcifications in a specimen radiograph and compare them with the detail of the same microcalcifications on the mammogram. The difference is nothing short of dramatic.

Even if one could differentiate benign from malignant with accuracy approaching 100 percent, this would still mean that those occult cancers obstructing ducts and causing benign lobular microcalcifications would be missed. If you, too, have been unable to confidently differentiate the benign from the malignant despite attending numerous lectures and reading many textbooks and articles, be comforted in knowing that you are not alone.

ASYMMETRIC DENSITY

An asymmetric density is a localizing sign of breast cancer. However, since very few breasts are symmetrical in appearance, single or multiple asymmetric densities are frequently present. This creates a dilemma because one cannot recommend biopsy for all asymmetric densities. The radiologist must constantly walk a fine line between trying to avoid overbiopsy of asymmetric densities (a majority of which are insignificant) and recognizing the occasional asymmetric density that does demand immediate biopsy. Even defining an asymmetric density is not simple because what one person calls an asymmetric density is called a mass by another.

Before worrying about an asymmetric density, one must be certain that it is not related to a prior breast biopsy. Postsurgical changes after a biopsy can create an asymmetric density in either the ipsilateral or contralateral breast. In the ipsilateral breast, postoperative fibrosis may cause an asymmetric density at the biopsy site (Fig. 6-30). A large enough biopsy may create a glandular defect at the site of excision and thereby cause the normal residual tissue in the contralateral breast to appear as an asymmetric density (Fig. 6-31).

Once it has been determined that previous surgery cannot explain the presence of an asymmetric density,

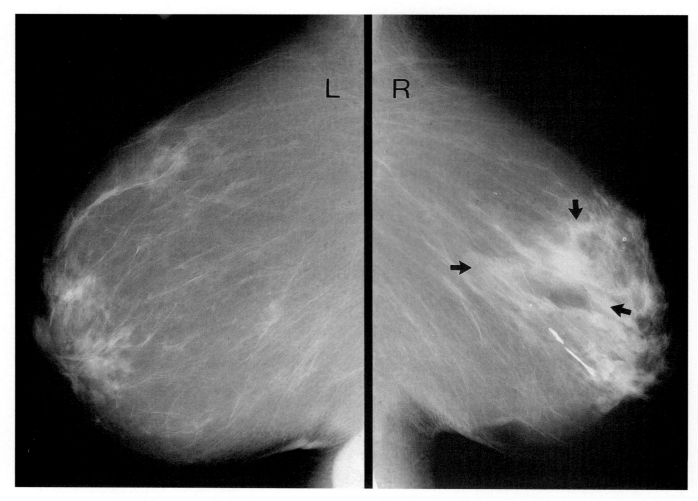

FIG. 6-30 *Increased density on right (arrows) is due to postoperative change from a previous biopsy in the area. (Reprinted by permission of the publisher from Homer MJ, Doherty FJ: Evaluation and Management of the Solitary Asymmetric Breast Density. Breast Disease 2:175–186, 1989. Copyright © 1989 by Elsevier Science Publishing Company, Inc.)*

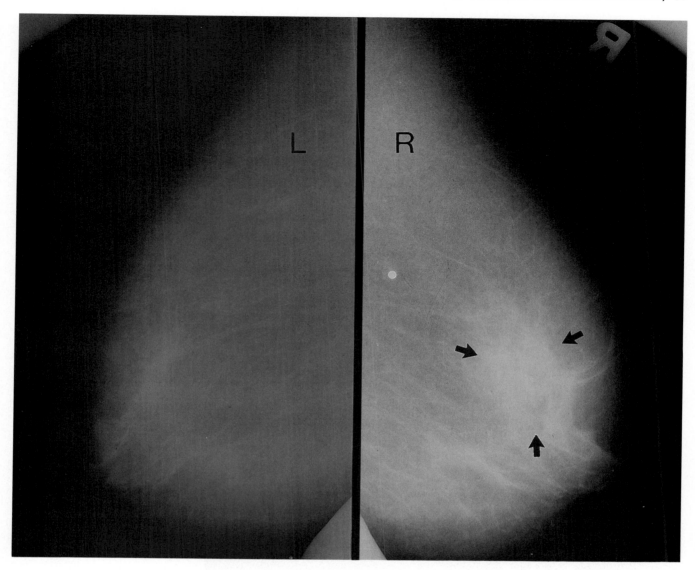

FIG. 6-31 *In the past, this patient had a previous left subareolar biopsy for a palpable mass which proved to be benign. This caused a glandular defect, making the normal contralateral right subareolar fibroglandular tissue (arrows) appear as an asymmetric density. (Reprinted by permission of the publisher from Homer MJ, Doherty FJ: Evaluation and Management of the Solitary Asymmetric Breast Density. Breast Disease 2:175–186, 1989. Copyright © 1989 by Elsevier Science Publishing Company, Inc.)*

there are guidelines that can be used to separate the majority of asymmetric densities that reasonably can be placed in a follow-up protocol from those few cases that require action.[29] The goal of this analysis is to decrease the number of needless biopsies performed for asymmetric densities. Under no circumstances should the guidelines be misinterpreted to mean that if an asymmetric density fulfills most or even all of the criteria, it can safely be ignored. These guidelines are not absolute guarantees that an asymmetric density is unimportant, but they are helpful in recognizing the asymmetric density that has a high likelihood of not representing malignancy (Fig. 6-32). The guidelines I use to analyze an asymmetric breast density reflect aspects of history, physical findings, and mammographic findings (Table 6-3).

History

The patient must be totally asymptomatic in the area of asymmetric density. In other words, she must admit to no knowledge of any problem in the region such as a feeling of fullness, thickening, or pain.

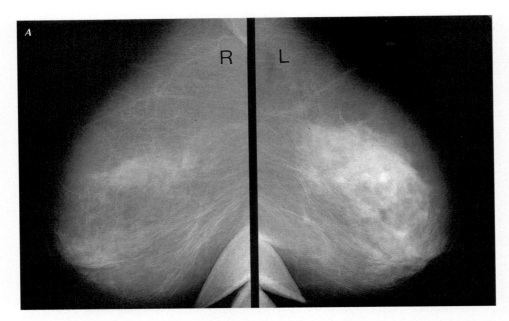

FIG. 6-32 A. *A routine screening mammogram was performed on this asymptomatic woman. OBL view shows a large area of asymmetric density in the upper half of the left breast. The area remained nonpalpable on directed breast repalpation. It is isodense compared to breast parenchyma in the same breast.*

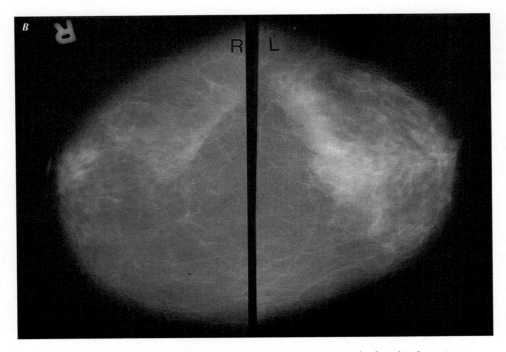

FIG. 6-32 (Continued)   B. *CC view shows that the asymmetric density is not volumetric and remains isodense relative to adjacent breast parenchyma. Fat is interspersed throughout the density. The asymmetric density remained stable throughout the follow-up, and biopsy was never performed.*

TABLE 6-3

CRITERIA FAVORING FOLLOW-UP FOR THE ASYMMETRIC DENSITY

HISTORY	PHYSICAL FINDINGS	MAMMOGRAPHIC FINDINGS
Asymptomatic	Negative breast repalpation	Multiplicity Located in upper outer quadrant in elderly patient Not volumetric in shape Contains fat Isodense relative to adjacent breast parenchyma Not a neodensity

Physical Findings

A normal breast palpation is important data pertaining to the analysis of an asymmetric density. A breast palpation directed toward an identified area of concern is much more sensitive than an undirected breast palpation. Therefore, the woman ideally should undergo a repeat breast palpation with special attention to the quadrant harboring the mammographic asymmetric density. In order to further optimize the sensitivity of the palpation, the woman should be repalpated as the clinician is viewing the mammogram. This guarantees a thorough examination of the correct location. The degree of confidence that should be placed on a normal breast palpation increases with large and superficially located asymmetric densities. In other words, the fact that a small asymmetric density located deep within a large breast is nonpalpable should not be considered an important factor in deciding patient management.

Mammographic Findings

MULTIPLICITY

Multiple asymmetric densities are a reassuring finding. When several areas of asymmetry vary only by size, there should be strong consideration for following the patient rather than arbitrarily excising one of the many densities. It makes no sense to excise the largest area of asymmetry when multiple areas exist. What is the guarantee that cancer lurks in the largest area of asymmetry? There is no rule stating that the largest asymmetric density is the one that is malignant. Often the fat-replaced breast contains multiple areas of asymmetry. The explanation for this is simply that as the woman ages and her breast parenchyma undergoes the normal evolutionary fat replacement, the process may not occur in a totally symmetrical fashion.

LOCATION

Location is a consideration in determining management of an asymmetric density. In general, the last place where breast tissue is replaced by fat is in the up-per outer quadrant. An asymptomatic woman with a very fat-replaced breast and a nonpalpable area of asymmetry in the upper outer quadrant is of less concern than one who has density in one of the other quadrants. Conversely, one should be more concerned if an asymmetric density is located in any of the other quadrants in a fat-replaced breast.

SHAPE

Breast cancer typically grows in a volumetric fashion, and normal breast parenchyma is characteristically more planar in appearance. Distinction between planar and volumetric can be reinforced by obtaining a third view (for example, a coned compression view or a third view taken at a different obliquity from the views already obtained). The demonstration of a planar, nonpalpable asymmetric density in an asymptomatic patient would make the option of follow-up a reasonable one. However, as with all the other guidelines used to analyze the asymmetric density, this distinction is not absolute, since on occasion breast cancer may indeed grow in a planar configuration.

FAT CONTENT

Another helpful guideline is that normal breast parenchyma often has fat traversing it. A volumetric breast cancer usually does not. The demonstration of a considerable amount of fat running through a large asymmetric density favors follow-up rather than biopsy.

DENSITY

When large enough, a breast cancer often appears whiter when compared to normal breast parenchyma. Therefore, when a large area of asymmetric density is not whiter than other densities in the ipsilateral or contralateral breast, in other words when it is isodense relative to other areas of parenchyma, consideration should be given to follow-up.

NOT A NEODENSITY

There is one final, very important point about the asymmetric density that must be stressed. The asymmetric density is not a neodensity. Each implies a different patient management. The guidelines used to analyze the asymmetric density should never be applied to the neodensity. As is emphasized in the upcoming section, development of a solitary neodensity is an ominous finding usually demanding further workup.

One common area of asymmetric density is the subareolar region. The asymmetry is most often caused by clinically unimportant subareolar fibrosis or ductal prominence. The probability of finding carcinoma with subareolar density alone, along with a normal breast palpation and without nipple changes such as discharge, eczema, or retraction, is very low. If the clinician opts for a biopsy of an asymmetric subareolar density located directly behind the nipple, preoperative localization is not required, since the surgeon can easily excise some tissue via a circumareolar incision, leaving little in the way of a biopsy scar.

An additional modality that may be used to evaluate the asymmetric density is ultrasound. The ultrasound of an insignificant asymmetric density will show no evidence of a cyst or mass. The asymmetric density will usually appear as an echogenic focus consistent with fibroglandular tissue.[29]

NEODENSITY

In the normal aging process, densities in the breast either remain stable or are gradually replaced by fat. The appearance of a new density in the breast, a neodensity, is viewed with great concern and usually requires further evaluation. None of the guidelines used to analyze an asymmetric density applies to the neodensity because the very appearance of a neodensity within the breast indicates that it is not a stable finding (Fig. 6-33). Of course, by definition there must be a prior mammogram for review in order to make the determination that the density is new. When multiple neodensities appear bilaterally, follow-up may be an option, since a reasonable working diagnosis would be fibrocystic change with development of multiple bilateral cysts. The patient should be questioned as to whether she is taking any medication such as estrogen, since it has been reported to cause increased breast density.[30] However, if multiple neodensities appear in only one breast (multiplicity but unilaterality), this would be somewhat unusual for typical fibrocystic change, and real consideration must still be given to biopsy in or-

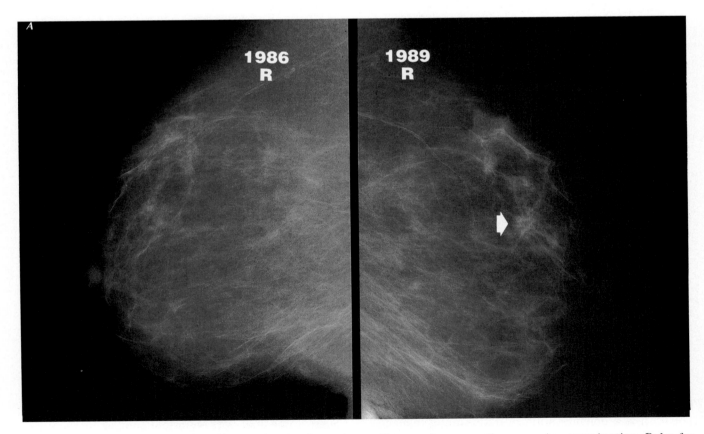

FIG. 6-33 A. *Between 8/86 and 1/89 a neodensity (arrow) was discovered on a routine screening examination. Rules for anaylzing this as an asymmetric density do not apply in this context.*

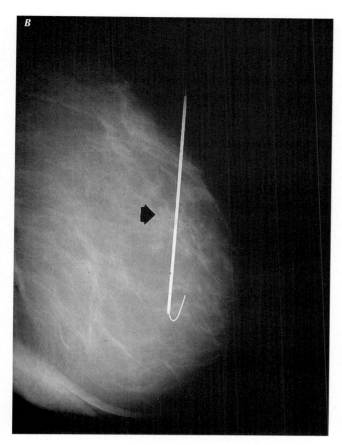

FIG. 6-33 (Continued) **B.** *Since the neodensity was nonpalpable, a preoperative needle localization was performed.*

der to establish the histologic etiology. There are no reliable rules for management in this situation so each case must be evaluated on an individual basis.

ARCHITECTURAL DISTORTION

Architectural distortion is a localizing sign of breast cancer produced by a desmoplastic reaction; its presence demands an explanation. Some benign etiologies for this finding, such as previous biopsy and inflammation can be suspected by history. If no explanation for the architectural distortion can be elicited, biopsy is often the next indicated procedure.

A difficult problem faced by the radiologist is how to manage an area of architectural distortion at the site of a previous biopsy for what was proven to be benign fibrocystic change. One cannot automatically assume that just because the woman has had a previous biopsy in the area, that must be the cause for the architectural distortion on the current mammogram. Unfortunately, an intramammary scar can mimic the appearance of carcinoma so each case must be evaluated on an individual basis.[31,32] Factors including the time interval between the prior biopsy and the current mammogram will contribute to the ultimate management decision.

Architectural distortion occurring at the interface between breast parenchyma and subcutaneous fat should be easily perceived (Fig. 6-34). Architectural distortion located more deeply within breast parenchyma may be a much more subtle finding and

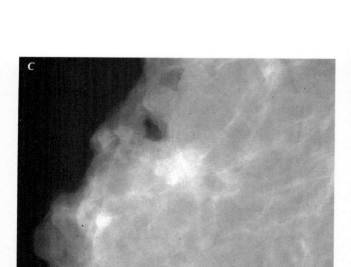

FIG 6-33 (Continued) **C.** *Specimen radiography confirmed excision of the neodensity. Histology revealed a 7-mm invasive ductal carcinoma.*

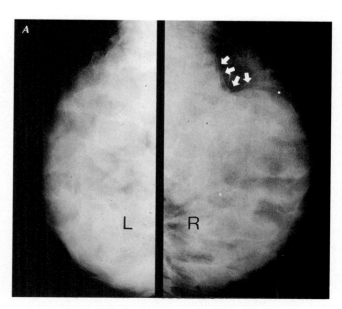

FIG. 6-34 A. *The architectural distortion at the parenchymal-subcutaneous fat interface (arrows) is caused by a late-stage palpable carcinoma.*

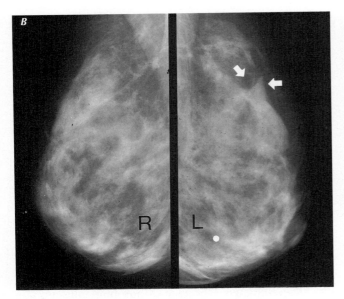

FIG. 6-34 *(Continued)* **B.** *The architectural distortion at the parenchymal-subcutaneous fat interface (arrows) is more subtle in this case but can be recognized by comparing the contour to the contralateral normal breast. Metallic marker is on incidental skin mole.*

may be better appreciated from a distance when comparing the overall stromal-parenchymal pattern of one side with the other. Magnification views or a coned compression view of the area may prove valuable in confirming the suspected findings (Fig. 6-35).

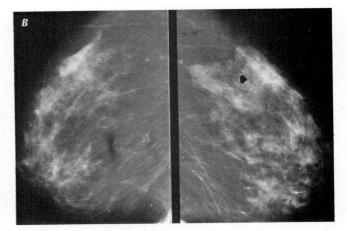

FIG. 6-35 *(Continued)* **B.** *LAT view confirms presence of the subtle area of architectural distortion (arrow).*

ENLARGED DUCTS

When comparing the symmetry of the breasts or the appearance of the same breast on two different examinations, not only must the radiologist compare the overall stromal-parenchymal pattern, but he or she should also assess ductal symmetry. Ductal asymmetry in a woman with nipple signs or symptoms such as retraction, eczema, or bloody or nonbloody discharge takes on great importance and often results in prompt excision of the mammographically abnormal ductal system. Management of the asymptomatic patient with ductal asymmetry is not as straightforward. The three

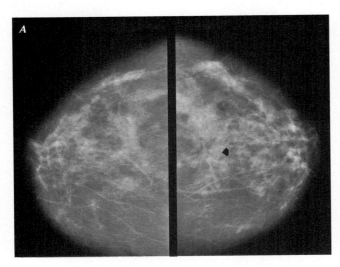

FIG. 6-35 **A.** *CC view shows architectural distortion (arrow).*

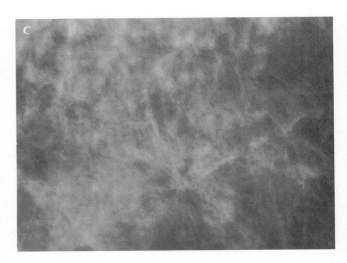

FIG. 6-35 *(Continued)* **C.** *Compression magnification view in CC projection clearly defines the architectural distortion.*

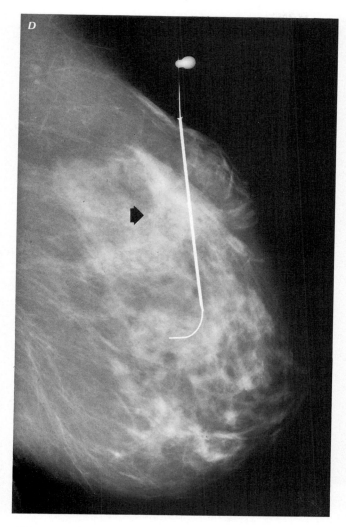

FIG. 6-35 *(Continued)* **D.** *Needle localization was performed because the breast palpation was normal. LAT view shows that the area of architectural distortion is directly posterior to the middle of the needle (arrow).*

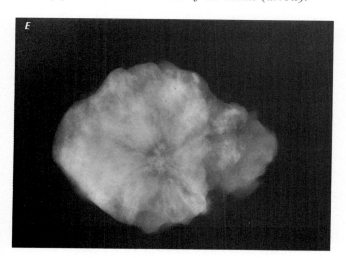

FIG. 6-35 *(Continued)* **E.** *Specimen radiograph confirms excision of the area. Histology revealed an infiltrating ductal carcinoma.*

situations encountered are prominence of a solitary duct, unilateral prominence of many ducts, and bilateral ductal prominence.

Enlargement of a single duct may be viewed as a solitary dominant geographic abnormality (Fig. 6-36). The mammogram cannot determine whether the duct is being enlarged by inspissated debris, blood, papilloma, or cancer, and biopsy is the only way to conclusively make this differentiation. Some place importance on the length of the duct and consider a solitary dilated duct that extends more than 3 cm into the breast to be especially suspicious for malignancy.[33] If the patient has had prior mammograms, every attempt should be made to obtain them to determine whether the solitary dilated duct is a new finding. Assuming there are no prior mammograms, the two management options are biopsy or follow-up. In many situations, we excise the dilated duct because surgery can be performed under local anesthesia on an outpatient basis, preoperative needle localization is not required, and the duct can be removed through circumareolar incision with excellent postoperative cosmesis. However, in the experience of many mammographers the solitary dilated duct in the asymptomatic woman with a normal breast palpation has a low probability of representing carcinoma[34,35] so follow-up is also an accepted option. My experience is similar, and I have yet to find one cancer manifesting itself as a solitary noncalcified dilated duct in the asymptomatic patient.

If the chance of finding occult carcinoma in the asymptomatic patient with a normal breast palpation is very low for the solitary dilated duct, then it is understandable that with multiple unilateral dilated ducts (Fig. 6-37) or bilateral ductal prominence, the chance of a malignancy is even less likely. My recommendation in these situations is follow-up. Biopsy is not offered as an option because the surgeon cannot know which of the many dilated ducts to biopsy. The alternative, which is excision of all ducts, would subject the woman to an extensive ductal resection.

One area of controversy regarding the workup of ductal enlargement is the role of ductography. At NEMCH ductography is not performed because although filling a duct with contrast will outline its contents, ultimately this will not change patient management, since the differentiation of benign from malignant cannot usually be made with contour evaluation. Ductography is discussed again in the section dealing with papilloma in Chap. 9.

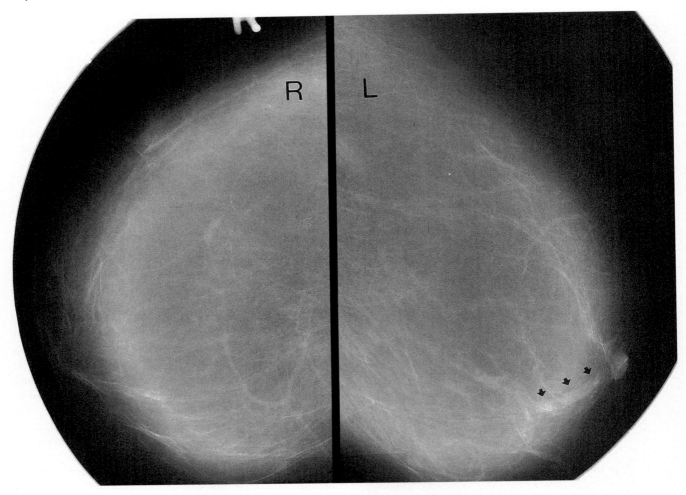

FIG. 6-36 *There is a unilateral enlarged duct (arrows) extending for 3.5 cm from the nipple. The patient was asymptomatic and had a negative breast palpation. She opted for excisional biopsy rather than follow-up. Histology revealed inspissated debris and ductal ectasia.*

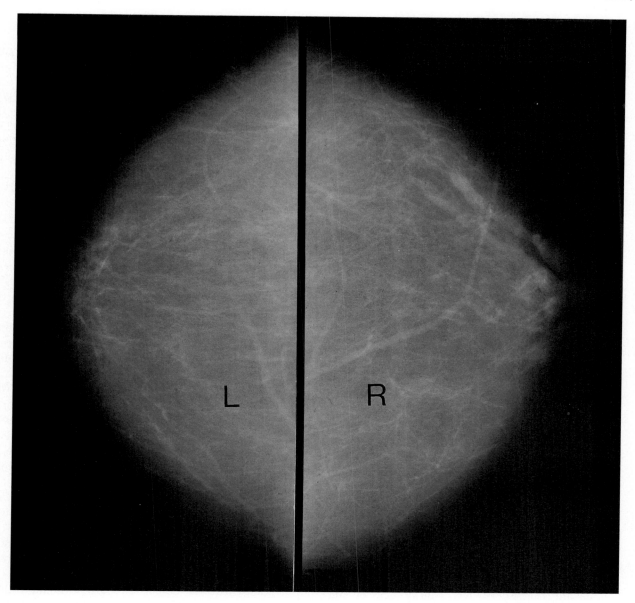

FIG. 6-37 *CC views from a routine screening examination revealed multiple dilated ducts extending from the right subareolar region. Since the patient was asymptomatic with a normal breast palpation, only follow-up was recommended. The ducts have remained stable through follow-up and biopsy was averted.*

REFERENCES

1. Swann CA, Kopans DB, Koerner FC, et al. The halo sign and malignant breast lesions. AJR **149**:1145–1147, 1987.
2. Gordenne WH, Malchiar FL. Mach bands in mammography. Radiology **169**:55–58, 1988.
3. Sickles EA. Breast masses: Mammographic evaluation. Radiology **173**:297–303, 1989.
4. Pennes DR, Rebner M. Layering granular calcifications in macroscopic breast cysts. Breast Disease **1**:109–112, 1988.
5. Sickles EA. Nonpalpable, circumscribed, noncalcified solid breast masses: Likelihood of malignancy based on lesion size and age of patient. Radiology **192**:439–442, 1994.
6. Homer MJ. Imaging features and management of characteristically benign and probably benign breast lesions. Radiol Clin North Am **25**:939–951, 1987.
7. Egan RL, McSweeney MB. Intramammary lymph nodes. Cancer **51**:1830–1842, 1983.
8. Jackson VP, Dines KA, Bassett LW, et al. Diagnostic importance of the radiographic density of noncalcified breast masses: Analysis of 91 lesions. AJR **157**:25–28, 1991.
9. Egan RL, McSweeney MB, Sewell CW. Intramammary calcifications without an associated mass in benign and malignant disease. Radiology **137**:1–7, 1980.
10. Sickles EA. Breast calcifications: Mammographic evaluation. Radiology **160**:289–293, 1986.
11. Lanyi M. Diagnosis and differential diagnosis of breast calcifications. Springer-Verlag, Berlin, 1986.
12. Homer MJ. Breast imaging: pitfalls, controversies, and some practical thoughts. Radiol Clin North Am **23**:459–472, 1985.
13. Colbassani HJ, Feller NF, Cigtay OS, et al. Mammographic and pathologic correlation of microcalcification in disease of the breast. Surg Gynecol Obstet **155**:689–690, 1982.
14. Murphy WA, DeSchryver-Keckskemeti K. Isolated clustered microcalcifications in the breast: Radiologic-pathologic correlation. Radiology **127**:335–341, 1978.
15. Homer MJ, Safaii H, Smith TJ, et al. The relationship of mammographic microcalcification to histologic malignancy: Radiologic-pathologic correlation. AJR **153**:1187–1189, 1989.
16. Homer MJ, Safaii H. Cancerization of the lobule: Implication regarding analysis of microcalcification shape. Breast Disease **3**:131–133, 1990.
17. Azzopardi JG. *Problems in Breast Pathology.* W.B. Saunders, London, 1979, pp. 203–212.
18. Homer MJ. Questions and answers. AJR **164**:1018, 1995.
19. Kopans DB, Meyer JE, Homer MJ, et al. Dermal deposits mistaken for breast calcifications. Radiology **149**:592–594, 1983.
20. Homer MJ, Marchant DJ, Smith TJ. The geographic cluster of microcalcifications of the breast. Surg Gynecol Obstet **161**:532–534, 1985.
21. Homer MJ, D'Orsi CJ, Sitzman SB. Dermal calcifications in fixed orientation: The tattoo sign. Radiology **192**:161–163, 1994.
22. Berkowitz JE, Gatewood OMB, Donovan GB, et al. Dermal breast calcifications: Localization with template-guided placement of skin marker. Radiology **163**:282, 1987.
23. Lanyi M. Differential Diagnose de Mikroverkalkungen: die verkalkte mastopathische Mikrocyste. Radiologe **17**:217–218, 1977.
24. Sickles EA, Abele JS. Milk-of-calcium within tiny benign cysts. Radiology **141**:655–658, 1981.
25. Kopans DB, Nguyen PC, Koerner FC, et al. Mixed form, diffusely scattered calcifications in breast cancer with apocrine features. Radiology **177**:807–811, 1990.
26. Homer MJ, Cooper AG, Pile-Spellman ER. Milk-of-calcium in breast microcysts: Manifestation as a solitary focal process. AJR **150**:789–790, 1988.
27. Homer MJ, Slowinski J. Spontaneously disappearing calcifications in the breast: Incidence, appearance, and implications. Breast Disease **5**:215–258, 1992.
28. Meybehm M, Pfeifer U. Vascular calcifications mimicking grouped microcalcifications on mammography. Breast Disease **3**:81–86, 1990.
29. Homer MJ, Doherty FJ. Evaluation and management of the solitary asymmetric breast density. Breast Disease **2**:175–186, 1989.
30. Berkowitz JE, Gatewood OMB, Goldblum LE, et al. Hormonal replacement therapy: Mammographic manifestations. Radiology **174**:199–201, 1990.
31. Sickles EA, Herzog KA. Intramammary scar tissue: A mimic of the mammographic appearance of carcinoma. AJR **135**:349–352, 1980.
32. Mendelson EB. Evaluation of the postoperative breast. Radiol Clin North Am **30**:107–138, 1992.
33. Martin JE, Moskowitz M, Milbrath JR. Breast cancer missed by mammography. AJR **132**:737–739, 1979.
34. Sickles EA. Mammographic features of 300 consecutive nonpalpable breast cancers. AJR **146**:661–663, 1986.
35. Moskowitz M. Minimal breast cancer redux. Radiol Clin North Am **21**:93–113, 1983.

NONLOCALIZING SIGNS OF BREAST CANCER

Nonlocalizing signs of breast cancer usually indicate advanced disease. Most of the signs can be recognized both clinically and with mammography. Their identification still does not indicate the location of the breast cancer so further investigation is required. These signs (Table 7-1) will now be reviewed in sequence.

ABNORMAL VEINS

Breast cancer, like other cancers, can recruit collateral flow to produce vascular asymmetry. Abnormal veins are defined as either more veins on one side when compared to the mirror image region in the contralateral breast, or veins that are much larger on one side than on the other. A venous diameter ratio of 1.4:1 or greater has been taken to indicate that a malignancy is responsible.[1] Unfortunately, abnormal veins are not a very helpful sign in the diagnosis of early breast cancer, since they usually appear late and by that time are often accompanied by other clinical or mammographic findings indicating cancer (Fig. 7-1). Benign processes can also cause abnormal veins to develop, further limiting their diagnostic importance (Fig. 7-2).

A problem arises when abnormal veins are present on a routine screening examination in the asymptomatic patient. Since difference in compression may produce the appearance of enlarged veins (not the appearance of an increased number of veins), one should be certain that the apparent enlargement is a reproducible finding and not an artifact of compression. The

TABLE 7-1
NONLOCALIZING SIGNS OF BREAST CANCER

1. Abnormal veins
2. Skin changes
3. Nipple and areolar abnormalities
4. Axillary lymph nodes

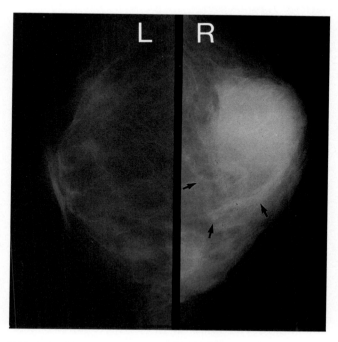

FIG. 7-1 *There is a late stage palpable carcinoma in the right breast with an abnormal vein adjacent to it (arrows).*

67

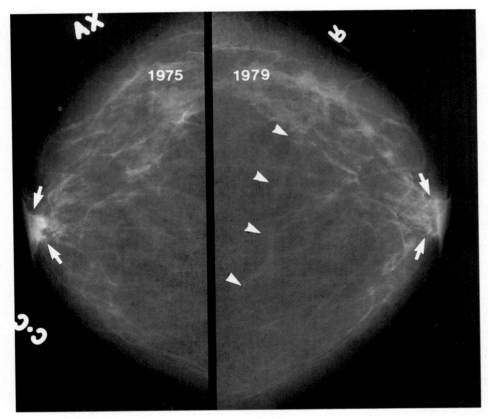

FIG. 7-2   *In 1975 this patient was put on antibiotics for an infection in the right subareolar area (arrows). On a routine examination in 1979, the postinflammatory subareolar changes (arrows) persist and in the interval an enlarged vein has developed (arrowheads).*

venous enlargement should be evident on every view of the breast. Venous channels of the breast, like venous channels in other parts of the body, may be recruited to bypass major obstructions,[2] and this possibility should be explored before assuming that primary breast pathology is the etiology for the venous asymmetry.

If no explanation can be found for venous asymmetry, I place the woman into a follow-up protocol. CT scan of the chest wall is a more aggressive and immediate way to pursue the possibility of a deep hidden cancer. However, I do not order this examination in the asymptomatic woman because venous asymmetry is most often a normal variation in the breast (Fig. 7-3). Since I have not yet found a cancer manifested by venous asymmetry alone in the asymptomatic woman that has escaped detection by ancillary mammographic views or repeat breast palpation, I do not routinely pursue the isolated finding of venous asymmetry more aggressively.

SKIN CHANGES

The mammographic skin changes caused by breast cancer can be divided into two major categories: retraction, or dimpling, and thickening. The etiology of these changes may be benign or malignant, chronic or acute. Mammography is such a sensitive examination that both retraction and thickening may be evident mammographically before they can be clinically detected. The skin may attain a thickness of 10 to 20 times normal before it can be perceived as abnormal by the palpating hand.[3] Flattening the breast by compression is the mammographic equivalent of examining the woman with her arms in different positions. Both maneuvers stretch the breast and accentuate subtle areas of retraction.

Since mammography can usually demonstrate retraction and thickening earlier than palpation, a corol-

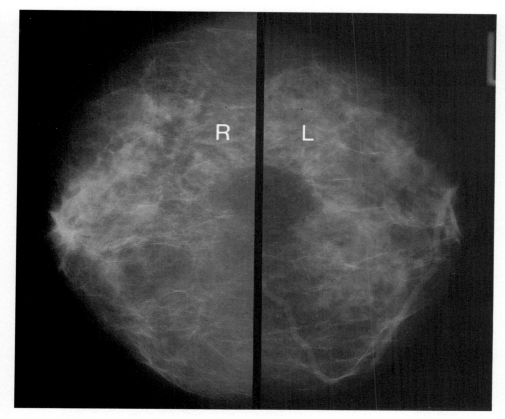

FIG. 7-3 *This routine screening mammogram reveals asymmetric veins on the left side. The patient was placed into a follow-up protocol and remained asymptomatic.*

lary is that when clinical retraction or thickening is present, it should be able to be identified by mammography. There is one exception: When the skin changes are focal, they will not be evident on the mammogram if they are not imaged in tangent. On the CC view, the only skin caught in tangent is on the 3 o'clock–9 o'clock plane of the breast. Similarly, only the 12 o'clock–6 o'clock plane is imaged tangentially on a true LAT view. Thus, if a focal area of dimpling is not located on these planes, it may not be identified on the mammogram even though it is visually apparent (Fig. 7-4).

Breast carcinoma may cause skin retraction or dimpling either by direct extension of tumor to the skin or by a desmoplastic reaction evoked by a deep malignancy causing shortening of Cooper's ligaments. It is most important to remember this latter mechanism because it explains why a breast cancer may be located at a considerable distance from the actual site of the skin retraction. When searching for the carcinoma on the mammogram, one's vision must not be telescoped to the immediate vicinity of the retraction.

Malignancy is not the only etiology of skin retraction, so before assuming that it is caused by a carcinoma, other etiologies such as trauma, biopsy, abscess, and burns must be investigated. A very helpful beginning to this process of exclusion is asking the woman, "Has anything ever happened to this area of your breast that has not happened to other areas in this breast or in the other breast?" A patient will often be able to remember the causal factor, thereby stopping a concern that would have been raised about an occult malignancy.

Thickening is the other skin change that a breast cancer may produce. The normal breast skin thickness is usually between 0.8 and 3 mm.[4] Numbers alone are not reliable because even skin of 3-mm thickness should be viewed with concern if the mirror-image region in the contralateral breast has thinner skin. Therefore, in addition to measurements, symmetry remains important. In the inframammary region, normal skin thickness may exceed 3 mm. This is a frequent occurrence, especially in older women. Inframammary skin thickening can be considered a normal variant in

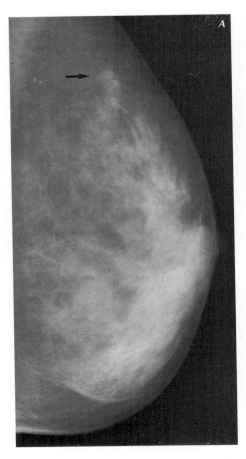

FIG. 7-4   A. *This 57-year-old patient was sent for mammography because of skin retraction in the right upper outer quadrant. No mass was palpable. A LAT view shows a 6-mm stellate mass (arrow) without associated skin changes.*

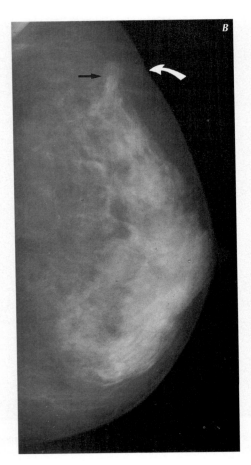

FIG. 7-4 *(Continued)*   **B.** *A view taken tangential to the skin retraction shows that the stellate mass (straight arrow) is indeed causing subtle focal skin retraction (curved arrow).*

the asymptomatic patient if it is bilateral, symmetrical, unassociated with any other mammographic findings in the region, and accompanied by a normal breast palpation (Fig. 7-5).

As with retraction, there are both benign and malignant etiologies for skin thickening. A useful approach to the evaluation of skin thickening is to classify it as either localized or generalized. Each category has a separate gamut of differential diagnostic possibilities. There is no absolute centimeter length that separates localized from generalized. This separation should be viewed as a concept which attempts to differentiate focal abnormalities from those which usually involve a larger surface area of the breast. Table 7-2 lists the primary differential diagnostic possibilities in each category.

Most causes of localized mammary skin thickening can be evaluated by either direct questioning of the patient or by careful inspection of the skin. When no explanation can be found for localized skin thickening,

TABLE 7-2
SKIN THICKENING

LOCALIZED
Prior biopsy
Abscess
Trauma
Dermatologic conditions
Nonsuppurative inflammation
Malignancy

GENERALIZED
Inflammatory carcinoma
Metastases to the breast
Pulmonary disease obstructing lymphatics
Acute mastitis
Anasarca
Radiation
Repeated thoracentesis

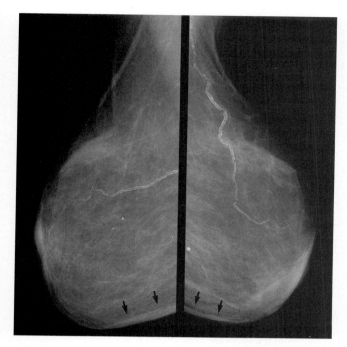

FIG. 7-5 *LAT views of each breast demonstrate normal inframammary skin thickening. Notice that it is bilateral, symmetric, and has no mammographic abnormality associated with it.*

biopsy is usually required to exclude the possibility of an underlying malignancy.

Generalized skin thickening may be unilateral or bilateral. In my experience, unilateral skin thickening is more common. Inflammatory carcinoma often pre-

sents with unilateral generalized skin thickening (Fig. 7-6). Labeling a cancer as inflammatory refers to clinical and pathologic features but not to its specific histologic type. Clinically, the redness, pain, and warmth mimic an inflammatory process. Pathologically, the diagnosis requires identification of tumor in the dermal lymphatics. On occasion an actual volumetric tumor mass or malignant microcalcifications may be completely obscured by the overall increased breast density and dilated lymphatic channels (Fig. 7-7). Diagnosis can often be made by superficial dermal punch biopsies obtained from the areas of skin thickening.

Metastases that produce blockage of lymphatic channels, either from a contralateral breast carcinoma or distant primary malignancy elsewhere in the body, may cause unilateral or bilateral generalized skin thickening and dilated lymphatic channels within the breast. In most cases, the primary cancer is already known, since metastatic spread to the breast usually occurs late.

The primary path of lymphatic drainage from the breast is toward the axilla. Other drainage routes are toward infraclavicular and supraclavicular nodes, subpectoral nodes beneath the pectoralis major muscle, intercostal and posterior mediastinal nodes. Lymphatic flow may be directed medially toward the anterior mediastinal and parasternal nodes as well as across the midline to the contralateral breast. An important concept that must always be remembered when evaluating a patient with generalized mammary skin thickening is that lymphatic obstruction anywhere along a drainage route may be the etiology. For instance, a pulmonary

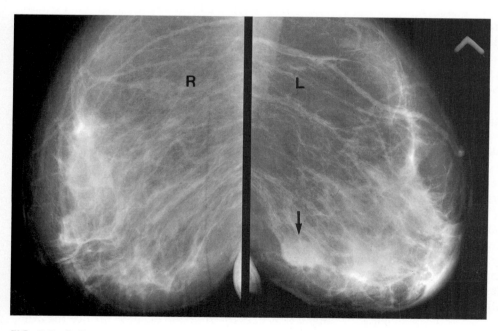

FIG. 7-6 *Inflammatory cancer presenting with unilateral generalized skin thickening. The primary site of tumor is evident (arrow).*

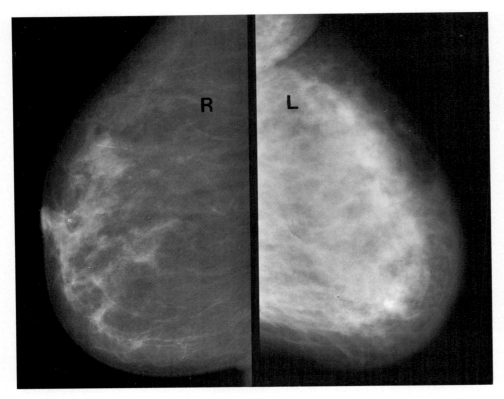

FIG. 7-7 *In this case of inflammatory breast cancer on the left, a tumor mass is not seen.*

problem obstructing central lymphatics may be mistaken for a primary breast process. Mesothelioma, lymphangitic spread of tumor to the chest from a distant primary site (often from the GI tract), bronchogenic carcinoma, actinomycosis of the chest wall, and bulky retrosternal adenopathy from lymphoma all can cause generalized mammary skin thickening by obstructing lymphatic channels (Fig. 7-8). Therefore, when a mammogram reveals generalized skin thickening, either unilateral or bilateral, the radiologist must be certain that the chest radiograph is normal before considering a breast process as the primary explanation for the findings.

The evaluation of the remaining differential diagnostic possibilities of generalized skin thickening, including acute mastitis, anasarca, radiation, and repeated thoracentesis, depends primarily on history and clinical findings.

The combination of generalized skin thickening and dilated lymphatics in the breast, whether filled by tumor or edema, causes diffuse increased density of the affected breast. An uncommon finding would be the presence of increased breast density without associated mammary skin thickening. On occasion, increased breast density due to increased tissue density within the breast may occur earlier than the skin thickening, but the skin thickening will eventually appear if the process continues unabated. However, there are a few conditions that can cause a diffuse increase in breast density without associated mammary skin thickening. One of these is extreme weight loss, caused either by diet or gastric bypass surgery. Another is iatrogenic in nature. Some drugs such as estrogen (Fig. 7-9) have been reported to cause increased breast density over time.[6]

NIPPLE AND AREOLAR ABNORMALITIES

Nipple and areolar abnormalities may be the only manifestations of a breast carcinoma. When there are signs or symptoms such as retraction, eczema, or discharge, the radiologist should very carefully scrutinize the nipple, areolar, and subareolar region. Even minor variations between sides take on potential significance with a history of nipple or areolar changes (Fig. 7-10).

Nipple retraction or flattening, either unilateral or bilateral, is often a normal variation. When a woman has unilateral or bilateral nipple retraction or flattening, it is necessary to obtain specific history regarding this finding, and in my practice the technologist is the one who obtains this information. Specifically, the pa-

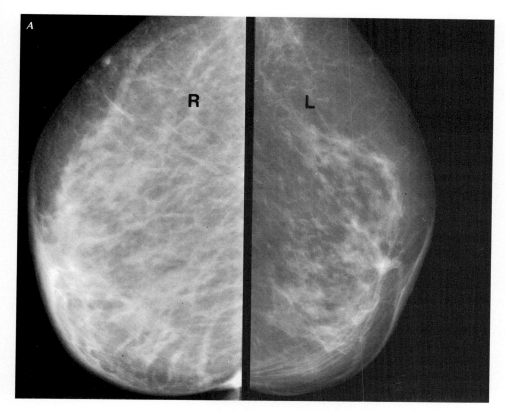

FIG. 7-8 A. *LAT view of each breast showing generalized skin thickening and increased markings on the right.*

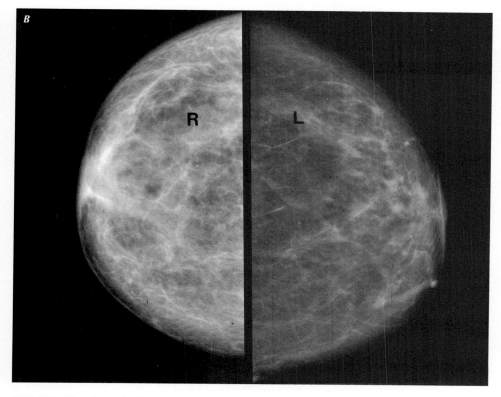

FIG. 7-8 *(Continued)* **B.** *CC views show same findings on the right side.*

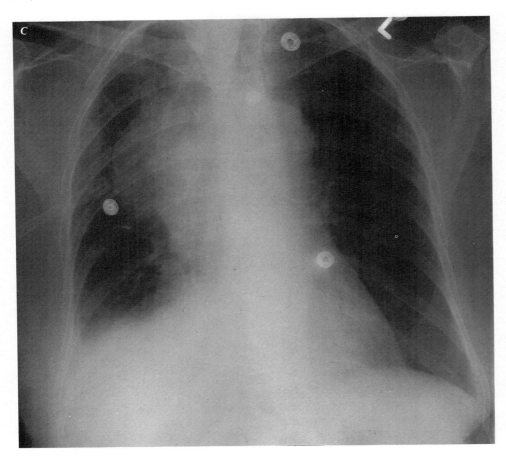

FIG. 7-8 *(Continued)* **C.** *The findings are caused by a late stage bronchogenic carcinoma obstructing the lymphatic drainage of the right breast.*

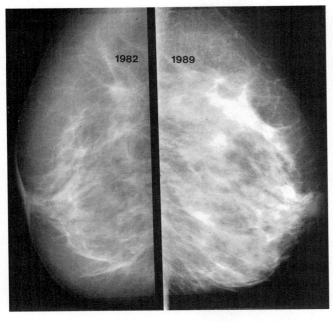

1982 1989

FIG. 7-9 *These LAT views of the right breast show a dramatic increase in density between 1982 and 1989. The skin thickness remains normal and unchanged. The left breast showed similar findings. This is the result of estrogen intake.*

tient is asked whether she has recognized that her nipple is flattened or retracted and if she has, for how long. The technologist usually receives one of three answers. Commonly the woman will state that her nipple (or nipples) has been retracted ever since she can remember. In this situation, the retraction probably represents a normal variation and there is no recommendation made on the mammogram report other than noting the presence of retraction and stating that the patient admits to having recognized its presence for years. The second possibility is that the patient does not know her nipple is retracted and cannot date its onset. The third possibility is that the woman knows that the nipple change is of recent onset. In these last two situations, even without breast palpation findings or mammographic abnormalities, subareolar biopsy must be considered. The only manifestation of a small subareolar carcinoma may be retraction or flattening of the nipple by tumor which either directly invades the nipple or causes shortening and retraction of Cooper's ligaments. This is one of the few situations in which blind biopsy is appropriate (although in reality, the biopsy is not really blind, since it is directed to the

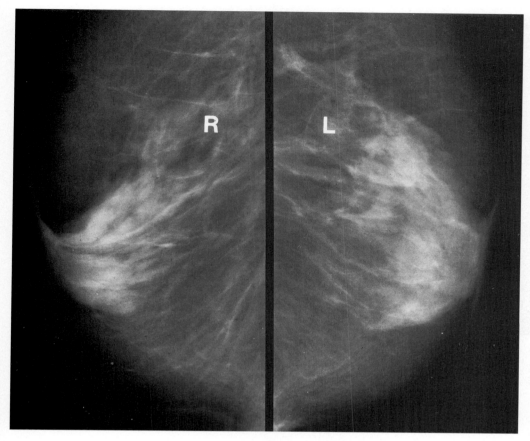

FIG. 7-10 *This patient complained of new bloody nipple discharge on the left. Nipple retraction was clinically evident. Notice the subtle increased left subareolar density, compared to the right. No mass was palpable. A subareolar biopsy on the left showed intraductal and invasive ductal carcinoma.*

immediate subareolar region). We have found breast carcinoma in this way (Fig. 7-11).

When the patient complains of nipple eczema, Paget's carcinoma should be a primary consideration. Initially, the clinician will usually attribute the skin changes to eczema and treat it with topical therapy. Nonhealing nipple eczema that is unresponsive to appropriate therapy must always warrant consideration of Paget's carcinoma as a distinct possibility. Nonhealing nipple eczema demands biopsy. Often there are no mammographic signs of Paget's carcinoma other than the localized skin condition (Fig. 7-12), and even this may be subtle or impossible to visualize mammographically. This is of little concern to the radiologist because the nipple eczema forces the woman to seek help from her physician, often her gynecologist, so the diagnosis of Paget's carcinoma is most commonly made by the clinician and not by the radiologist.

Paget's carcinoma is not just a ductal carcinoma that involves the nipple and causes eczema. In order to make the diagnosis, a unique intraepidermal cell, the Paget cell, must be identified. Paget cells are relatively

large cells having clear or light-colored cytoplasm and contain a large round or polymorphic nucleus. The origin of the Paget cell is still debated. Some believe it to be a neoplastic cell that migrates from an underlying carcinoma to the nipple epidermis. Others believe that the Paget cell actually arises in the nipple, totally independent from the underlying carcinoma. It is assumed that this occurs either through malignant transformation or degeneration from existing cells. What is important is that Paget's carcinoma has a high association with deep tumor foci, which are often not in anatomic continuity with the epidermis. The deeper carcinoma may either be intraductal or invasive. The presence of this deeper tumor is the reason that some consider local excision and breast-conserving therapy an unacceptable option for treatment of Paget's carcinoma.[7]

Nonlactational nipple discharge may be a manifestation of either benign or malignant disease. Nipple discharge may be either physiologic or pathologic. Physiologic discharge is typically bilateral, arising from multiple ducts, and is not spontaneous. Pathologic dis-

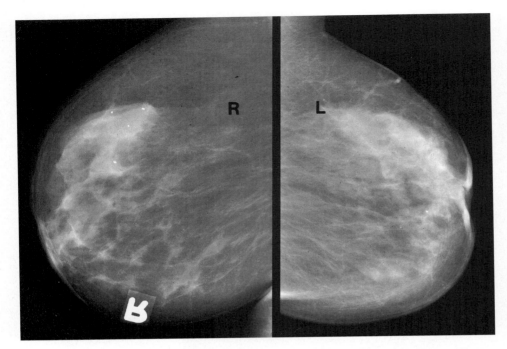

FIG. 7-11 *LAT view shows obvious nipple retraction on the left. The patient stated this was new but was not getting worse. At no time was a mass palpable. A subareolar biopsy was performed, which confirmed the presence of an invasive ductal carcinoma.*

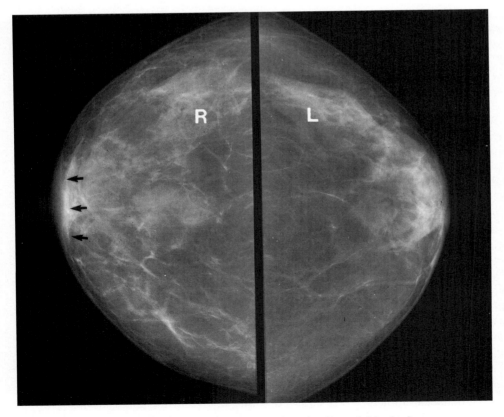

FIG. 7-12 *This patient had a biopsy because of nonhealing right nipple eczema. Notice the periareolar skin thickening (arrows). Biopsy revealed Paget's carcinoma.*

charge is characteristically spontaneous, persistent, and arises from a single duct. The most common cause of a bloody nipple discharge is a benign intraductal papilloma. Malignant discharge need not be bloody.

It is beyond the scope of this text to discuss the evaluation and management of nipple discharge. Obviously when a mammographic finding or clinically palpable abnormality accompanies the discharge, the surgeon knows where to perform the diagnostic biopsy. Confusion arises when the discharge is unaccompanied by any other clinical or mammographic findings. At NEMCH the quadrant containing the offending ductal system is identified by careful palpation. The dilated ducts are visualized during surgery and excised. This is a commonly accepted practice.[8] We do not perform galactography to identify the abnormal ductal system. Our practice is at variance with those who believe in the importance of galactography for evaluation of nipple discharge.[9,10] Galactography is discussed again in Chap. 9.

AXILLARY LYMPH NODES

Abnormal axillary lymph nodes are a nonlocalizing sign of breast cancer and reflect late stage disease. Occasionally, axillary lymph nodes may be the only manifestation of an occult breast carcinoma, and therefore unexplained unilateral axillary adenopathy is a definite indication for mammography.[11] As a general rule, normal lymph nodes do not exceed 1.5 cm in greatest diameter unless they are replaced by fat.[12] However,

normal lymph nodes can be much larger than 1.5 cm. With vigorous compression normal axillary lymph nodes may be seen extending inferiorly from the axillary region down to the plane of the nipple or may even appear intramammary in location (Fig. 7-13). Fat-

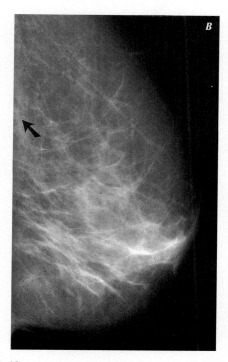

FIG. 7-13 (Continued) **B.** OBL view from a different patient. Notice the normal axillary lymph node (arrow).

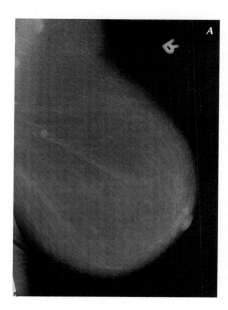

FIG. 7-13 **A.** An OBL view with vigorous compression demonstrates normal axillary lymph nodes extending caudad, approaching the plane of the nipple.

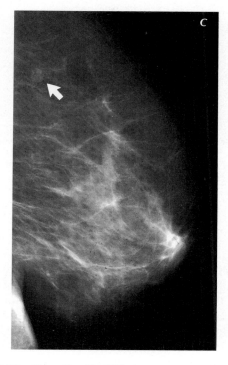

FIG. 7-13 (Continued) **C.** OBL from same patient 3 years later. Vigorous compression makes the axillary lymph node (arrow) appear intramammary in location.

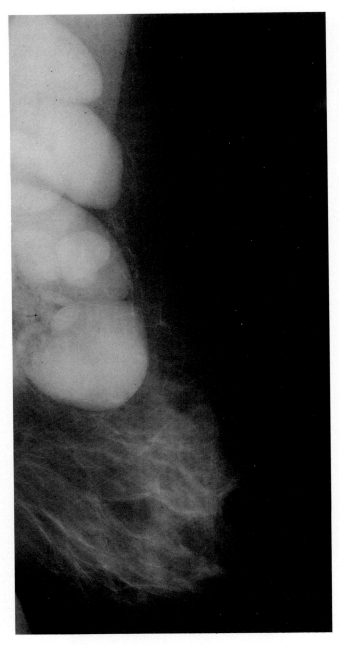

FIG. 7-14 *Huge axillary lymph nodes are obvious in this patient with lymphoma. Notice their oval shape.*

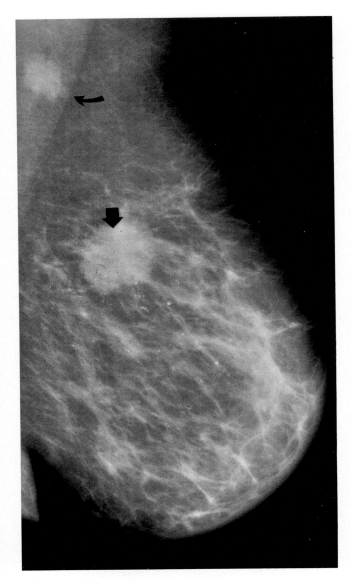

FIG. 7-15 *This is a case of late stage breast carcinoma (straight arrow) with lymphatic obstruction causing generalized skin thickening. There is palpable axillary adenopathy. The irregular margins of the lymph node (curved arrow) suggest capsular invasion, which was confirmed histologically. (Courtesy of Murray Dimant, M.D., Fall River, MA).*

replaced nodes are easily recognized on mammography by their lucent centers. The observation that nodes involved by lymphoma or lymphoid hyperplasia tend to be oval (Fig. 7-14), while malignant or postinflammatory nodes tend to be faceted, is usually of little practical help in patient management, since a diagnostic biopsy will be necessary in any case.[13] As with lymph nodes elsewhere in the body, a normal size lymph node does not exclude the possibility that it contains malig-

nancy, since microscopic metastatic deposits may not enlarge the node. On occasion, it will be hard to clinically differentiate an enlarged axillary node from a mass in the tail of Spence, which can extend high into the axilla. This is not really a management problem, since in either situation the mass will require biopsy. In a patient with known breast carcinoma and palpable adenopathy, demonstration of a poorly marginated lymph node suggests capsular invasion (Fig. 7-15).

REFERENCES

1. Dodd GD, Wallace JD. The venous diameter ratio in the radiographic diagnosis of breast cancer. Radiology **90**:900–904, 1968.
2. McLean GK, Friedman AK. Detection of a venous collateral pathway by mammography: superior vena cava syndrome. JAMA **239**:2022–2023, 1978.
3. Egan RL. Mammography. Am J Surg **106**:421–429, 1963.
4. Willson SA, Tucker AK. Patterns of breast skin thickness in normal mammograms. Clin Radiol **33**:691–693, 1982.
5. Dershaw DD, Moore MP, Liberman L, et al. Inflammatory breast carcinoma: Mammographic findings. Radiology **190**:831–834, 1994.
6. Berkowitz JE, Gatewood OMB, Goldblum LE, et al. Hormonal replacement therapy: mammographic manifestations. Radiology **174**:199–201, 1990.
7. Ikeda DM, Helvie MA, Frank TS, et al. Paget disease of the nipple: Radiologic-pathologic correlation. Radiology **189**:89–94, 1993.
8. Urban JA, Egeli RA. Non-lactational nipple discharge. CA A cancer journal for clinicians **28**:130–140, 1978.
9. Cardenosa G, Doudna C, Eklund GW. Ductography of the breast: Technique and findings. AJR **162**:1081–1087, 1994.
10. Tabar L, Dean PB, Pestek Z. Galactography: the diagnostic procedure of choice for nipple discharge. Radiology **149**:31–38, 1983.
11. Abrams RA, Homer MJ, O'Connor T, et al. Breast cancer presenting as an axillary mass: A case report and review of the literature. Breast Disease **3**:39–46, 1990.
12. Kalisher L, Chu AM, Peyster RG. Clinicopathological correlation of xeroradiography in determining involvement of metastatic axillary nodes in female breast cancer. Radiology **121**:333–335, 1976.
13. Kalisher L. Xeroradiography of axillary lymph node disease. Radiology **114**:67–71, 1975.

FIBROCYSTIC CHANGE: THOUGHTS

WHAT IS FIBROCYSTIC DISEASE?

It is readily apparent from the literature that the term *fibrocystic disease* connotes different things to different people. At NEMCH we have been uncomfortable with that term for several reasons. Perhaps it should not be considered a disease in the usual sense if a majority of women have it. At our institution, virtually every breast biopsy contains some focus of histologically evident fibrocystic disease. Love et al.[1] proposed the question, Is it reasonable to define as a disease any process that occurs clinically in 50 percent and histologically in 90 percent of women? From a psychological point of view, it can be unsettling for an asymptomatic woman to be told that she has a disease. This anxiety can become exacerbated further if she reads in the lay press that fibrocystic disease may be premalignant. In fact, the article is usually referring to a small subgroup of fibrocystic disease, the epithelial hyperplasias with marked atypia,[2] but often the woman does not realize this or the article does not make this clear. Another problem with using the term *fibrocystic disease* relates to the difficulty that it may create with insurance carriers. When a woman applies for life insurance and is asked whether she has any known disease, should the answer be yes because a radiologist has diagnosed fibrocystic disease by mammography? If she says no and develops a breast cancer later in life, does that mean that she was not honest at the time of filling out her insurance forms? The radiologist should understand the consequences of making the mammographic diagnosis of fibrocystic disease before using the term.

The concept of fibrocystic disease that has evolved at NEMCH is not unique to our institution. We believe that fibrocystic disease is not a single disease at all but is composed of several entities grouped under this term, often in a rather indiscriminate fashion. In most cases, physicians who use this term, both clinicians and radiologists, are probably describing a normal physiologic spectrum of breast change. Some women at the far end of the spectrum are symptomatic from their particular form of fibrocystic problem. The term *fibrocystic disease* has been totally abandoned at NEMCH and the term *fibrocystic change* has been substituted. Support for this concept is shared by many others.[3]

DYSPLASIA AND MAMMOGRAPHY

The term *dysplasia* refers to alterations in the appearance of adult cells. This alteration is characterized by variation in size, shape, and organization. This term can be used after cellular structure is analyzed and determined to be abnormal. As a radiologist, I do not see cells on the mammogram but only densities and calcifications. Dysplasia is not synonymous with cystic disease. If microcysts and macrocysts are lined with regular-appearing cells, there is no dysplasia present. Dysplasia is not synonymous with fibrosis. Though there may be fibrosis present in a dense breast, if there are no cells present whatsoever within the fibrotic areas, or if the few cells present are regular in appearance, there is no dysplasia. Indeed, the term is not necessarily synonymous with any mammographic pattern of fibrocystic change. Even if a woman has florid sclerosing adenosis with hundreds of diffuse bilateral scattered microcalcifications, she does not necessarily have dysplasia. If the areas of sclerosis are acellular, then there is no dysplasia present. If in the areas of adenosis all of the glands are lined by regular-appearing cells, then there is no dysplasia present.

An association between dysplasia and breast density (the breast parenchymal pattern) has been proposed,[4] but others are of the opinion that the dense mammogram is in no way reflective of dysplasia. In fact, there may be nothing abnormal with the dense mammogram other than that it is difficult to interpret.[5,6] The breast density varies during the lifetime of a woman, changing throughout childhood and adolescence. Initially, the breast appears rather dense in the young woman and eventually becomes fat-replaced as she ages and enters the menopausal and postmenopausal periods. When in this normal evolutionary cycle does the denseness of the breast become abnormal? While probably few would argue that a dense breast in the 70-year-old woman is abnormal because by that time most of the breast should be replaced by fat, who can be certain whether this density is abnormal in the transition years of 40 to 60?

My personal feelings about the relationship between breast density, dysplasia, and parenchymal patterns are quite straightforward. Since 1976, the issue has not yet been resolved and respected mammographers are still in disagreement. Regardless of personal bias, the concept is not universally accepted and, to quote Tabar, parenchymal patterns "should not be used to guide screening programs."[7] Even if there is a correlation between breast density and dysplasia, labeling a woman who has dense breast tissue as having dysplasia is not justified. The term *dysplasia*, when used correctly by the knowledgeable pathologist diagnosed by histologic tissue analysis, has definite meaning and potentially important consequences. Severe dysplasia is recognized by some to possibly be premalignant. I do not believe that this is what most radiologists intend to diagnose when they see a breast that is dense in a 40-year-old and call it dysplastic.

I believe that since a diagnosis of dysplasia can only be made by the pathologist, the word *dysplasia* does not belong in the mammography report.[8] The amusing thing is that our clinicians do not even demand that we use the word. If you do not believe this, stop using the word in your reports and nothing will happen to you except perhaps suffering an occasional joke from a clinician who states that he noticed that you stopped seeing dysplasia in all his patients. If we use the word, then I think that it is reasonable for our colleagues to expect us to know the objective criteria upon which this diagnosis is based. When a radiologist reads a stack of mammograms and sees dysplasia in case after case, he should eventually stop, look in the mirror, and say, "Maybe I don't really know what I'm talking about! How can everyone have dysplasia? What are the criteria I use to make this diagnosis?"

Some clinicians have told me that they know that when a mammogram is given to one radiologist, they can always expect a diagnosis of dysplasia, but if another radiologist interprets the same mammogram, it is read as normal. These areas of subjective perception probably do more harm than good to the patient and also serve to diminish the respect of our referring clinicians regarding our mammographic interpretation. If one continues to use the word *dysplasia* in the mammographic report, then one should realize that it is being used incorrectly. In 1981 I stopped using the word *dysplasia* in my reports and no one objected. From that moment on I was able to easily divest myself from a concept which I had never truly understood and which troubled me because of the consequences that its use created.

METHYLXANTHINE AND MAMMOGRAPHY

Dr. John Minton suggested that there is a relationship between methylxanthine intake and fibrocystic change.[9-11] This concept has received considerable publicity in the lay press, and review of this topic as well as the biochemical basis for it are beyond the scope of this text. What is important is that the relationship remains controversial and largely unsubstantiated by others. Many clinicians have failed to duplicate Minton's findings and believe that there is no relationship whatsoever between methylxanthine and the breast. The important concern from the radiologist's point of view is whether there should be any restriction on methylxanthine intake prior to the performance of the mammogram. In Minton's own work, patients were taken off methylxanthine for months. I am unaware of any reproducible scientific evidence documenting that tighter compression can be applied to the breast if the patient is off methylxanthine for several days prior to having a mammogram. In my practice I have no such restriction. When a woman is told that she needs a routine screening mammogram, her anxiety level almost invariably increases and I believe that the examination should be performed as quickly as feasible. I am not inclined to delay a routine examination in order to achieve an unproven theoretical benefit of better compression based on anecdotal experience.

REFERENCES

1. Love SM, Gelman RS, Silen W. Fibrocystic "disease" of the breast—a nondisease? N Engl J Med **307**:1010–1014, 1982.

2. Dupont WD, Page DL. Risk factors for breast cancer in women with proliferative breast disease. N Engl J Med **312**:146–151, 1985.

3. Hutter RVP. Goodbye to "fibrocystic disease." N Engl J Med **312**:179–181, 1985.

4. Wolfe JN, Albert S, Belle S, et al. Breast parenchymal patterns and their relationship to risk for having or developing carcinoma. Radiol Clin North Am **21**:127–136, 1983.

5. Page DL, Winfield AC. The dense mammogram. AJR **147**:487–489, 1986.

6. Egan RL, McSweeney MB. Mammographic parenchymal patterns and risk of breast cancer. Radiology **133**:65–70, 1979.

7. Tabar L, Dean PB. Mammographic parenchymal patterns. JAMA **241**:185–189, 1982.

8. Homer MJ. The mammography report. AJR **142**:643–644, 1984.

9. Minton JP, Foecking MK, Webster DJT, et al. Caffeine, cyclic nucleotides and breast disease. Surgery **86**:105, 1979a.

10. Minton JP, Foecking MK, Webster DJT, et al. Response of fibrocystic disease to caffeine withdrawal and correlation of cyclic nucleotides with breast disease. Am J Obstet Gynecol **135**:157, 1979b.

11. Minton JP, Abou-Issa H, Reiches N, et al. Clinical and biochemical studies on methylxanthine-related fibrocystic breast disease. Surgery **90**:299, 1981.

Chapter 9

BENIGN LESIONS IN THE BREAST

This chapter reviews the mammographic features of benign breast lesions. Emphasis will be placed upon whether mammographic features are helpful in differential diagnosis. While in some cases the mammographic features of a lesion are virtually pathognomonic of the process, in others they are quite nonspecific, and the benign nature of the lesion is ultimately diagnosed by aspiration, biopsy, or stability on follow-up examinations.

FIBROADENOMA

The fibroadenoma is a tumor which develops under the hormonal influence of estrogen. It typically appears after puberty. Clinically, it is a smooth, firm, freely mobile mass within the breast. Sometimes its lobulated borders can be perceived by the palpating fingers (Fig. 9-1). The histologic differentiation of fibroadenoma into intracanalicular (where there is a proliferation of connective tissue within the lumen of the duct) and pericanalicular (where this proliferation occurs in the outer margin of duct) has no mammographic correlate. Fibroadenomas tend to regress with menopause. As they involute, their noncalcified appearance changes and microcalcifications develop. These eventually grow more numerous and increase in size to become macrocalcifications (Fig. 9-2). The typical degenerating fibroadenoma contains popcornlike macrocalcification, which is easily recognized by mammography. Since fibroadenomas are commonly found in association with normal breast parenchyma, as well as with various forms of benign fibrocystic change, their sharp margins are often not demonstrated by mammography (Fig. 9-3).

Differentiation of a cyst from a noncalcified fibroadenoma can be made by ultrasound or aspiration. However, unless the classic macrocalcifications are present, recognition by mammography that a solid mass is a benign fibroadenoma is impossible. When the fibroadenoma has certain features, it is one of the few breast lesions that can be recognized with enough confidence to avoid biopsy. However, in situations in which all these features are not present, either follow-up or biopsy is indicated. These features relate to margin and calcium content. When all the margins are clearly visible by mammography and can be judged to be sharp and when the entire volume of the mass is replaced by dense macrocalcification and rim calcium, its appear-

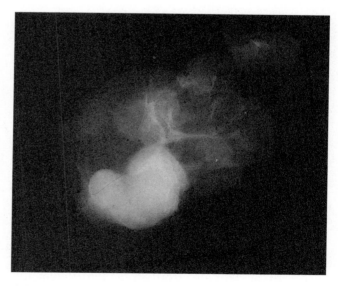

FIG. 9-1 *Specimen radiograph of a lobulated fibroadenoma.*

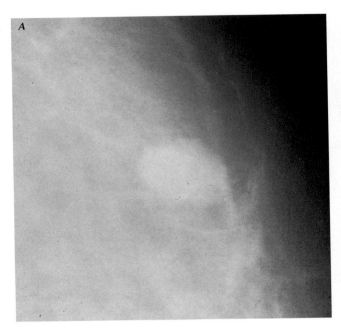

FIG. 9-2 A. Noncalcified fibroadenoma.

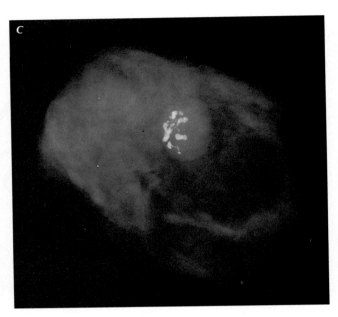

FIG. 9-2 (Continued) C. Fibroadenoma containing macrocalcifications.

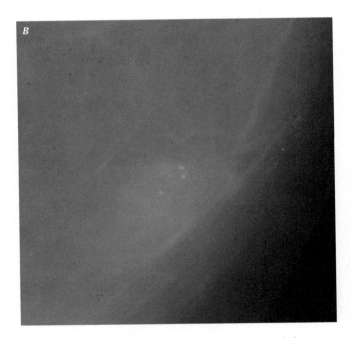

FIG. 9-2 (Continued) B. Fibroadenoma containing microcalcifications. Notice its irregular margins.

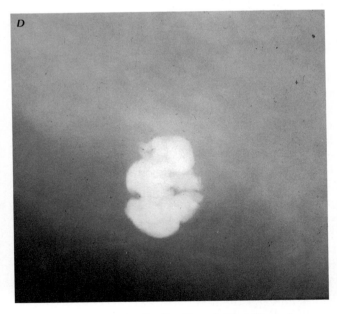

FIG. 9-2 (Continued) D. Totally calcified fibroadenoma.

ance can be considered to be pathognomonic. Similarly, when sharp margins are identified and the calcium present is dense macrocalcification or rim calcium, it can still be recognized as a fibroadenoma. When all the borders cannot be declared to be sharply marginated, or when in addition to macrocalcifications, microcalcifications are present within the mass, the level of confidence that the lesion is a fibroadenoma is de-

creased (Fig. 9-4). In these cases, the choice is between follow-up and biopsy. Other information such as the patient's age, risk factors, multiplicity, and bilaterality weigh into the option chosen.

The fibroadenoma may enlarge in a premenopausal woman, a postmenopausal woman taking exogenous estrogen, and on occasion in a postmenopausal woman receiving no hormonal replace-

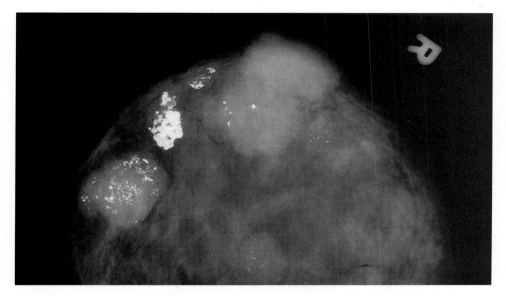

FIG. 9-3 *This breast contains numerous fibroadenomas showing the full spectrum of appearance from noncalcified to dense, popcornlike macrocalcifications. Many of the fibroadenomas do not have sharp margins.*

ment.[1,2] When a fibroadenoma grows to a very large size, it is called a *giant fibroadenoma* (Fig. 9-5). The giant fibroadenoma is histologically similar to the smaller fibroadenoma, and there is no higher incidence of malignant transformation. A young woman with a fibroadenoma does not have a higher risk for developing breast carcinoma. But some believe that an active fibroadenoma developing in the peri- or postmenopausal age group is associated with a higher risk for the development of breast cancer.[3]

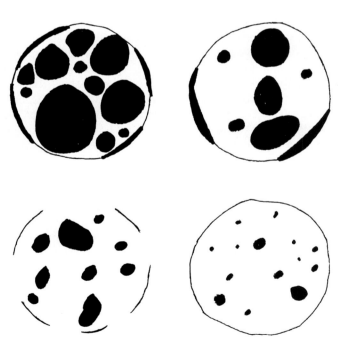

FIG. 9-4 *The two top panels represent fibroadenomas with sharp margins, dense macrocalcifications, and rim calcium. Masses illustrated in the bottom panels are likely to be fibroadenomas but because the margins are not sharply defined, or because there is a mixture of macrocalcification and microcalcification, the certainty is decreased and either follow-up or the obtaining of tissue is recommended.*

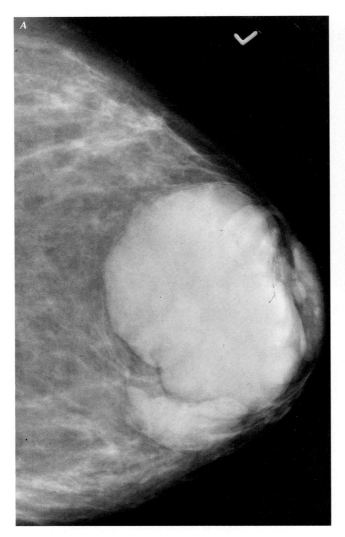

FIG. 9-5 A. *This 11.5-cm palpable mass is a giant fibroadenoma.*

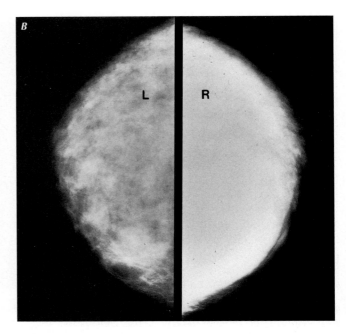

FIG. 9-5 *(Continued)* **B.** *This 30-year-old woman saw her physician because her right breast was firmer and was enlarging more rapidly than her left. Mammography revealed a large space-occupying mass in the right breast. There was no evidence of skin retraction or thickening. Histology revealed a giant fibroadenoma.*

BREAST CYST

The enlargement and dilatation of lactiferous ducts give rise to breast cysts. These simple cysts are typically multiple and occur primarily in women 30 to 50 years of age. Though they are found less frequently in the younger and older age groups, cysts are by no means an uncommon occurrence at either end of the spectrum. Simple breast cysts are lined by a single layer of epithelial cells and contain clear or yellow transudate fluid. Typically, their size increases and decreases over time.

Simple breast cysts usually contain no calcium. On occasion, rim calcium may be present,[4] or there may be centrally located tiny punctate microcalcifications within a benign cyst.[5] These are recognized by

their positional change when they fall to the most dependent portion of the cyst on a true lateral view. Tiny microcysts may also contain a form of calcium called *milk of calcium*. These may have a diffuse or focal distribution.[6,7] Layering calcium and rim calcium have already been discussed in Chap. 6.

Although traditional teaching emphasizes the reliance upon the presence of sharp borders to differentiate between benign and malignant, this sign is not always reliable in a specific patient. The border of a benign cyst may appear poorly defined when overlapped by areas of normal breast parenchyma. As mentioned previously, the presence of a halo sign, or partial halo sign, is not pathognomonic of a benign mass. Breast cysts commonly undergo spontaneous regression.[8] If the mammogram is performed during this process, the cyst may have angular borders.

Perhaps the most direct and cost-effective way to confirm that a palpable breast mass is a cyst is by needle aspiration. Depending upon one's practice, this procedure can be performed by the clinician or radiologist. The aspiration is both diagnostic and therapeutic. If the mass totally disappears on palpation and the fluid has a benign appearance according to the experience of the physician performing the aspiration, the diagnosis of benign simple cyst can be made. Handling aspirated fluid is controversial, and while some clinicians send all aspirated fluid for cytologic analysis, others routinely discard fluid that appears unremarkable. It would be wise for the radiologist and clinician to have an established policy for management of aspirated fluid. When the radiologist assumes the primary responsibility for aspiration of a palpable mass presumed to be a cyst, the aspiration is usually preceded by an ultrasound examination. The criteria we rely on to diagnose a simple cyst by ultrasound include demonstration of an anechoic mass, sharp margins, good through transmission of sound, compressibility, and a well-defined posterior wall. When we aspirate a breast cyst, we obtain a postaspiration mammogram to serve as a new baseline for the patient. We can judge whether the mammographic abnormality has totally disappeared and will also know if the cyst recurs at a future examination (Fig. 9-6).

Ultimately, the management of a palpable mass is the responsibility of the clinician. However, the radiologist assumes the primary responsibility for management of the nonpalpable mass. When a mass does not meet ultrasound criteria for a simple cyst, the differential diagnosis includes possibilities such as a complex cyst and a solid lesion, either benign or malignant. In this situation, we usually do not attempt aspiration, since the surgeon prefers to excise the entire mass without the area being violated by a needle.

Sometimes a palpable simple benign cyst will have a thick fibrous capsule. Although aspiration by the clinician may have failed, a repeat aspiration may be successful under ultrasound guidance, thereby saving the woman from a biopsy.

It is not our practice to perform pneumocystograms despite the claim by some that replacing cyst

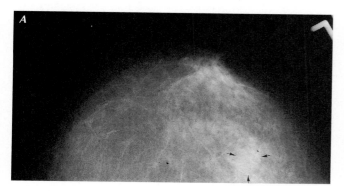

FIG. 9-6 **A.** *CC view from a routine screening mammogram reveals a nonpalpable 1.5-cm mass in the outer half of the left breast (arrows). It contains no definite calcifications.*

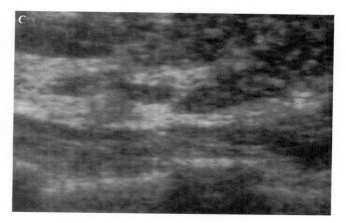

FIG. 9-6 *(Continued)* **C.** *Postaspiration ultrasound confirms that the mass has disappeared.*

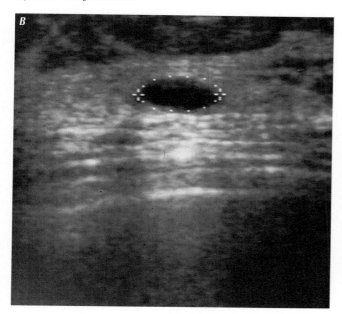

FIG. 9-6 *(Continued)* **B.** *Ultrasound revealed features consistent with a simple cyst.*

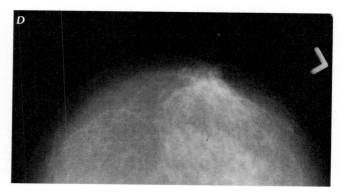

FIG. 9-6 *(Continued)* **D.** *Postaspiration mammogram obtained immediately after the aspiration now serves as the new baseline mammogram. The mass has disappeared.*

fluid by air reduces cyst recurrence. We do not believe that performing pneumocystograms routinely to find the rare entity of intracystic carcinoma is justified, especially when considering the added time and repeat mammograms this would require in every patient undergoing a routine cyst aspiration. Intracystic carcinoma accounts for approximately 0.3 percent of all breast cancer.[9] Usually, when this rare lesion is present, there will be clues to suspect its presence such as an abnormal mammogram, an abnormal ultrasound examination or abnormal fluid if the mass has been aspirated. Also, regrowth of the same cyst after aspiration, even if the fluid has a benign cytology, is a well-accepted surgical indication for careful follow-up or excision.

Superficially located simple cysts, especially in the small-breasted woman, may be ruptured by vigorous compression during mammography.[10] The radiologist should be aware of this possibility as an explanation for why a mass might "disappear" between routine views taken during the same examination.

PHYLLODES TUMOR

This tumor, originally referred to as cystosarcoma phyllodes, is usually classified as either benign or malignant. Differentiation between these two categories is made by histologic criteria including the number of mitoses per high-power field, stromal pleomorphism, the presence of cellular atypia, and evidence of invasion. The mammographic appearance of a benign phyllodes tumor may be indistinguishable from that of a giant fibroadenoma (Fig. 9-7). It is typically large, noncalcified, and has smooth or lobulated rather sharply marginated borders. There are usually no associated secondary signs of invasion such as skin thickening or retraction. Prominent vascularity can be seen with either a benign or malignant phyllodes tumor, so this is of very little help in differential diagnosis (Fig. 9-8). Many pathologists are of the opinion that a benign phyllodes tumor is not synonymous with a giant fibroadenoma. If not completely excised, a benign phyllodes tumor may recur locally. Interestingly, the histologic features do not always correlate with the biologic behavior of the tumor.[11]

INTRAMAMMARY LYMPH NODE

A normal lymph node usually measures less than 1.5 cm in greatest diameter, is noncalcified, and has sharp margins.[12] However, now that more axillary contents

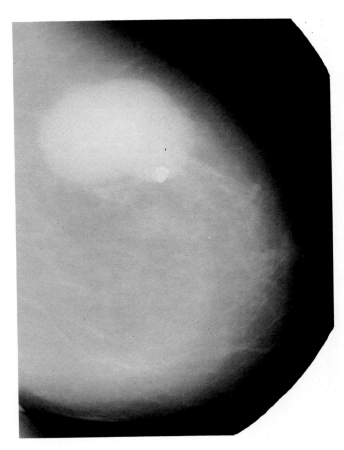

FIG. 9-7 *This 7-cm palpable mass was a benign phyllodes tumor. Differential diagnosis includes a giant fibroadenoma.*

are routinely visualized on the oblique view, most radiologists realize that normal nonpalpable axillary lymph nodes can exceed more than 1.5 cm in greatest diameter. When lymph nodes are located in the axilla, they should be recognized as part of normal anatomy. With good compression, normal lymph nodes may be seen along the chest wall down to the plane of the nipple, as illustrated in Chap. 7. Diagnostic problems occur when a lymph node is in an intramammary location. Typically intramammary lymph nodes are located in the upper outer quadrant, but they may occur in other quadrants of the breast.[13] In this situation, the node may trigger a localization and biopsy, since it will be interpreted as an occult breast mass.[14] When the node contains the additional mammographic features of a hilus and central fat (Fig. 9-9), it is our policy not to recommend biopsy but to place the patient in a follow-up protocol for what is a lesion with a high probability of being benign.[15] Magnification is often helpful in demonstrating these characteristics. While these findings are not pathognomonic of a lymph node, since other benign entities such as fibroadenomas and hemangiomas may have similar findings,[16] the chance of

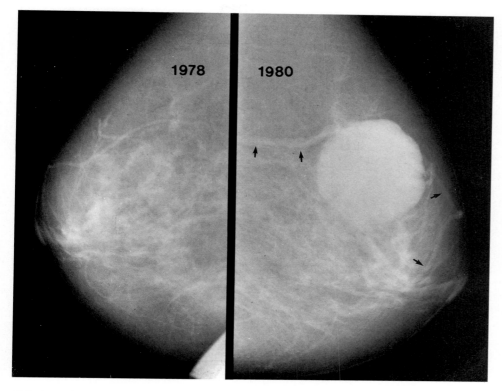

FIG. 9-8 *LAT views of the left breast demonstrate that a 6-cm mass has developed over a two-year interval. Notice the enlarged vein that is present (arrows). Histology revealed a benign phyllodes tumor.*

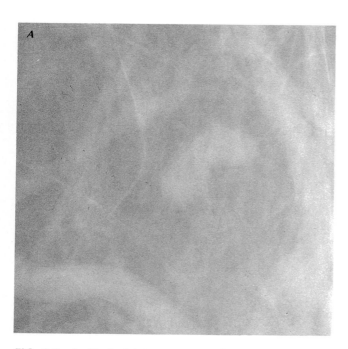

FIG. 9-9 A. *Typical intramammary lymph node containing central hilus. It has remained stable throughout the follow-up.*

FIG. 9-9 *(Continued)* **B.** *This 6-mm sharply marginated noncalcified mass was discovered on a routine screening mammogram. The patient opted for needle localization and excision rather than follow-up. Histology revealed an intramammary lymph node.*

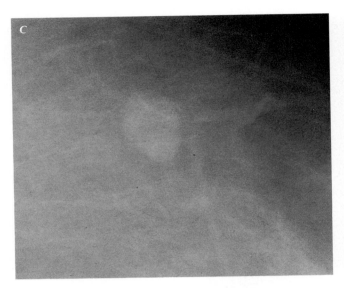

FIG. 9-9 (Continued) C. This nonpalpable 1.2-cm noncalcified sharply marginated mass was discovered on a routine screening mammogram.

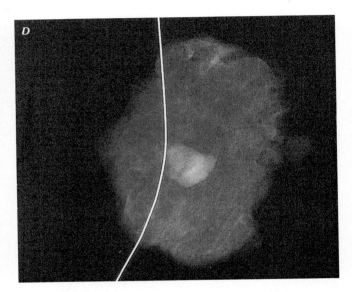

FIG. 9-9 (Continued) D. Needle localization and excision were performed. Specimen radiography confirmed excision of the mass. Notice its well-defined lobulated margins. Histology revealed a normal lymph node.

the mass being a carcinoma still remains extremely low. In fact, some mammographers choose to ignore the mass altogether because of the extremely low probability of it being anything clinically significant. When the notch and central fat are absent, I manage the finding as I do a sharply marginated noncalcified mass less than 1 to 1.5 cm in greatest diameter and the woman is placed into a follow-up protocol. For reasons stated in Chap. 6, we do not use ultrasound on these small masses.

Normal intramammary lymph nodes may appear or enlarge in the breast. They may be reacting to inflammatory conditions of the skin.[17] However, when a lymph node appears or enlarges, whether it is intramammary or axillary, a determination must be made as to why it is growing. The concern, of course, is that it is enlarging because of infiltration by a neoplastic process such as lymphoma or metastatic disease from an adjacent breast carcinoma.[18] However, even in the presence of a breast malignancy, enlarging lymph nodes may not reflect metastatic involvement. Some breast malignancies such as medullary carcinoma cause the development of reactive adenopathy.[19] No rules can be given as to when to force biopsy in this situation, since every case must be evaluated individually.

LIPOMA

Just as in other parts of the body, when a lipoma occurs in the breast, its appearance is characteristic and it should not be necessary to perform a biopsy to establish its benign nature.[20] The lipoma is a lucent,

space-occupying mass surrounded by a capsule. It displaces the surrounding normal parenchyma (Fig. 9-10). Calcifications of fat necrosis may be contained inside the lipoma. The typical lipoma is soft, freely mobile, and occurs most commonly in the postmenopausal age group. A lipoma is excised either because it is palpable and the woman finds it annoying or because it has grown so large that the breast becomes asymmetric, creating a cosmetic problem (Fig. 9-11). Radiologists commonly mistake a lipoma for normal fatty tissue in the breast. The breast is composed of a honeycomb structure and when white glandular tissue is replaced by fat in the normal evolutionary process, the fat naturally assumes a circular shape. The differentiation of normal fat from lipoma rests upon the presence of a capsule which surrounds the true lipoma and displacement of the adjacent breast parenchyma.[21]

The liposarcoma is a rare lesion of the breast which should not be confused with a lipoma. This malignant tumor is rapidly growing and contains soft tissue elements. If differentiation is not obvious by either mammographic or clinical criteria, then it is prudent to perform a biopsy to obtain tissue for histologic diagnosis.

HAMARTOMA

A hamartoma is a rare benign lesion of the breast. Synonyms include lipofibroadenoma and fibroadenolipoma. As these names suggest, the lesion is com-

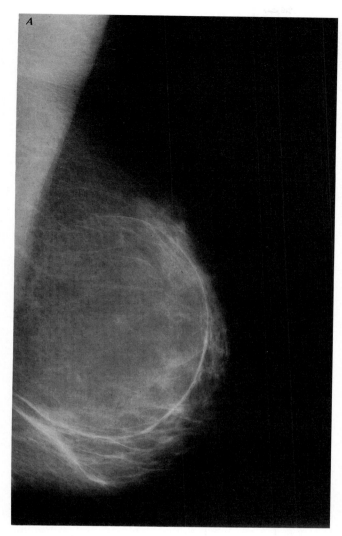

FIG. 9-10 A. *This is the characteristic appearance of a lipoma in the breast. It is a lucent space-occupying lesion surrounded by a capsule.*

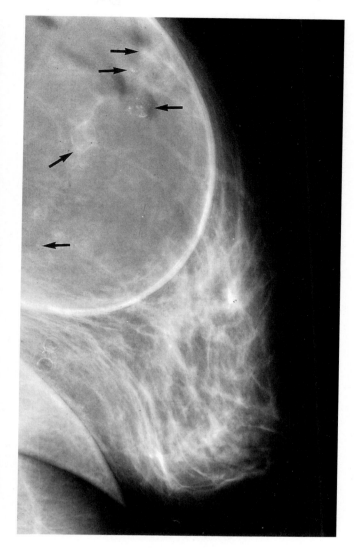

FIG. 9-11 *This 39-year-old woman was admitted for resection of a 1.5-kg lipoma. Notice its thick capsule and how it displaces normal breast parenchyma. Numerous areas of fat necrosis are present within the lipoma (arrows).*

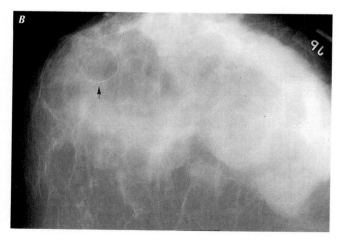

FIG. 9-10 (Continued) B. *This is a smaller lipoma of the breast. Part of its capsule is calcified (arrow).*

posed of lipid, glandular, and fibrous tissue. It is one of the few breast lesions to characteristically contain both fat and water density substances (Fig. 9-12). Although mammographically it appears to have a capsule, hamartomas do not possess a true capsule but are surrounded by a thin layer of fibrous tissue (Fig. 9-13). While the features of a breast hamartoma are considered to be virtually pathognomonic, because of its rarity it is unlikely for anyone to have had sufficient experience to recognize it and confidently diagnose it, thereby avoiding a biopsy. In fact, a breast hamartoma may have variable features, including a homogenous density and irregular margins.[22] A liposarcoma could also be confused with this lesion, since it may contain fat and soft tissue density. However, the key differential feature be-

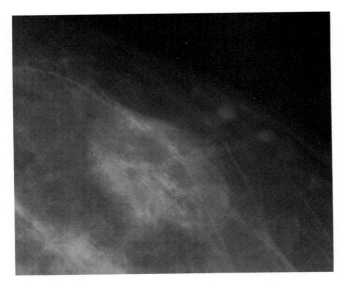

FIG. 9-12 *This breast hamartoma contains both fat and soft tissue elements.*

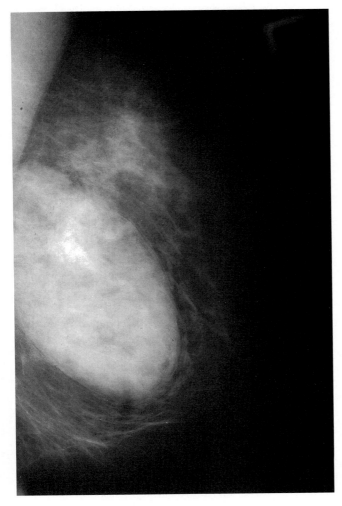

FIG. 9-13 *This breast hamartoma also contains fat and soft tissue components. It is surrounded by a thin layer of fibrous tissue having the appearance of a capsule.*

tween this malignant lesion and the benign breast hamartoma is that the sarcoma is a rapidly growing firm lesion, while the adenolipofibroma is a soft, often nonpalpable lesion not displaying rapid growth. Although the radiologist may be firm in suggesting the diagnosis of benign breast hamartoma when characteristic mammographic features are present, because of its rarity a surgeon might still demand histologic confirmation of its benign nature.

GALACTOCELE

The galactocele is one of the few breast lesions with a benign nature that can be readily recognized by mammography because of its fat content. A galactocele is a benign breast cyst that contains thick, inspissated, milky fluid. It is commonly found in the retroareolar region and typically appears during or shortly after lactation. It is hypothesized that a galactocele results when lactation is abruptly suppressed. Since mammography is not usually performed in this age group, radiologists may be unfamiliar with the mammographic features of this entity. Like a lipoma, it can be a lucent lesion (Fig. 9-14) that requires no further workup, since carcinoma is composed of soft tissue density. However, a galactocele need not be lucent. It may contain calcium density, and on horizontal beam mammography a fat calcium level will be produced.[23] Galactoceles may contain a fat fluid level, which similarly would be demonstrated only by horizontal beam mammography. If the water density of a galactocele is greater than its lipid content, the galactocele can appear as a soft tissue density, and when the contents are not in the liquid state, a fat fluid level will not be produced. It will have the appearance of a mottled density with a mixture of fat and water, not too dissimilar from a breast hamartoma.[24]

RADIAL SCAR

The radial scar is a proliferative breast lesion containing a central core of elastosis and entrapped ductal elements. The lesion is often surrounded by areas of adenosis, epithelial hyperplasia, and papillomatosis. The elastosis component of the lesion obliterates the normal ductal-lobular anatomy of the breast. Radial scar has also been described by other terms such as indurative mastopathy,[25] focal fibrous disease,[26] and benign sclerosing ductal proliferation.[27] This entity is more commonly diagnosed on the histologic level and infrequently presents as a clinically palpable mass or a mammographic abnormality in an asymptomatic patient. The radial scar is of more interest to the pathol-gist's role is more straightforward, since the mammographic features of radial scar are those of an irregular noncalcified mass often associated with architectural distortion (Fig. 9-15). Since these features are indistinguishable from carcinoma, their recognition will trigger recommendation for an immediate biopsy. There are no reliable mammographic features to help differentiate carcinoma from radial scar.[29–31]

PAPILLOMA

The papilloma is a proliferation of epithelial tissue attached to the duct wall by a fibrovascular stalk. It may occur anywhere in the ductal system. The solitary papilloma is commonly located centrally in the subareolar ducts. Some believe that it may be associated with a slightly increased risk of breast cancer.[32] Multiple papillomas are located peripherally in the breast. They are more likely to be associated with atypia and epithelial hyperplasia and therefore they are associated with a moderate increased risk of cancer.[33] Multiple

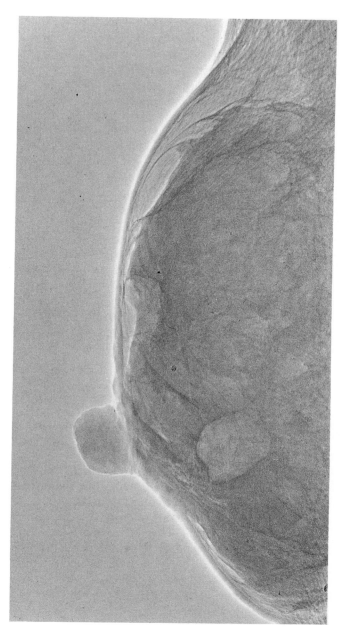

FIG. 9-14 *This 42-year-old woman had just stopped nursing and developed a palpable mass corresponding to the lucent lesion seen on this xerogram. The mass was aspirated and yielded milky yellow material. The palpable mass disappeared and did not recur. The clinical presentation, mammographic findings, and aspiration material are all characteristic of a galactocele. (Courtesy of Edward A. Sickles, M.D., San Francisco, CA.)*

ogist than the radiologist because of its controversial nature. Some believe that this lesion slowly progresses to tubular carcinoma and that the pathologist must carefully examine it because of the tendency toward malignant transformation.[28] However, the belief that radial scar is a benign process with malignant potential is not universally accepted. In contrast, the radiolo-

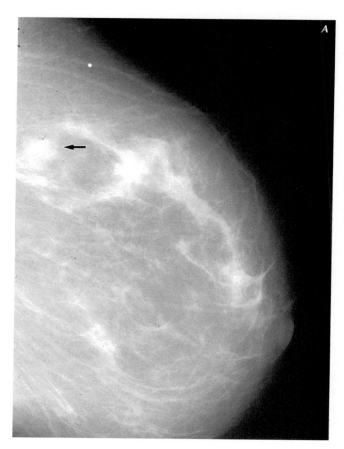

FIG. 9-15 A. *A routine screening mammogram in this 53-year-old woman revealed a poorly defined noncalcified mass (arrow).*

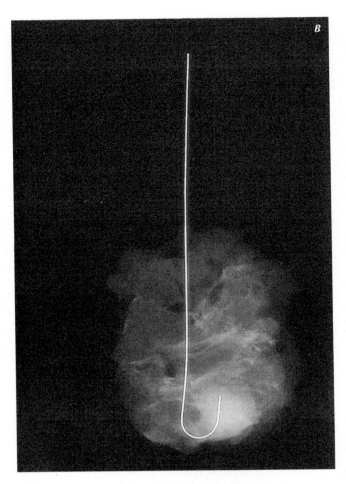

FIG. 9-15 *(Continued)* **B.** *Needle localization and biopsy were performed. Specimen radiography confirmed excision of the mass. Histology revealed focal fibrosis.*

papillomas are not synonymous with the term *papillomatosis*, which will be discussed in the next section.

The symptomatic papilloma is most likely to be located in the subareolar region. A papilloma may cause either a serous or sanguineous nipple discharge and it is the most common etiology of a bloody nipple discharge. Rarely, the papilloma may be intracystic rather than intraductal, and in this case a discharge will occur only if the cyst communicates with a duct.[34]

Papillomas are commonly so small that they are neither visible by mammography nor clinically palpable. They can grow large enough to obstruct the duct, and then the mammographic sign of duct dilation will be evident. Large papillomas may even present as a mass on mammography (Fig. 9-16). Infrequently, papillomas may contain small punctate microcalcifications (Fig. 9-17).

The role of ductography in the evaluation of a woman with a nipple discharge is controversial. Some advocate ductography as the procedure of choice.[35]

Successful ductography requires identification and cannulation of the precise ductal orifice which drains the pathologic ductal system. This usually requires that the discharge be spontaneous and of the exudative type in order to sufficiently enlarge the ductal orifice for identification and cannulation. Some advocate that ductography be performed immediately prior to surgery so that the abnormal ductal system can be injected with a dye such as methylene blue to aid the surgeon in identifying the location of the pathologic ductal system.

In many hospitals, including NEMCH, ductography is not performed. In most cases, the surgeon is able to identify the quadrant of the abnormal ducts by noting where palpation causes the discharge to be expressed. In some instances, an actual trigger zone causing the nipple discharge is identified by palpation. With this knowledge, the surgeon will make a circumareolar incision and identify the pathologic ductal system by direct inspection. If a ductogram is required, the surgeon can inject dye and directly visualize the duct. The procedure is easily tolerated by the already anesthetized patient.

PAPILLOMATOSIS

Papillomatosis is a proliferative epithelial disorder. This proliferation occurs within the ducts rather than the lobules. It is one of the forms of fibrocystic change that is believed to carry an increased risk of developing carcinoma, especially when marked atypia is present. This entity is not synonymous with multiple papillomas.[36] Mammographically, it most often presents as a solitary geographic cluster of microcalcifications or an irregular mass, usually indistinguishable from carcinoma (Fig. 9-18). Biopsy is required to establish the benign etiology of the calcifications. When the area of papillomatosis is nonpalpable, as is often the case, needle localization is required.

ACUTE MASTITIS

Acute mastitis most often occurs during lactation. Since it is an infection, the breast appears tender, swollen, and red. The patient may be febrile with an elevated sedimentation rate and a leukocytosis. Enlarged, painful, axillary lymph nodes may be palpable. Treatment consists of appropriate antibiotic therapy. If a focal abscess is present, it may require surgical drainage. Rarely, the abscess may be indolent and differentiation from carcinoma will be impossible except by excisional biopsy (Fig. 9-19). Infectious agents that may cause an indolent abscess include tuberculosis.[37]

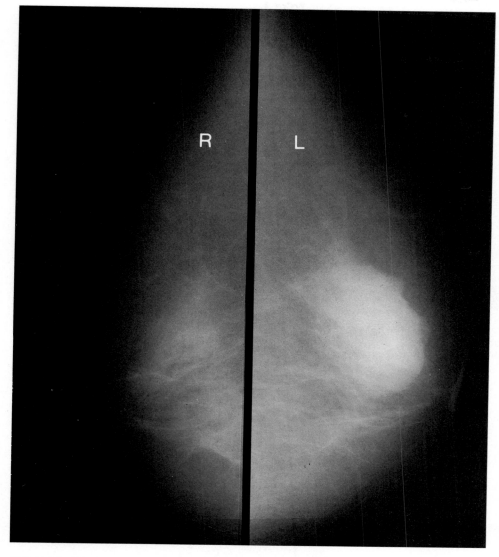

FIG. 9-16 *The increased left subareolar density was palpable. Excisional biopsy revealed a giant benign papilloma.*

The mammographic features of acute mastitis are usually indistinguishable from those of inflammatory breast cancer and include generalized skin thickening, increased markings throughout the affected breast, and an overall increase of breast density when compared to the normal contralateral side (Fig. 9-20). However, clinically there is usually less of a problem differentiating acute mastitis from inflammatory breast cancer because the latter disease occurs in older women who do not have other evidence of infection such as fever and leukocytosis. We do not obtain a mammogram on a patient with acute mastitis unless there is an unusual circumstance such as atypical presentation or failure of the presumed mastitis to resolve after appropriate therapy.

CHRONIC MASTITIS/PLASMA-CELL MASTITIS

Chronic mastitis is a process that causes aseptic inflammation in the breast. Typically, chronic mastitis occurs in the elderly woman. It is an entirely different entity than acute mastitis and does not represent an end stage or an indolent form of that disease. Chronic mastitis is probably a sequela of secretory disease and is often asymptomatic. It has been theorized that as the woman ages, there is a stasis of ductal secretion leading to eventual inspissation. The ducts lose their integrity and their contents leak into the breast

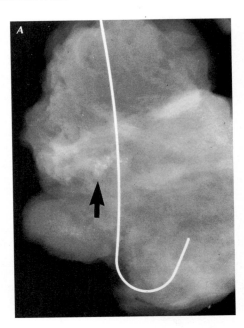

FIG. 9-17 A. *This woman underwent needle localization for excision of a small mass containing microcalcifications. Specimen radiograph confirms excision of the lesion (arrow).*

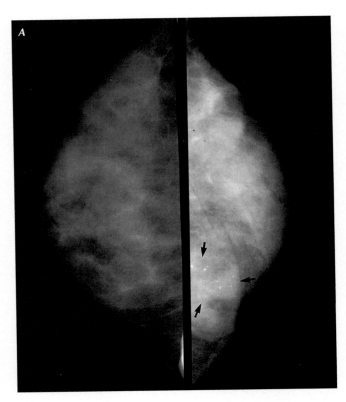

FIG. 9-18 A. *This woman presented for evaluation of a palpable mass in the lower portion of her right breast. Mammogram revealed a mass (arrows) in the inferior portion of the left breast. It contained microcalcifications.*

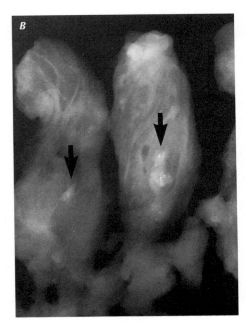

FIG. 9-17 (Continued) **B.** *Radiography of the sectioned tissue was required to isolate the lesion (arrows), since nothing was visually evident. Histology revealed an intraductal papilloma containing microcalcifications.*

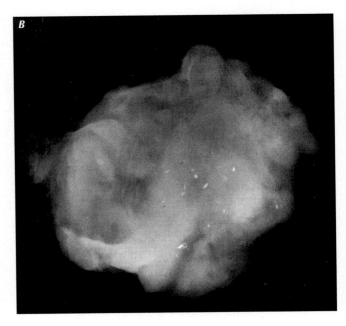

FIG. 9-18 (Continued) **B.** *The mass with microcalcification was excised. Histology revealed papillomatosis.*

parenchyma. As this occurs, a reaction to the material is evoked, which can be likened to a chemical mastitis. The breast tissue tries to wall off the secretions with dense macrocalcifications. There are no clinical signs of acute inflammation, and palpation is usually normal. Occasionally, a firm nodularity or even a mass may be palpable when the disease is predominantly focal in nature. However, focality need not be present, since the ductal ectasia is often bilateral. When the process occurs focally in the subareolar area, nipple retraction and even a discharge may be present. If it is superficially located, focal skin thickening and retraction may be present. When the fibrotic element predominates, an irregular mass indistinguishable from carcinoma may be evident both by palpation and mammography (Fig. 9-21).

The histologic hallmarks of chronic mastitis are ductal ectasia and heavily calcified ductal secretions. Numerous eosinophils and plasma cells are present. The latter cell type gives rise to the term *plasma-cell mastitis*, which is a synonym for this entity.[38]

The mammogram usually reveals dense round or oval macrocalcifications with lucent centers (Fig. 9-22), but they may be more linear in appearance (Fig. 9-23). Since the calcifications evoked by chronic mastitis are related to the ducts, they have polarity with orientation toward the nipple. Chronic mastitis can be considered a form of nontraumatic fat necrosis so the appearance of macrocalcifications is identical in these two entities. When the disease manifests itself as large macrocalcifications with polarity, it should be recog-

FIG. 9-18 *(Continued)* **C.** *This solitary geographic cluster of microcalcifications proved to be a focus of papillomatosis.*

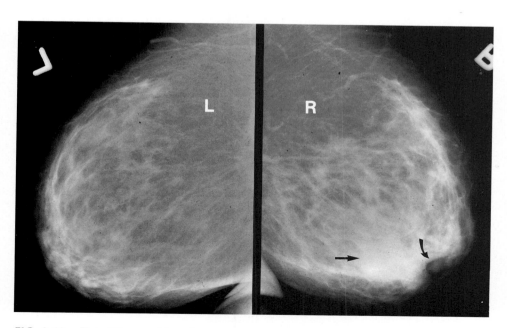

FIG. 9-19. *This 47-year-old patient presented with a painless mass (arrow) and skin retraction (curved arrow) in the right breast. Excision revealed a large abscess cavity with severe acute and chronic inflammation. The skin contained focal chronic inflammation. There was no evidence of malignancy.*

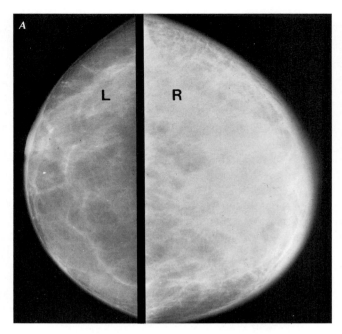

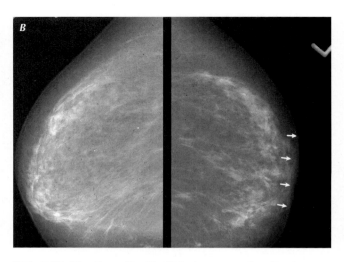

FIG. 9-20 (Continued) **B.** *This is a more localized example of acute mastitis confined to the periareolar region. Notice the skin thickening (arrows).*

FIG. 9-20. **A.** *The generalized skin thickening and increased density in the right breast is being caused by an acute mastitis. The mammographic appearance is identical to inflammatory carcinoma.*

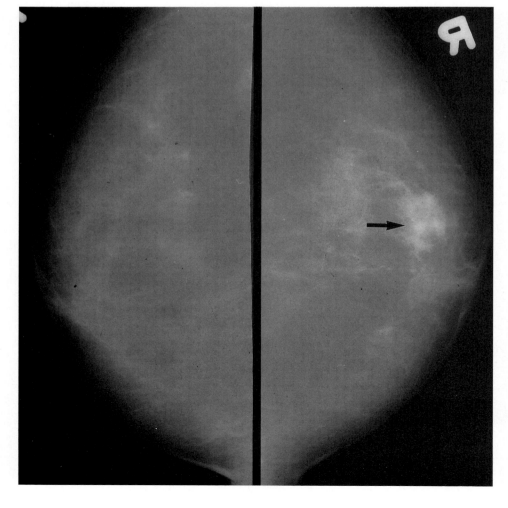

FIG. 9-21 *This 46-year-old woman underwent excisional biopsy for a firm palpable mass in the right breast (arrow). Mammography demonstrated that it was a noncalcified irregular mass. Histology revealed focal fat necrosis.*

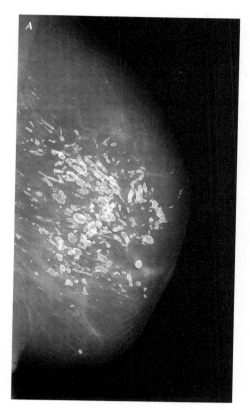

FIG. 9-22 A. *These are characteristic calcifications of chronic mastitis. They were present bilaterally. The patient was asymptomatic and had a normal breast palpation.*

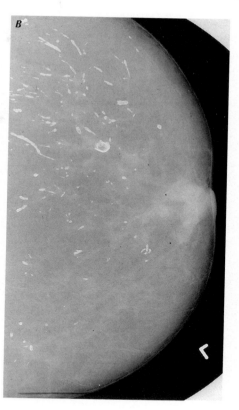

FIG. 9-22 *(Continued)* **B.** *This is another asymptomatic patient with chronic mastitis. The process was present bilaterally. The enlarged subareolar ducts were excised, and they revealed ductal ectasia and inspissated debris.*

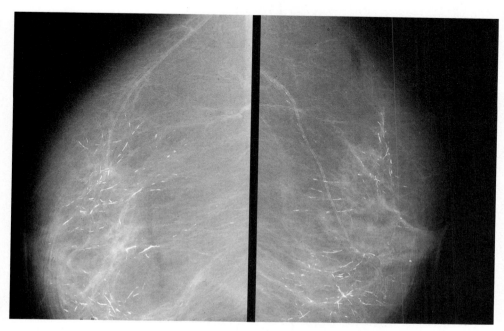

FIG. 9-23 *This woman, who was also asymptomatic, has chronic mastitis from secretory disease. The calcifications are more linear in appearance. Notice the polarity of the calcifications toward the nipple.*

nized as a benign process. Chronic mastitis may be bilateral, unilateral (Fig. 9-24), or focal.

It is not considered a premalignant condition and when it can be recognized by mammographic features, biopsy is not necessary. However, when the disease is focal and has features of a mass or microcalcification making it indistinguishable from carcinoma, biopsy is usually unavoidable.

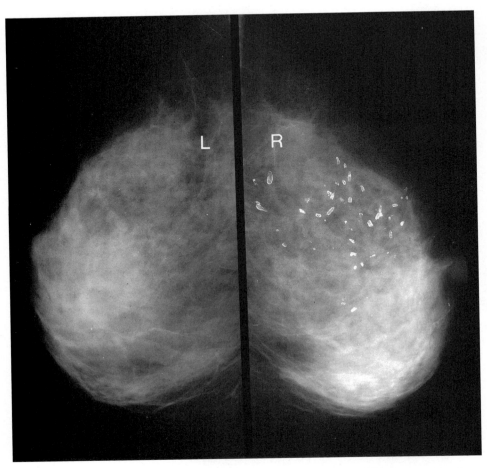

FIG. 9-24 *In this asymptomatic woman, chronic mastitis was present only in the right breast.*

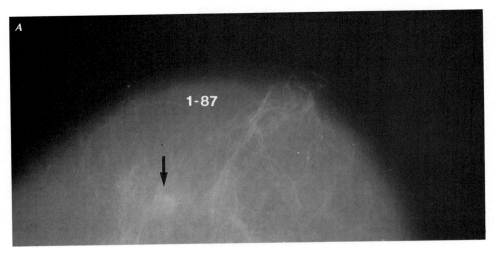

FIG. 9-25 A. *This patient underwent excisional biopsy for this palpable irregular mass (arrow). It was benign.*

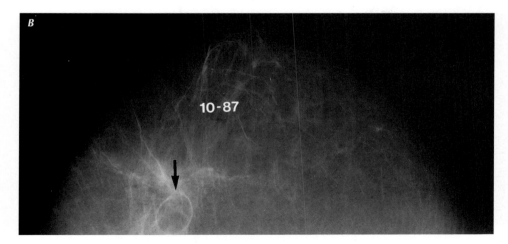

FIG. 9-25 *(Continued)* **B.** *Nine months later, a lipid cyst has developed at the biopsy site. (Courtesy of Jon Pitman, M.D., Lewston, ME.)*

FAT NECROSIS

Fat necrosis is a nonsuppurative lesion characterized by histiocytic giant cells containing foamy cytoplasm, lipid-laden macrophages, and fibrous proliferation. Depending upon the age and etiology of the lesion, there may also be acute or chronic inflammatory cells, hemorrhage, and calcification. Various etiologies can cause the development of fat necrosis such as direct external trauma,[39] breast biopsy (Fig. 9-25) and reduction mammoplasty[40] (Fig. 9-26), irradiation[41] (Fig. 9-27), systemic diseases such as nodular panniculitis[42] (Fig. 9-28), and ductal ectasia seen in chronic mastitis.[43]

The mammographic features of fat necrosis vary greatly from those of a pathognomonic appearance,

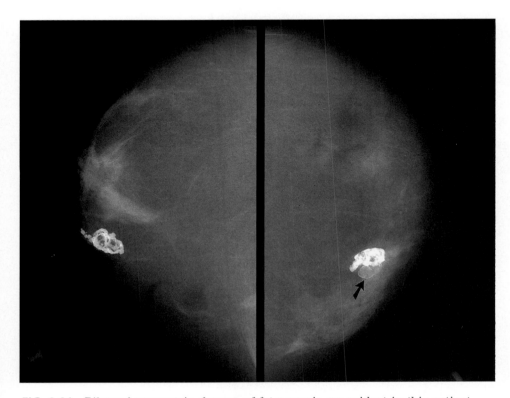

FIG. 9-26 *Bilateral symmetric changes of fat necrosis are evident in this patient who underwent reduction mammoplasty. Notice the lipid cyst with rim calcium (arrow).*

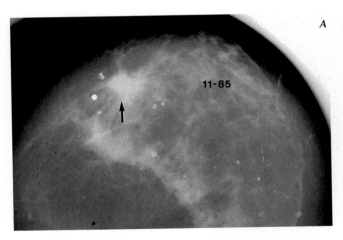

FIG. 9-27 **A.** *A nonpalpable stellate mass (arrow) was discovered on routine screening mammography.*

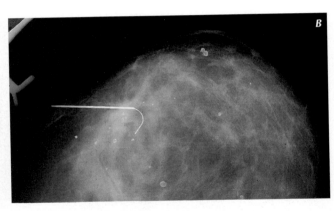

FIG. 9-27 *(Continued)* **B.** *Needle localization and biopsy revealed an invasive ductal carcinoma. The patient was treated with lumpectomy and radiation.*

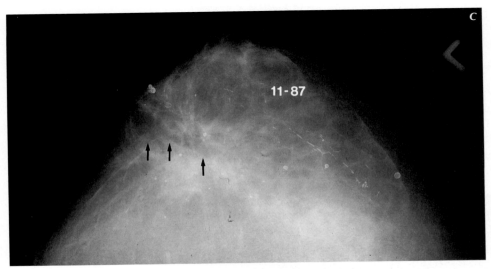

FIG. 9-27 *(Continued)* **C.** *A film 2 years later shows that several lipid cysts (arrows) have developed at the biopsy site.*

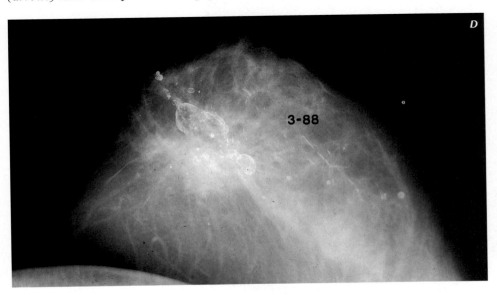

FIG. 9-27 *(Continued)* **D.** *A film 4 months later shows the characteristic appearance of calcification in lipid cysts.*

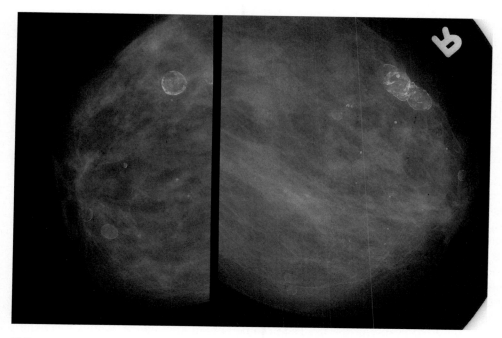

FIG. 9-28 *This patient has nodular panniculitis (Weber-Christian disease). The mammogram shows numerous areas of fat necrosis.*

which allows its benign nature to be easily recognized, to an appearance indistinguishable from carcinoma.[44] In this latter situation, the lesion can appear as a stellate mass, sometimes containing microcalcifications, with possible associated focal skin retraction and thickening. It is also clinically indistinguishable from carcinoma. The typical benign appearance is that of a rounded lesion containing central fat (lipid) surrounded by a fibrous pseudocapsule. The capsule may calcify in an "egg-shell" fashion (Fig. 9-29). The central lipid material may also calcify and can exhibit different appearances, ranging from dense macrocalcification

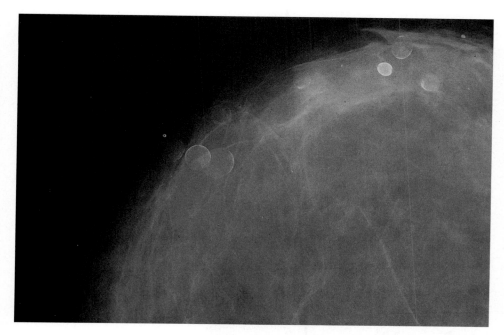

FIG. 9-29 *Notice the typical rim, or "egg-shell," calcium seen in this case of fat necrosis. The patient was asymptomatic, and the cause for the fat necrosis is unknown.*

(Fig. 9-30) to branching, angular, or rodlike microcalcifications similar to tumor calcium.

The radiologist faces a difficult decision when fat necrosis does not appear in its typical benign form. Excision is often required to exclude the presence of malignancy. Multiplicity and bilaterality may indicate follow-up rather than biopsy when areas of presumed fat necrosis are present. This is often the case with ductal ectasia. A prior breast biopsy or reduction mammoplasty as an explanation for fat necrosis may also allow the follow-up option (Fig. 9-31). In cases of bilaterality and multiplicity, the random selection of one focus to excise may be less reasonable than follow-up.

One difficult problem is the management of microcalcification developing at the site of a lipid cyst of fat necrosis in a patient who has undergone biopsy and irradiation for breast conservation therapy. The development of calcium may be either the first sign of treatment failure or the normal evolution of calcification seen in this setting. Our rule is that if the calcium develops within or at the margin of the lipid cyst, we follow it because this is what is expected to happen in areas of fat necrosis (Fig. 9-32). If, however, microcalcification is developing outside the area of previous fat necrosis, biopsy is usually performed.

SCLEROSING ADENOSIS

The term *sclerosing adenosis*, a form of fibrocystic change, appropriately describes the histologic features of this entity. It is a process that contains areas of lobular hyperplasia (adenosis) interspersed with bands of connective tissue fibrosis (sclerosis). Mammographically, this process may have a focal or diffuse presentation. When it is a focal process, it appears as a mass or a solitary cluster of microcalcifications with or without an associated mass density. The calcifications can vary greatly in appearance from round, regular punctate forms to very irregular pleomorphic shapes. In this focal presentation, differentiation from malignancy is usually impossible without biopsy (Fig. 9-33).

The second mode of presentation is the diffuse type, where both breasts contain numerous bilateral microcalcifications without a dominant cluster or associated mass (Fig. 9-34). Often, these breasts are quite dense and magnification views will help confirm the presence of the diffuse bilateral microcalcification. When the woman is asymptomatic, biopsy is hard to justify, since it would be random. If the biopsy proves the lesion to be benign, the woman would still require follow-up, since the presence of carcinoma is not ruled out for the remaining ipsilateral or contralateral breast calcifications. In addition, the biopsy would make follow-up mammography more difficult to interpret, since resulting postbiopsy changes such as architectural distortion or parenchymal scar could incorporate the residual microcalcifications, creating the appearance of carcinoma and leading to yet another biopsy. Still another reason for not biopsying diffuse bilateral microcalcifications is that the probability of the extensive bilateral process representing carcinoma is extremely

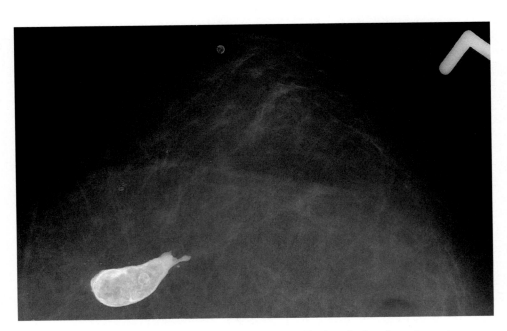

FIG. 9-30 *This woman underwent biopsy and irradiation for her breast carcinoma. Fat necrosis with dense macrocalcification has developed.*

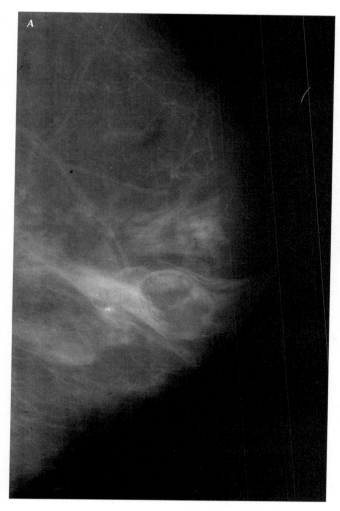

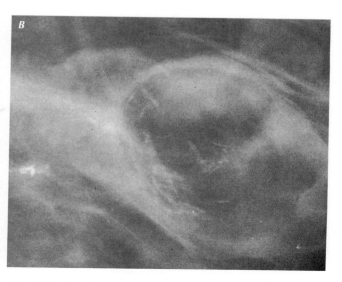

FIG. 9-31 (Continued) *B. Close-up shows a lipid cyst with central linear pleomorphic calcifications. The patient wanted it excised because it felt rock hard compared to her contralateral breast. Histology revealed fat necrosis.*

FIG. 9-31 *A. This patient had bilateral reduction mammoplasties 2 years earlier. She presented for evaluation of a palpable subareolar mass.*

low. What is the likelihood of an asymptomatic patient with normal breast palpation having both breasts universally involved with diffuse tumor? For this reason we put all patients with diffuse bilateral microcalcifications into our standard follow-up protocol beginning at 6 months and lasting for a minimum of $2\frac{1}{2}$ to 3 years.

I follow sclerosing adenosis not because of the fear that it represents carcinoma, but because of the possibility that hiding amidst the benign calcifications is a malignant cluster of microcalcifications that cannot be recognized on mammography because of the background noise from the diffuse calcifications. When

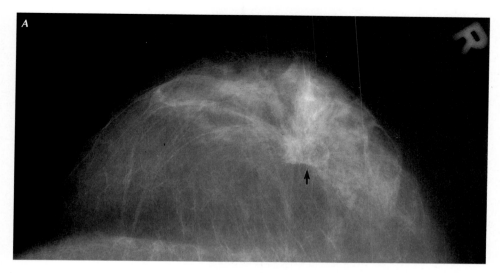

FIG. 9-32 *A. This patient undergoes annual mammography because she has had a previous carcinoma treated by lumpectomy and radiation. Her original tumor was completely excised with clear margins, and she has received appropriate radiation therapy to her tumor bed (arrow).*

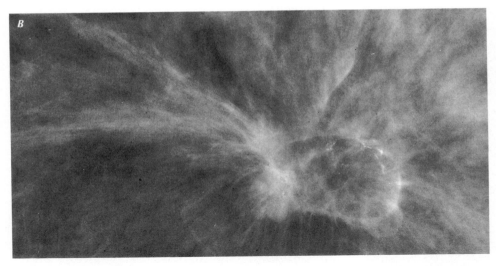

FIG. 9-32 (Continued) **B.** *Close-up view of tumor bed. All findings are consistent with postbiopsy scar and traumatic lipid cyst. Although the calcifications are linear and pleomorphic, they do not extend beyond the margins of the area of fat necrosis and biopsy was not recommended.*

sclerosing adenosis is evaluated on follow-up mammography, if any focal area changes, such as by developing an associated mass or more calcifications, a biopsy will be recommended.

Follow-up of diffuse bilateral sclerosing adenosis will either reveal stability or the progressive development of more bilateral microcalcifications. Biopsy is not performed in the latter situation because although

the mammographic pattern is indeed changing, it is doing so in a bilateral, uniform pattern, and this is normal for the progression of sclerosing adenosis. Biopsy is reserved only for a focal geographic change.

It is imperative to remember that the diffuse form of sclerosing adenosis is bilateral. If a woman has unilateral, extensive, diffuse microcalcifications, this cannot be assumed to be sclerosing adenosis. Since the

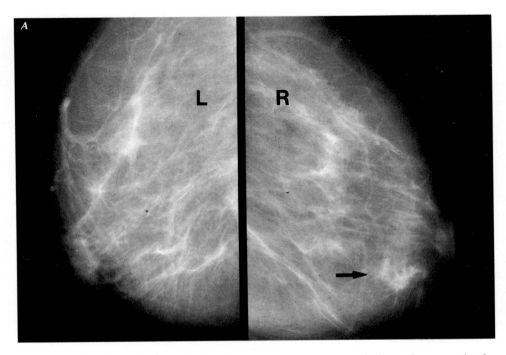

FIG. 9-33 **A.** *This 48-year-old patient presented with a palpable irregular mass in the right breast (arrow). Biopsy revealed sclerosing adenosis.*

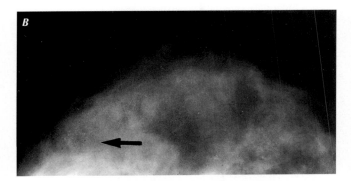

FIG. 9-33 *(Continued)* **B.** *A solitary geographic cluster of microcalcifications (arrow) was discovered on this routine screening mammogram.*

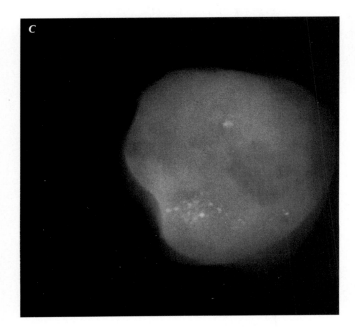

FIG. 9-33 *(Continued)* **C.** *Specimen radiograph confirmed excision of the microcalcifications. Histology revealed focal sclerosing adenosis.*

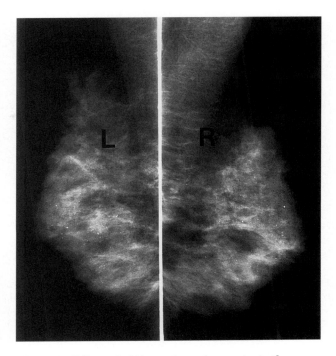

FIG. 9-34 *Bilateral oblique views demonstrate the presence of diffuse bilateral calcifications in dense breasts.*

TRAUMA TO THE BREAST

The most common cause for breast hemorrhage is usually trauma. In many ways breast trauma is analogous to trauma to the lung. Trauma to the lung can cause a hematoma or contusion. Just as when laceration of the lung interstitium with hemorrhage creates a pulmonary hematoma, laceration of breast stroma with hemorrhage is the mechanism for formation of a breast hematoma. The hematoma usually appears as a well-defined, ovoid mass with relatively sharp margins. It decreases in size with time and either totally resolves without any mammographic residual, resolves leaving a residual area of architectural distortion, or never completely resolves, leaving the patient with an organizing hematoma appearing as a mammographic mass density (Fig. 9-35). In the latter two cases, unless a clear relationship between the initial trauma and the mammographic findings of architectural distortion or mass is established, biopsy may be required to determine the histology.[45]

As in the lung, where pulmonary contusion assumes the appearance of an alveolar process which slowly resolves over time, so too does breast contusion appear as an increased density which resolves with time. The contusion initially appears as an asymmetric

contralateral breast is not involved, the pattern should be viewed as a solitary geographic abnormality (only half of the organ is involved), and biopsy is indicated even with a normal breast palpation. I have seen several cases such as these, and the histologic diagnosis is usually diffuse intraductal carcinoma, which explains why the breast palpation is often normal. Our protocol is to perform an incisional biopsy where the postoperative cosmesis should be the best, and specimen radiograph the biopsied tissue to be certain it contains calcium. If the process is benign, we assume the remaining calcifications in the breast are benign and place the woman into follow-up.

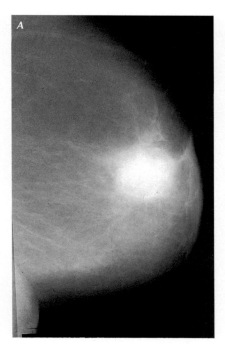

FIG. 9-35 A. *This is a postoperative breast hematoma.*

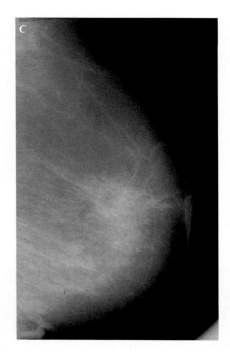

FIG. 9-35 *(Continued)* **C.** *Two years later only increased breast markings remain at the site of the hematoma.*

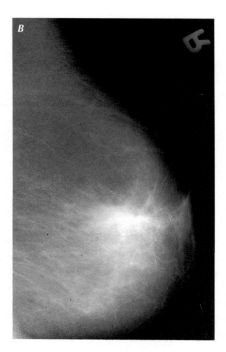

FIG. 9-35 *(Continued)* **B.** *One year later the hematoma shows some resolution.*

or increased density. Since it represents blood within the parenchyma, its margins are poorly defined. Skin thickening localized to the contusion may also be present. Although the mammographic presence of asymmetric breast density with associated skin thickening is an ominous finding suggestive of carcinoma, in the context of significant breast trauma, a repeat mammogram within 1 to 2 weeks rather than biopsy is recommended. If the mammographic findings show regression, follow-up until complete resolution is an appropriate management option (Fig. 9-36).

All of the above mammographic features are not necessarily related to trauma alone, but they can be seen in patients with a bleeding diathesis. However, without a history of significant trauma or a medical condition resulting in a bleeding diathesis, spontaneous breast hemorrhage is a worrisome finding, since it may be caused by an underlying occult carcinoma, and in this situation immediate workup should be considered.

PSEUDO-LESIONS

On occasion, normal developmental variants, or normal anatomic structures, may be confused with benign or malignant processes. Accessory breast tissue may occur anywhere along the mammary streak which extends from the axilla to the groin. Since this accessory tissue may manifest as an asymmetric density, it may raise the question of the presence of malignancy. Accessory breast tissue (Fig. 9-37) has been reported to occur in the axilla[46] and in the caudal aspect of the breast.[47] Since accessory breast tissue may harbor a benign or malignant lesion, it must be evaluated as carefully as all other areas of the breast.

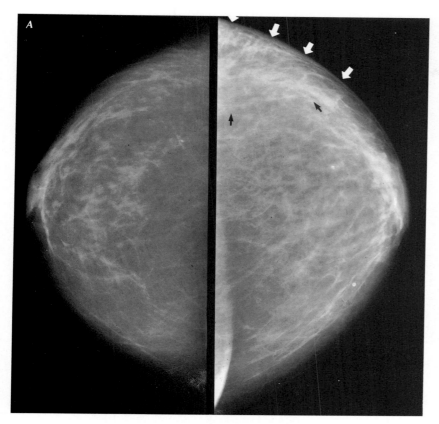

FIG. 9-36   A. *This patient was in an automobile accident and sustained a massive contusion involving the right side of the chest, including her breast. The mammogram was obtained during her recovery in the hospital because she had never had one before. Compared to the normal left breast, the right breast revealed increased density with associated skin thickening laterally (arrows). (A and B: From Homer MJ, Mammary Skin Thickening. Contemporary Diagnostic Radiology 4(15):1–5, 1981. Copyright © 1981 by Williams & Wilkins. With permission.)*

Normal muscles may occasionally be mistaken for a breast mass. On the craniocaudal view, the sternal insertion of the pectoral muscle may be misinterpreted as a medial mass.[48] This medial insertion can be seen when the technologist has vigorously pulled and compressed, with the breast in slight external rotation (Fig. 9-38). The demonstration of this structure bilaterally indicates its etiology. It is never seen on the oblique or true lateral view. If the radiologist suspects this as the cause of a medial density but is not certain, placing the patient into follow-up will document its stability. The sternalis muscle, which is a variant of the musculature of the chest wall, has been reported to be the cause of

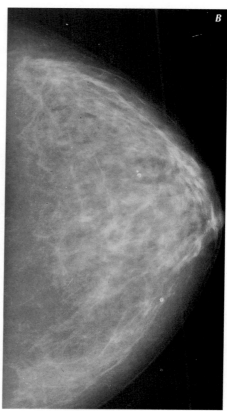

FIG. 9-36 (Continued)   B. *Repeat mammogram of the right breast 3 weeks later showed complete resolution of the process. This is characteristic of a breast contusion.*

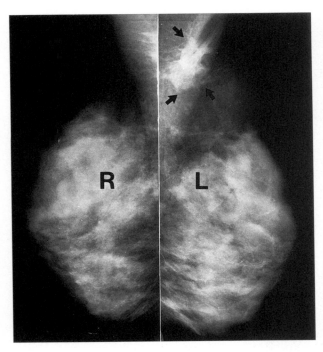

FIG. 9-37 *The asymmetric density in the left axilla (arrows) represents accessory breast tissue.*

a rounded or irregular density located medially on the craniocaudal view.[49] Prominence of the inferior portion of the pectoralis muscle may be mistaken for a mass on the oblique view.[50]

REFERENCES

1. Meyer JE, Frenna TH, Polger M, et al. Enlarging occult fibroadenomas. Radiology **183**:639–641, 1992.

2. Swisher FC, Gade NR, Suk JJ, et al. Enlarging fibroadenoma in a postmenopausal woman: Case report. Radiology **184**:425–426, 1992.

3. Moskowitz M, Gartside P, Wirman JA, et al. Proliferative disorders of the breast as risk factors for breast cancer in a self-selected screened population: pathologic marker. Radiology **134**:289–291, 1980.

4. Paulus DD. Benign diseases of the breast. Radiol Clin North Am **21**:26–29, 1983.

5. Pennes DR, Rebner M. Layering granular calcifications in macroscopic breast cysts. Breast **1**:109–112, 1988.

6. Homer MJ, Cooper AG, Pile-Spellman ER. Milk-of-calcium in breast microcysts: manifestation as a solitary focal process. AJR **150**:789–790, 1988.

7. Linden SS, Sickles EA. Sedimented calcium in benign breast cysts: the full spectrum of mammographic presentations. AJR **152**:967–971, 1989.

8. Brenner RJ, Bein ME, Sarti DA, et al. Spontaneous regression of internal benign cysts of the breast. Radiology **193**:365–368, 1994.

9. Hoeffken W, Lanyi M, *Mammography*. W. B. Saunders, Philadelphia, 1977, p 174.

10. Pennes DR, Homer MJ. Disappearing breast masses caused by compression during mammography. Radiology **165**:327–328, 1987.

11. Liberman L, Bonaccio E, Hamele-Bena D, et al. Benign and malignant phyllodes tumors: Mammographic and sonographic findings. Radiology **198**:121–124, 1996.

12. Egan RL, McSweeney MB. Intramammary lymph node. Cancer **55**:1838–1842, 1983.

13. Meyer JE, Ferraro FA, Frenna TH, et al. Mammographic appearance of normal intramammary lymph nodes in an atypical location. AJR **161**:779–780, 1993.

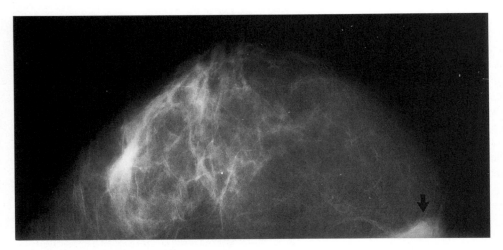

FIG. 9-38 *The density seen far medially on this CC view (arrow) represents the sternal insertion of the pectoral muscle.*

14. Meyer JE, Kopans DB, Lawrence WD. Normal intramammary lymph nodes presenting as occult breast masses. Breast 8:30–32, 1982.

15. Homer MJ, Pile-Spellman ER, Marchant DJ, et al. The normal intramammary lymph node: mammographic appearance and management. Applied Radiology 14:115–122, 1984.

16. Homer MJ. Imaging features and management of characteristically benign and probably benign breast lesions. Radiol Clin North Am 25:939–951, 1987.

17. Kopans DB, Meyer JE, Murphy GF. Benign lymph nodes associated with dermatitis presenting as breast masses. Radiology 137:15–19, 1980.

18. Lindfors KK, Kopans DB, McCarthy KA, et al. Breast cancer metastasis to intramammary lymph nodes. AJR 146:133–136, 1986.

19. Neuman ML, Homer MJ. The association of medullary carcinoma with reactive axillary adenopathy. AJR 167:185–186, 1996.

20. Homer MJ. Imaging features and management of characteristically benign and probably benign breast lesions. Radiol Clin North Am 25:940–941, 1987.

21. Hoeffken W, Lanyi M. *Mammography*. W. B. Saunders, Philadelphia, 1977, p 128.

22. Helvie MA, Adler DD, Rebner M, et al. Breast hamartomas. Variable mammographic appearance. Radiology 170:417–421, 1989.

23. Sickles EA, Vogelaar PW: Fluid level in a galactocele seen on a lateral projection mammogram with a horizontal beam. Dis Breast 7:22–23, 1981.

24. Gomez A, Mata JM, Donoso L, et al. Galactocele: three distinctive radiographic appearances. Radiology 158:43–44, 1986.

25. Cohen MI, Matthies HJ, Mintzer RA, et al. Indurative mastopathy: a cause of false-positive mammograms. Radiology 155:69–71, 1985.

26. Hermann G, Schwartz IS. Focal fibrosis disease of the breast: mammographic detection of an unappreciated condition. AJR 140:1245–1246, 1983.

27. Fenoglio C, Lattes R. Sclerosing papillary proliferation in the female breast: a benign lesion often mistaken for carcinoma. Cancer 33:691–700, 1974.

28. Linnell F, Ljungberg O, Andersson I. Breast carcinoma. Aspects of early stages, progression and related problems. Acta Pathol Microbiol Immunol Scand. (A) 272 (suppl):14–62, 1980.

29. Adler DD, Helvie MA, Oberman HA, et al. Radial sclerosing lesion of the breast: Mammographic features. Radiology 176:737–740, 1990.

30. Orel SG, Evers K, Yeh IT. Radial scar with microcalcifications: radiologic-pathologic correlation. Radiology 183:479–482, 1992.

31. Ciatto S, Morrone D, Catarzi S. Radial scars of the breast: review of 38 consecutive mammographic diagnoses. Radiology 187:757–760, 1993.

32. Woods ER, Helvie MA, Ikeda DM, et al. Solitary breast papilloma: comparison of mammographic, galactographic, and pathologic findings. AJR 159:487–491, 1992.

33. Cardenosa G, Eklund GW. Benign papillary neoplasms of the breast: mammographic findings. Radiology 181:751–755, 1991.

34. Hoeffken W, Lanyi M, *Mammography*. W. B. Saunders, Philadelphia, 1977, pp 120–127.

35. Jones MK. Galactography: procedure of choice for evaluation of nipple discharge. Sem Interventional Rad 9:112–119, 1992.

36. Love SM, Schnitt SJ, Connolly JC, et al. Benign breast disorders, in Harris JR, Hellman S, Henderson IC, Kinne DW (eds): *Breast Diseases*. Lippincott, Philadelphia, 1987, p 42.

37. D'Orsi CJ, Feldhaus L, Sonnenfeld M. Unusual lesions of the breast. Radiol Clin North Am 21:67–80, 1983.

38. Hoeffken W, Lanyi M, *Mammography*. W. B. Saunders, Philadelphia, 1977, pp 139–143.

39. Minagi H, Youker JE. Roentgen appearance of fat necrosis in the breast. Radiology 90:62–65, 1968.

40. Baber CE, Libshitz HI. Bilateral fat necrosis of the breast following reduction mammoplasties. AJR 128:508–509, 1977.

41. Bassett LW, Gold RH, Mirra JM. Nonneoplastic breast calcifications in lipid cysts. AJR 138:335–338, 1982.

42. Bernstein JR. Nonsuppurative nodular panniculitis. JAMA 238:1942–1943, 1977.

43. Paulus DD. Benign diseases of the breast. Radiol Clin North Am 21:38–40, 1983.

44. Bassett LW, Gold RH, Cove HC. Mammographic spectrum of traumatic fat necrosis: the fallibility of "pathognomonic" signs of cancer. AJR 130:119–122, 1978.

45. Frates MC, Homer MJ, Robert NJ, Smith TJ. Noniatrogenic breast trauma. Breast Dis 5:11–19, 1992.

46. Adler DD, Rebner M, Pennes DR. Accessory breast tissue in the axilla: mammographic appearance. Radiology 163:709–711, 1987.

47. Scanlon KA, Propeck PA. Accessory breast tissue in an unusual location. AJR 166:339–340, 1996.

48. Britton CA, Baratz AB, Harris KM. Carcinoma mimicked by the sternal insertion of the pectoral muscle. AJR 153:955–956, 1989.

49. Bradley FM, Hoover HC, Hulka CA, et al. The sternalis muscle: an unusual normal finding seen on mammography. AJR 166:33–36, 1996.

50. Meyer JE, Stomper PC, Lee RR. Pectoralis muscle simulating a breast mass. AJR 152:481–482, 1989.

CHAPTER 10

IMAGING THE AUGMENTED AND RECONSTRUCTED BREAST

Kathleen M. Harris

It is estimated that 1.5 to 2 million women in the United States have had augmentation to increase breast size or have had reconstruction following mastectomy. Widely publicized concerns about the safety of the silicone polymer and health issues related to implant failure have led physicians (and sometimes attorneys) to refer women for breast imaging evaluation. Patients with symptoms related to their breasts or with symptoms of autoimmune disease are referred for possible implant rupture.

This chapter will review definitions and terminology associated with augmentation and reconstruction, the various types of implants, and the imaging characteristics that distinguish normal implants from those that are damaged. The advantages and limitations of mammography, ultrasound (US), and magnetic resonance imaging (MR) will be addressed with regard to the woman who has had breast augmentation or reconstruction. Special problems with technique and interpretation will be discussed.

DEFINITIONS AND TERMINOLOGY

Implants can be placed for augmentation of breast size (usually bilateral) or for reconstruction following mastectomy (usually unilateral).

Position

Implants, either silicone or saline, can be placed in the prepectoral or retropectoral positions. When implants are placed in the prepectoral (retroglandular) position, the pectoral muscle lies posterior to the implant, and the glandular tissue is anterior and adjacent to the implant. With retropectoral implants (submuscular), the pectoral muscle is anterior and overlies the implant.

Fibrous Capsule

All implants, whether silicone or saline, will be surrounded by a fibrous capsule (Fig. 10-1*A*) which forms in an attempt to wall off the foreign material. On close mammographic inspection, the fibrous capsule can be seen as a thin, soft tissue line adjacent to the implant, measuring between 0.5 and 1.0 mm.[1] Typically, the fibrous capsule does not adhere to the implant, and the implant can "move around" to some extent within the pocket created by the surrounding capsule.

Elastomer Shell (Envelope)

The elastomer shell or envelope (Fig. 10-1*A*) of all silicone and saline implants is a semipermeable membrane of variable thickness and consists of long polymer chains of polydimethylsiloxane with methyl cross-linkages (silicone polymer) that create an elastic "solid" shell. The outer surface of the shell can be smooth (shiny) or rough (dull). The dull-surfaced envelopes may be textured (a permanent textured pattern imbedded within the shell) or may be "fuzzy" (a coating of polyurethane applied to the outer surface of the shell). The textured surface and polyurethane-coated implants were developed to increase the outer surface area and thus decrease the likelihood of for-

mation of the tight fibrous capsule associated with capsular contracture. Polyurethane-coated implants have been discontinued because of breakdown of the polyurethane into toluene diamine, a potentially carcinogenic substance. Mammographically, the elastomer shell is visible in saline implants but cannot be seen in silicone implants because of the radiodense gel.

Bulge

A bulge (Fig. 10-1*B*) consists of an outpouching of both the intact implant and the overlying intact fibrous capsule and does not represent implant failure.

Hernia

A hernia (Fig. 10-1*C*) consists of an outpouching of an intact implant through a tear in the fibrous capsule and does not represent implant failure. A hernia, however, may continue to enlarge and develop a rupture at its apex.

Intracapsular Leak

An intracapsular leak (Fig. 10-1*D*) occurs when silicone gel escapes through tears in the envelope, resulting in partial or complete collapse of the elastomer shell. The fibrous capsule remains intact, confining the silicone gel within.

INTACT IMPLANT

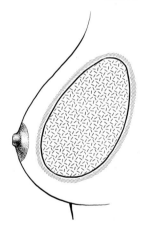

☐ Fibrous Capsule
— Silicone Envelope
▨ Silicone Gel

FIG. 10-1   A. Implants consist of a thin silicone envelope (elastomer shell) that contains the silicone gel in silicone implants or the saline in saline-filled implants. The fibrous capsule (see Fig. 10-3D) is often visualized as a thin band of soft tissue measuring 0.5 to 1.0 mm adjacent to the implant.

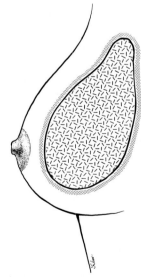

FIG. 10-1   (Continued) B. A bulge is an outpouching of the intact implant within an intact fibrous capsule (see Fig. 10-3A).

HERNIA

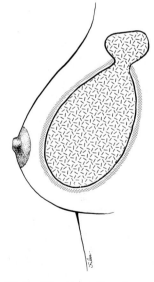

FIG. 10-1   (Continued) C. A hernia occurs when a portion of the intact implant protrudes through a tear in the fibrous capsule (see Fig. 10-3B).

Confined Leak

A confined leak (Fig. 10-1*E*) consists of free silicone gel that has escaped through tears in both the envelope and the fibrous capsule. The silicone remains confined to the area adjacent to the implant by a new fibrous capsule which prevents its migration.

Gross Leak

A gross leak (Fig. 10-1*F*) occurs when free silicone migrates into the breast tissue, axilla, or beyond. A gross leak can take the form of large confluent collections, small discrete globules, or a combination of both.

IMPLANT TYPES AND PERCUTANEOUS INJECTIONS

Various implant types have been developed, consisting most commonly of silicone or saline, or a combination of both. Implants are oval in configuration and are soft and pliable, with associated wrinkles, folds, and undulations (Fig. 10-2*A*). In the mediolateral oblique (MLO) view, the implant assumes an oval or "teardrop" configuration (largest diameter superior to inferior), and in the craniocaudal (CC) view, it appears more round. Less commonly seen are sponge implants, single lumen (silicone and saline) mixed implants, and direct silicone injections.

Saline Implants

Saline implants (Fig. 10-2*B*) consist of an outer silicone shell (envelope) that has been inflated with normal saline injected through a permanent valve. Saline is more radiolucent than silicone, allowing for visualization of wrinkles and folds of the silicone envelope. The valve and sometimes a ring used to surgically position the implant can be seen mammographically. Occasionally, with overpenetrated views, breast masses or breast calcifications can be imaged through the saline implant.

Silicone Implants

Silicone implants (Fig. 10-2*C*) consist of an outer silicone shell (envelope) filled with a semiviscous silicone

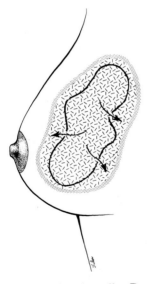

INTRACAPSULAR LEAK

FIG. 10-1 *(Continued)* **D.** *In an* intracapsular leak, *silicone gel escapes through tears in the envelope causing the envelope to collapse inwardly. The intact fibrous capsule, however, contains the intracapsular leak. A leak of this type cannot be seen with film-screen mammography but is detectable with US and MRI (see Figs. 10-7B, 10-7C, and 10-8A).*

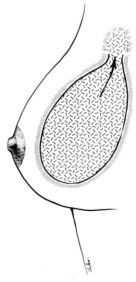

CONFINED LEAK

FIG. 10-1 *(Continued)* **E.** *A* confined leak *consists of a tear in both the implant envelope and the fibrous capsule. The free silicone becomes walled off by a fibrous reaction and remains confined to the area of the implant. A confined leak may be difficult to distinguish from a bulge or hernia unless ultrasound is employed (see Figs. 10-3C and 10-7E).*

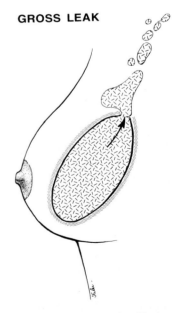

GROSS LEAK

FIG. 10-1 *(Continued)* **F.** *A gross* leak *occurs when free silicone extrudes into the breast, axilla, or beyond. Extruded silicone can appear as large confluent collections, small discrete globules, or a combination of both (see Figs. 10-3D and 10-3E).*

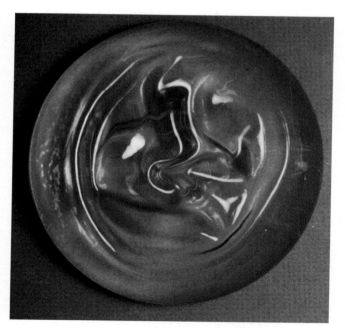

FIG. 10-2 *A. This photograph of a silicone-gel-filled implant shows the shiny, smooth surface of the silicone envelope. Wrinkles and folds are common in this soft, pliable implant.*

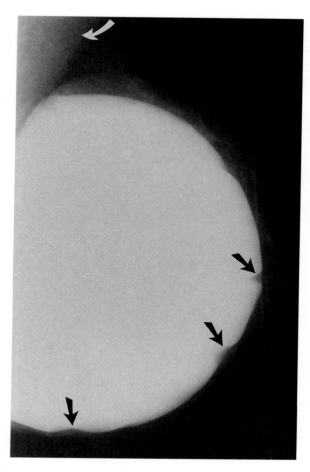

FIG. 10-2 *(Continued) C. Wrinkles (black arrows) can be seen in this prepectoral silicone implant on the overpenetrated MLO view. Note the pectoral muscle which is posterior to the implant (white arrow).*

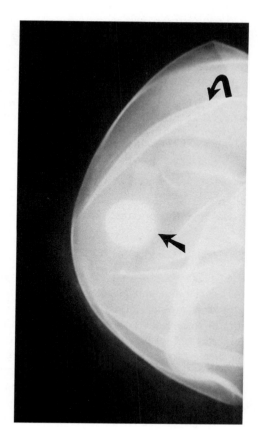

FIG. 10-2 *(Continued) B. The valve used to fill the saline implant can be seen on the overpenetrated CC view (straight arrow). Note the wrinkles (curved arrow) which are more easily visualized in the relatively less radiodense saline implant.*

gel (consisting of variously sized shorter polymer chains of polydimethylsiloxane) which is permanently sealed within the envelope. Because of the marked radiopacity of the silicone gel, wrinkles are less often seen and breast lesions adjacent to the implant can be obscured.

Double-Lumen Implants

Most commonly, double-lumen implants (Fig. 10-2D) consist of an outer saline implant that surrounds an inner silicone implant. This provides a second elastomer shell and is thought to decrease the likelihood of silicone gel extrusion into the breast tissue if the inner silicone implant fails. Often the outer saline bag will deflate with no known clinical or cosmetic consequences, since the saline is resorbed and the inner silicone implant persists.

Reverse double-lumen implants, consisting of an inner saline implant surrounded by a thick outer rim of silicone, are less commonly seen.

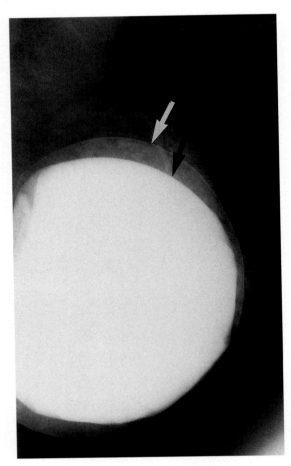

FIG. 10-2 *(Continued)* **D.** *The double-lumen implant is in the prepectoral position. The outer saline compartment is more radiolucent (white arrow) and surrounds the more radiopaque inner silicone implant (black arrow).*

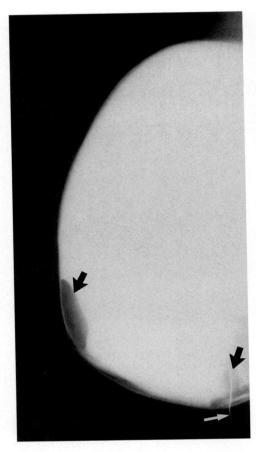

FIG. 10-2 *(Continued)* **E.** *A mixed implant is a single-lumen silicone implant into which saline has been injected at the time of surgery to adjust size. The saline (black arrows) is more radiolucent and is seen inferiorly in the upright MLO view. Silicone is an oil and floats superiorly, whereas saline gravitates inferiorly. A metal wire (white arrow) marks the cutaneous scar inferiorly at the surgical site of implant insertion.*

Mixed Implants

A mixed implant (Fig. 10-2E) consists of a single-lumen silicone implant into which saline has been inserted at surgery for adjustment of the implant size.

Sponge Implants (Figs. 10-2F, G)

In the 1950s, Ivalon sponge implants (constructed of a polyvinyl alcohol-formaldehyde polymer) and, in the early 1960s, Etheron sponge implants (a polyether) were the mainstay for augmentation mammoplasty.[2] The sponge material could be carved to the desired shape at surgery. Unfortunately, sponge implants became extremely hard and painful after a few years because the fibrous capsule thickened excessively (measuring 4 to 5 mm), which constricted the implant and diminished its size. The sponge material was found to cause sarcomas in animals and was discontinued. Surgical explantation of sponge implants requires re-moval of the entire fibrous capsule since the fibrous tissue grows into the openings of the porous sponge.

Other Implant Types

Over the past 30 years, hundreds of different types of implants have been manufactured. *Multicompart-mental* silicone implants consist of more than one silicone compartment. *Expander* type implants can be repeatedly injected with saline to gradually stretch the overlying tissues to create a pocket for placement of an implant following mastectomy. *Stacked* implants consist of two separate implants placed on top of each other to obtain a larger breast size.

Percutaneous Injections

In the 1950s, methods for breast augmentation included percutaneous injections of foreign substances such as

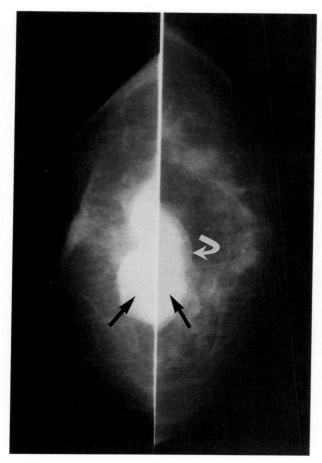

FIG. 10-2 *(Continued)* *F. Prepectoral sponge implants (straight arrows) are seen in these side-by-side right and left CC views. The sponges were placed 40 years earlier and have become hard and contracted. Note the thickened fibrous capsule (curved arrow) that surrounds and constricts the implant.*

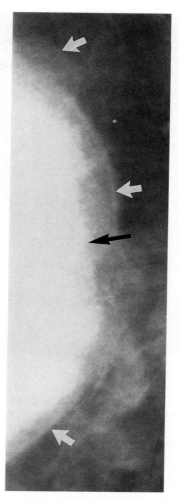

FIG. 10-2 *(Continued)* *G. The thickness of the fibrous capsule (white arrows) and its interdigitation with the opaque sponge material (black arrow) is better seen on this close-up view of the left sponge implant shown in 10-2F.*

paraffin or liquid silicone, or the injection or implantation of the patient's own adipose tissue. The disadvantage of using adipose tissue was its tendency to shrink and necrose due to lack of a blood supply.

Percutaneous injection of synthetic material (Figs. 10-2*H, I*) into the breast tissue has been associated with complications including hard, painful, granulomatous masses and migration of the foreign material into the axilla or elsewhere in the body. Evaluation of the breasts mammographically or by clinical examination for possible malignancy is extremely difficult once a woman has had silicone injections. Typical rim calcifications are seen mammographically surrounding the opaque silicone granulomas. Sonography is not useful, since the free silicone creates a "snowstorm" pattern that obliterates all detail of the underlying tissues. Direct injections of silicone have been prohibited in the United States but are still performed in some Asian countries.

MAMMOGRAPHIC IMAGING AND TECHNIQUES

Women with implants should not have a two-view phototimed "screening" mammogram, since manual exposure settings (kVp and MAS) and additional implant displacement (ID) views are required. In our practice, while the woman is in the breast center, the radiologist reviews the mammograms and obtains any additional special views or US as required for each individual case.

Normal implants (silicone or saline) are soft and pliable, smooth in contour, and oval in configuration. Wrinkles are more commonly seen in the relatively less

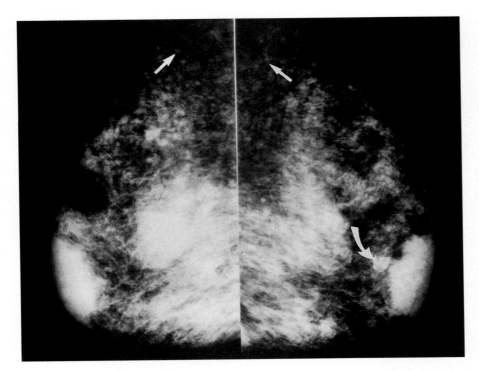

FIG. 10-2 *(Continued)* **H.** *The extensive large and small radiopacities seen throughout both breasts in these side-by-side right and left MLO views are silicone granulomas from prior percutaneous silicone injections into the breasts. Note silicone migration superiorly toward the axillary regions (straight arrows). Rim calcifications surround the silicone granulomas (curved arrow) (see Fig. 10-2I).*

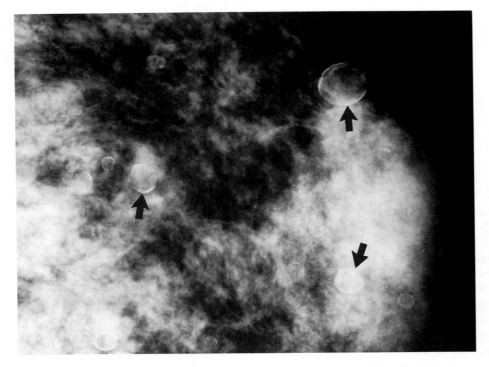

FIG. 10-2 *(Continued)* **I.** *This close-up of the same breast as Fig. 10-2H better demonstrates the rim calcifications (arrows) that surround the silicone granulomas.*

radiodense saline implants (see Fig. 10-2B) but can be seen in silicone implants with overpenetrated views (see Fig. 10-2C). Wrinkles or folds are seen in over 50 percent of implants (silicone and saline).[1,3]

Contour deformities of the implants are common. Implant *bulges* (outpouching of the intact implant with an intact overlying fibrous capsule) and *hernias* (outpouching of an intact implant through a tear in the fibrous capsule) are difficult to distinguish mammographically and sonographically. A hernia, however, may progressively enlarge and eventually rupture. Deformities associated with a bulge (Fig. 10-3A) or hernia (Fig. 10-3B) are not a sign of implant rupture. Overpenetrated mammographic views can help distinguish a bulge or hernia from a *confined leak* (Fig. 10-3C).

Mammographically, a *confined leak* is less radiodense compared to the adjacent implant. A line of demarcation may be visible between the free silicone and the implant. Confined leaks are walled off by a fibrous reaction and therefore often have smooth margins. With *gross leaks*, the greater radiopacity of extruded silicone, compared to most breast masses, can help to differentiate a silicone granulomatous mass from a breast parenchymal mass (Fig. 10-3D). Ring calcifica-

tions (see Fig. 10-2I) can form around the older silicone granulomas. Larger amounts of extruded silicone (Fig. 10-3E) are characteristically radiopaque and may appear as large, confluent collections as well as smaller, rounded globules.

Extruded silicone elicits a foreign-body granulomatous response. Fibroblasts encase the silicone, and giant cells attempt to break up and phagocytize it. The silicone granulomas will remain indefinitely encased in the fibrous tissue. Therefore, it is impossible to differentiate an old silicone leak from a new leak without a history and prior films. In the case of a new silicone implant surrounded by residual silicone from a previously ruptured implant, MR imaging can best evaluate the integrity of the new implant.

The presence of an implant poses special imaging problems including compaction of the breast tissue and obscuration of breast lesions by the radiopaque implant. Additional problems arise because one cannot use phototimed technique or compress over the implant. There is the possible risk of causing an implant rupture with compression.

To overcome the problems of visualizing the breast tissue, for implant patients *four views* are required of each breast. The standard craniocaudal (CC) and mediolateral oblique (MLO) views of each breast include the implant and breast tissue while minimal compression is applied (just enough to hold the breast in place and to prevent motion). Next, the implant displacement views (ID), described by Eklund and colleagues,[4] are performed in the CC and MLO projections, whereby the implant is displaced posteriorly and only the breast tissue anterior to the implant is optimally compressed. Because of the radiopacity of the implant, the phototimer cannot be used with the standard CC and MLO views. Use of the phototimer positioned under the radiopaque implant would result in a prolonged exposure with overpenetration of the breast parenchyma and excessive radiation to the patient. Therefore, the technologist first obtains a single film using a manual setting for the KV and MAS and checks the technique of the processed film before proceeding with the other standard CC and MLO views. Phototiming is useful for the ID views since the radiopaque implant is not included in the image.

For women with retropectoral implants or for those with a larger amount of breast tissue anterior to the implant, more breast tissue can be imaged with the ID views. Conversely, it may be impossible to perform implant displacement views with stiff, noncompliant implants associated with capsular contracture or whenever very little breast tissue overlies the implants. In these difficult cases, a 90-degree lateral (ML) view can image additional tissue that may be obscured on the MLO view. Despite the use of 4-view mammography of each breast, an average of 25 percent of the parenchyma can be obscured by the implant.[4] In the

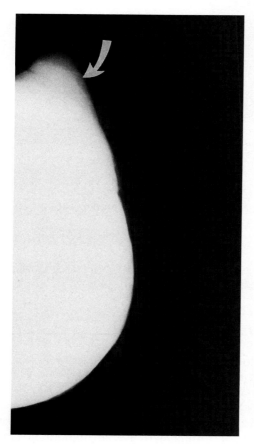

FIG. 10-3 *A. MLO view of a bulge (arrow) of a prepectoral silicone implant.*

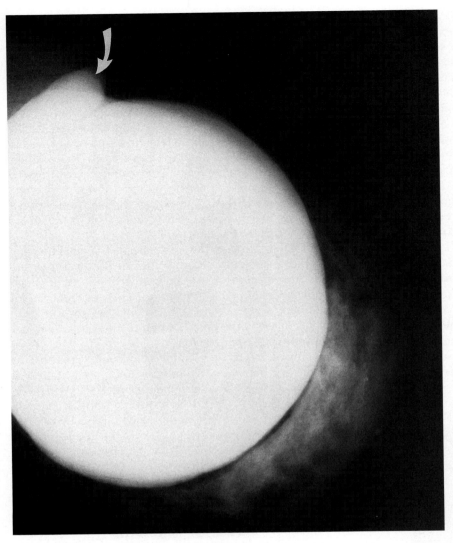

FIG. 10-3 *(Continued)* **B.** *A* hernia *is seen superiorly (arrow) on the MLO view of a prepectoral silicone implant.*

implant displacement views, breast tissue adjacent to the implant will be displaced along with the implant and will not be visualized. Therefore, a mass in the periprosthetic space adjacent to an implant may be excluded on the ID view and may be better evaluated with ultrasound.

The same indications for obtaining special mammographic views that would apply for women without implants apply for implant patients. Tangential views for palpable abnormalities, cone-down compression spot films (with implant displacement), and magnification views for microcalcifications can be performed with special care.

The posterior wall of the implant cannot be imaged with standard film-screen mammographic views. Xeroradiographs, special high-kVp film-screen chest wall technique (visualizing the ribs), CT scans, or MR can image the posterior implant wall. Ultrasound can image the posterior wall in smaller implants placed in smaller-sized breasts.

ULTRASOUND OF IMPLANTS AND SONOGRAPHIC TECHNIQUE

Ultrasound (US) is useful to evaluate breast masses detected mammographically or by clinical examination or whenever implant rupture is suspected.

Both silicone and saline implants appear anechoic and are not distinguishable by their US features unless a valve or tubing of a saline implant is detected. Sonographically, there is a thin echogenic interface between the breast and the implant in prepectoral im-

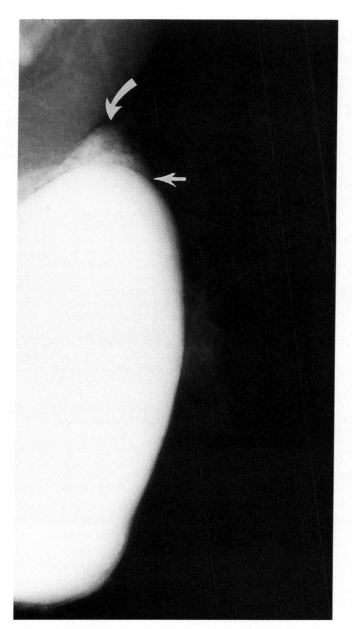

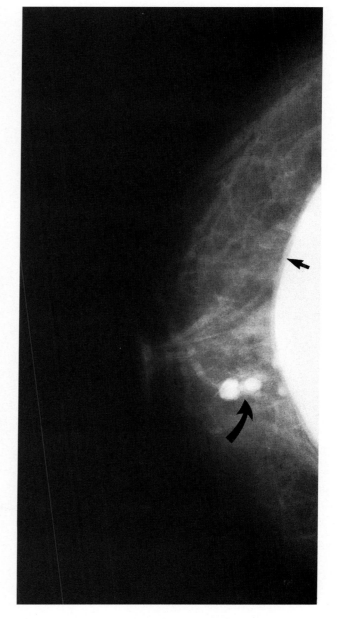

FIG. 10-3 *(Continued)* **C.** A confined leak *can mimic a bulge or hernia. Free silicone has been walled off by a fibrous reaction and appears slightly less radiodense (curved arrow) than the superior aspect of the adjacent prepectoral silicone implant on the MLO view. Note the line of demarcation between the confined leak and the adjacent implant (straight arrow).*

FIG. 10-3 *(Continued)* **D.** A gross leak *can consist of discrete silicone globules (curved arrow) within the breast. The silicone globules seen on the CC view are residual granulomas from a previous rupture that occurred 10 years earlier. The present silicone implant was intact. A normal-appearing, thin, fibrous capsule (straight arrow) measuring one mm in thickness, is seen adjacent to the silicone implant.*

plants (Figs. 10-4*A, B*) and between the pectoral muscle and the implant in retropectoral implants (Fig. 10-4*C*). Reverberation echoes (Figs. 10-4*B, C*), normally seen in the anterior aspect of silicone and saline implants, appear as horizontal echoes that run parallel to the anterior echogenic interface. Wrinkles can appear as an undulating surface (Fig. 10-4*D*). Radial folds (Fig. 10-4*E*) appear as echogenic bands that extend from the

implant surface into the implant but do not cross the entire implant. With US it may be difficult to distinguish radial folds from the complicated internal bands associated with intracapsular leaks.

Because the radiopaque implant can obscure lesions mammographically, palpable abnormalities and periprosthetic lesions can be evaluated by US, which allows visualization of all the breast tissue overlying

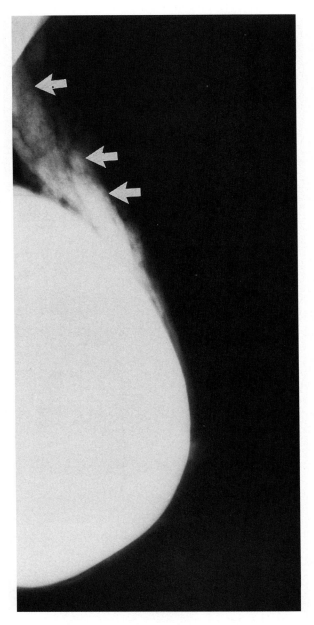

FIG. 10-3 *(Continued)* **E.** *Gross leakage can consist of a combination of larger confluent collections plus smaller globules (arrows). Free silicone extends toward the axilla superiorly on the MLO view.*

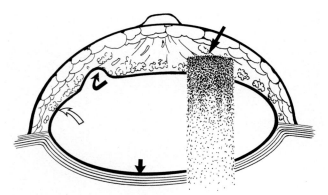

FIG. 10-4 **A.** *This line drawing illustrates pertinent sonographic features. An echogenic line (open arrow) demarcates the tissue/implant interface of silicone and saline implants. The posterior wall of all silicone implants is artifactually displaced posteriorly (short black arrow), due to the slower speed of sound in silicone than in breast tissue. Thus, the implant appears to be 1.5 times larger in its AP diameter than its true size, which may contribute to difficulty in imaging the posterior implant wall in larger-sized implants. A bulge or hernia (curved arrow) is contiguous with the implant and has an anechoic appearance similar to the rest of the implant (see Fig. 10-4D). Free silicone microglobules mixed within the tissues have a characteristic highly echogenic "snowstorm" appearance (long black arrow), with obliteration of all the underlying structures as the echogenic "noise" propagates posteriorly (see Figs. 10-7E, 10-7F, and 10-7G).*

the implant. US can distinguish palpable portions of the implant, such as wrinkles, bulges, valves, or silicone granulomas from breast lesions. Occasionally, US can image fluid in the periprosthetic space, which is an incidental finding unrelated to implant failure. Fluid collections are common surrounding polyurethane-coated implants.

The same 7.5- to 10-MHz transducers used in breast US can readily image all the overlying breast tissue as well as the implant. A limitation of US is its inability to visualize calcifications. Thus, US is useful for problem solving but cannot be used to screen for occult microcalcifications. The posterior wall of the implant may be difficult to visualize in larger-sized breasts with larger implants because of artifactual posterior displacement of the posterior wall (Fig. 10-4A) of the implant, due to the slower speed of sound in silicone.[5,6] Occasionally, a 5-MHz transducer can be used to visualize the posterior implant wall if a posterior rupture is suspected.

During US examination, the entire circumference of the implant, as well as the entire overlying breast tissue and the axilla, can be imaged. In women with capsular contracture, the breast may be stiff and noncompliant, making it difficult to maintain good contact of the transducer with the breast. The use of a standoff device (Kitecko, 3M) "softens" the interface between the transducer and breast and improves transducer "contact." By rotating the patient medially and laterally, the entire breast and implant can be imaged.

In our practice, the same radiologist who interprets the mammogram personally performs the US examination. Using real-time visualization, the radiologist can place a finger on a palpable abnormality, which can aid in distinguishing a true breast lesion from a palpable portion of the implant. A metal marker placed on the patient's skin over a breast lesion detected sonographically can facilitate mammographic visualization with additional special mammographic views.

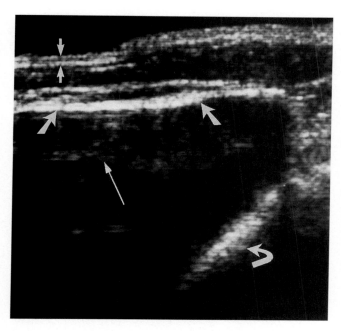

FIG. 10-4 *(Continued)* **B.** *Sonographically, the intact implant is anechoic compared to breast tissue. The echogenic interface (slanted arrows) can be seen between the breast and the underlying silicone implant in this prepectoral silicone implant. Reverberation echoes (long thin arrow) are normally seen in the anterior aspect of both silicone and saline implants. Note the skin (opposed short arrows), which appears as a double line when the standoff pad is used. Also note the small amount of overlying breast tissue. The lateral wall of the implant (curved arrow) can be seen, but the posterior wall was not imaged.*

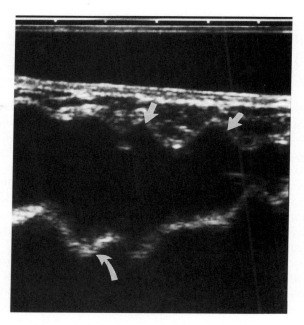

FIG. 10-4 *(Continued)* **D.** *Wrinkles, bulges (straight arrows), or hernias are anechoic and contiguous with the rest of the implant. Note the small amount of breast tissue between the skin and the implant in this prepectoral silicone implant. Wrinkles, bulges, or hernias may be palpable when close to the skin surface. The posterior wall of the implant (curved arrow) is imaged in this smaller-sized implant.*

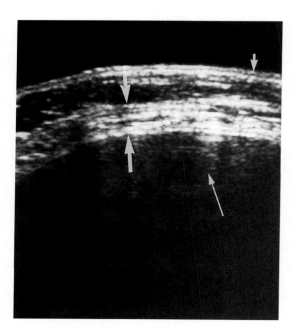

FIG. 10-4 *(Continued)* **C.** *The pectoral muscle (opposed arrows) overlies this silicone implant. Note the skin (short arrow) and the normal reverberation echoes (long thin arrow) in the anterior aspect of the implant. The posterior implant wall was not imaged.*

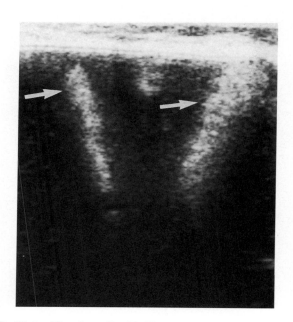

FIG. 10-4 *(Continued)* **E.** *The echogenic bands (straight arrows) represent radial folds within this silicone implant. Folds originate from the implant edge, extend inward, and do not cross the entire implant. Sonographically, it may be difficult in some cases to differentiate radial folds from the bizarre internal echoes associated with intracapsular leaks (see Fig. 10-7C). Note that the posterior implant wall is partially seen (curved arrows).*

CONCOMITANT BREAST PARENCHYMAL ABNORMALITIES

Although it has been shown that the presence of implants does not increase the likelihood of developing breast cancer, it may be more difficult to detect subtle signs of malignancy such as microcalcifications (Fig. 10-5A) or masses (Fig. 10-5B), due to suboptimal visualization of the breast tissue mammographically. Therefore, a meticulous search of the 4-view mammogram of each breast and follow-up of any abnormal physical finding are necessary. In patients with implants, benign and malignant breast lesions require a workup similar to one that would be performed for patients without implants, except that the implant itself poses special imaging problems. Additional evaluation may include spot compression views, magnification views, or US for masses suspected mammographically or by clinical examination (Fig. 10-5C).

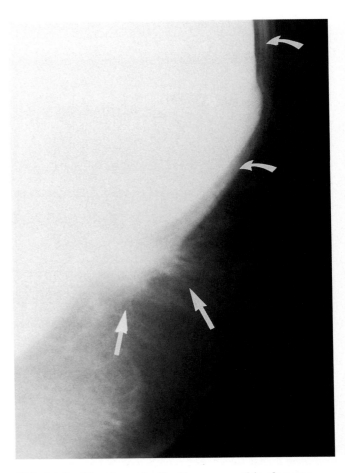

FIG. 10-5 (Continued) **B.** Mammographic close-up view reveals an area of architectural distortion with spiculated margins (straight arrows) adjacent to the silicone implant in this patient who had a subtle thickening on physical examination. The silicone implant had been placed in the retropectoral position following a left mastectomy 13 years earlier. Note the overlying pectoral muscle (curved arrows). This represented a recurrence of the carcinoma which had the identical histologic appearance as the original malignancy.

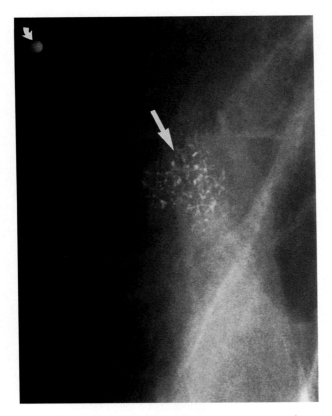

FIG. 10-5 **A.** Magnification ID view of a cluster of microcalcifications (arrow) was obtained with compression after the implant was displaced posteriorly. This represented a ductal carcinoma-in-situ that presented as a clinically palpable focal thickening. A metal marker (short arrow) had been placed on the skin over the palpable area. This patient was fearful that mammography might rupture her implant and allowed us to take only the ID view.

COMPLICATIONS RELATED TO THE FIBROUS CAPSULE

Capsular calcifications are an incidental finding detectable on overpenetrated mammographic views (Fig. 10-6A). These plaquelike calcifications may be focal or diffuse. Capsular calcifications are associated with older implants (silicone or saline) and are of no known clinical significance. Capsular calcifications are not a sign of implant failure, although there may be a coex-

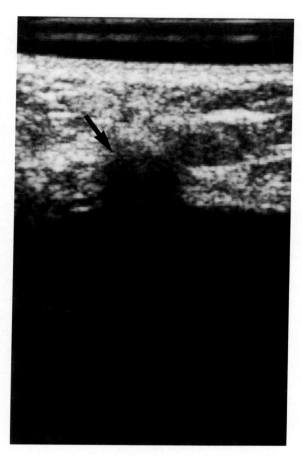

FIG. 10-5 (Continued) C. Ultrasound performed to evaluate the area of concern of the patient in Fig. 10-5B reveals an irregularly marginated hypoechoic mass (arrow) adjacent to the implant. At surgery, this was an infiltrating ductal carcinoma that was adherent to the implant.

istent rupture in an implant with a calcified capsule. Also, capsular calcifications are not a sign of capsular contracture.

Capsular contracture is the most common clinical entity resulting in patient dissatisfaction. Capsular contracture develops when the surrounding fibrous capsule constricts, resulting in rounding and increased firmness of the implant as it is squeezed into a smaller space. The diagnosis is made clinically, based on firmness, tenderness, and lack of compressibility of the breast. Occasionally a thickened fibrous capsule (1.5 mm or greater) and rounding of the implant can be seen mammographically (Fig. 10-6B). Most patients with clinical capsular contracture, however, have no mammographic signs. Sonographically, the anterior-to-posterior (A-P) diameter of the implant may be increased as the implant becomes more rounded, protuberant, and noncompliant. The etiology of capsular contracture is unknown, but it is speculated that it is related to a foreign-body reaction to microscopic gel bleed or to other inflammatory processes. Treatment

consists of closed or open capsulotomy or surgical capsulectomy. During closed capsulotomy, the breast is externally squeezed forcibly between the plastic surgeon's hands to break up the tight fibrous capsule. Complications from this procedure, including herniation and gross implant rupture, have resulted in its discontinuation.

COMPLICATIONS RELATED TO THE IMPLANT

Gel Bleed

The phenomenon of *microscopic gel bleed* occurs to some extent in all silicone gel implants and is not a sign of implant failure. The shorter polymer chains of the silicone gel can readily traverse spaces between

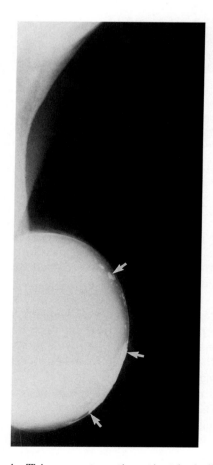

FIG. 10-6 A. This asymptomatic patient had silicone implants placed 20 years earlier. Extensive calcified plaques (arrows) are seen overlying the left implant on the overpenetrated MLO view. Capsular calcifications are seen with older implants (silicone or saline) and are unrelated to implant rupture.

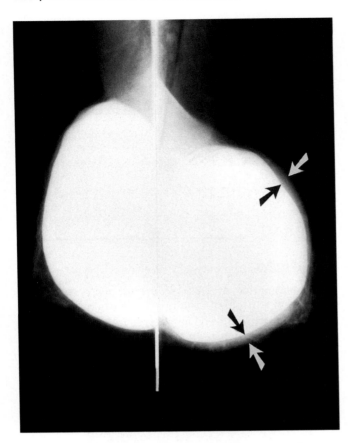

FIG. 10-6 (Continued) B. This patient presented clinically with a firm, tender, protuberant left breast. Side-by-side right and left MLO views reveal prepectoral silicone implants bilaterally. There is rounding of the left implant and thickening of the fibrous capsule (opposed white and black arrows) associated with capsular contracture. The normal oval-shaped right implant is shown for comparison.

the longer polymer chains of the intact elastomer shell (envelope). The fibrous capsule surrounding the implant confines the microscopic gel bleed in most cases. Occasionally, however, microscopic droplets of silicone can enter the lymphatic system and be deposited remotely. Asymptomatic silicone lymphadenopathy can be found serendipitously when one performs US of the axilla. This may be associated with microscopic gel bleed without implant failure. When microscopic gel bleed remains within the confines of the fibrous capsule, it is not recognizable by mammography, US, or MR imaging.

Occasional amounts of *excessive gel bleed* can be detected with MR imaging as a "noose" sign or "inverted teardrop" sign.[7] At surgical explantation, excessive gel bleed can appear as a thick, sticky material overlying the implant, without an obvious tear in the envelope. Some believe a small tear or "microhole" of the envelope always exists and can be found with a meticulous search of the explanted implant in cases of

excessive gel bleed.[8] Others debate whether "excessive gel bleed" represents implant failure. Excess gel bleed found serendipitously by MR imaging or a thick, sticky material overlying the implant at the time of surgical explantation is categorized as implant failure by some[9,10] but not by other[11] authors. Various terms have been published in the literature that refer to larger collections of silicone gel outside the envelope when there is no obvious tear in the envelope and without envelope collapse; these include "thick gel bleed," "gel leakage," "profound gel bleed," and "extensive gel bleed."

Saline Implant Collapse

Tears in the silicone envelope of a saline implant can result in rapid deflation of the implant over a period of hours or a few days. Fatigue fractures can occur with continued abrasion of wrinkles within the envelope or in areas of the valve or seams. The saline is resorbed with no complications except for diminished breast size. The collapsed saline envelope usually remains within the breast (Fig. 10-7A).

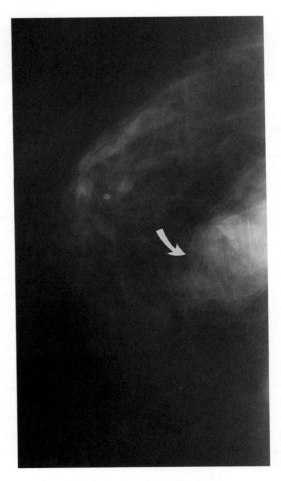

FIG. 10-7 A. Mammographically, this saline implant (arrow) has completely deflated. The collapsed silicone envelope, folded upon itself, is seen posteriorly in the prepectoral position on this overpenetrated CC view.

Intracapsular Leak of Silicone Implants

With an intracapsular leak, one or more tears occur in the silicone envelope, allowing the internal silicone gel to traverse the openings to the outer side of the envelope. Depending on the size of the envelope tear and the viscosity of the silicone gel, the envelope may or may not collapse inwardly. The intact surrounding fibrous capsule contains the intracapsular leak. Film screen mammography cannot image intracapsular leaks. Sonographically, the collapsed envelope has the appearance of short segments of double lines called "doublets" or the "stepladder" sign. MR imaging reveals the characteristic "linguine" sign of the collapsed envelope[12,13] which is analogous to the "stepladder sign"[14] or "doublets"[15] seen with ultrasound. The US signs of intracapsular leak include diffuse, homogeneous internal echoes throughout the implant[15–17] (Fig. 10-7B), linear or curvilinear horizontal lines[14,15,18] (Fig. 10-7B), and/or complicated, bizarre, echogenic patterns extending across the entire implant[17,18](Fig. 10-7C). The curvilinear collapsed envelope floating within the gel can be occasionally imaged with xeroradiographs or CT scans.

Caution must be used in diagnosing intracapsular leaks by US and MR imaging. There are reports in the literature of false positives (e.g., folds mistaken for a collapsed envelope) and false negatives (e.g., intracapsular leak without collapse of the envelope) with both modalities. MR imaging has been reported to be the most sensitive, however, in detecting intracapsular leaks, with US being the next most sensitive modality, and mammography being the least sensitive.[19] The sensitivity of US improves with the experience of the radiologist performing the scan. In our clinical practice, because of reports of false positives and false negatives with the sonographic signs of intracapsular leak, we recommend MR imaging for confirmation before suggesting surgical explantation whenever an intracapsular leak is suspected sonographically.

Intracapsular leaks may be more frequent than previously suspected. Many are found serendipitously during breast US or MR imaging or at surgical explantation. Many women with intracapsular leaks are asymptomatic, although some experience a change in the size, contour, or consistency of their implants.

Extracapsular Leak of Silicone Gel

An extracapsular leak occurs whenever silicone gel traverses tears in both the silicone envelope and the fibrous capsule. The free silicone may remain confined to the area adjacent to the implant, or it may extrude into the tissues of the breast, axilla, or beyond.

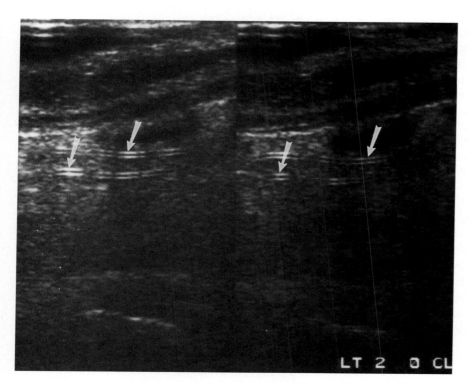

FIG. 10-7 *(Continued)* **B.** *Side-by-side transverse sonographic images of an intracapsular leak reveal the horizontal parallel lines of the collapsed envelope (arrows) called "doublets" or the "stepladder sign," as well as low-level internal echoes throughout the implant.*

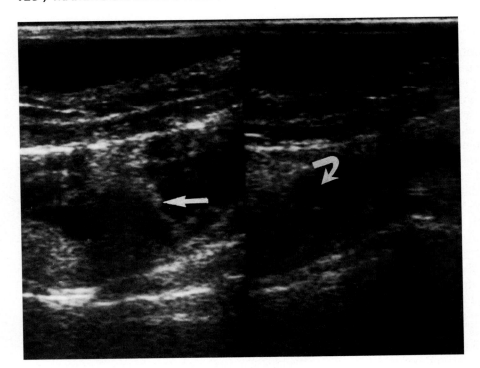

FIG. 10-7 *(Continued)* **C.** *Sonogram of this intracapsular leak shows bizarre internal echoes, including irregular hypoechoic areas (curved arrow) and bands (straight arrow) crossing the entire implant in the side-by-side transverse images. Note the increased echogenicity of the implant.*

A *confined leak* (Figs. 10-1*E* and 10-3*C*) occurs when the free silicone remains adjacent to the implant and is resealed by a new fibrous capsule. Mammographically, the smooth contour of a confined leak may be indistinguishable from a bulge or hernia. Sonographically, however, the free silicone of a confined leak has the characteristic highly echogenic "snowstorm" pattern which is easily distinguishable from a bulge or hernia, which are anechoic and contiguous with the implant.

Gross leaks (Figs. 10-1*F*, 10-3*D*, *E*, and 10-7*D*) occur when free silicone is deposited within the breast, axilla, or beyond (infraclavicular area, pectoral muscle, chest wall, upper extremity, or even the inguinal area). Mammographically, radiopaque silicone granulomas may mimic breast masses. The silicone, however, is usually more radiodense and may have a calcified rim. Sonographically, free silicone creates a characteristic highly echogenic "snowstorm" pattern, with loss of all detail posteriorly (Figs. 10-4*A* and 10-7*E*). This

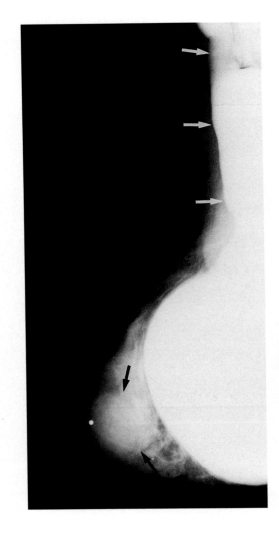

FIG. 10-7 *(Continued)* **D.** *This silicone implant has ruptured into the axilla (white arrows). A metal marker has been placed over a palpable mass (black arrows) which was a simple cyst at ultrasound.*

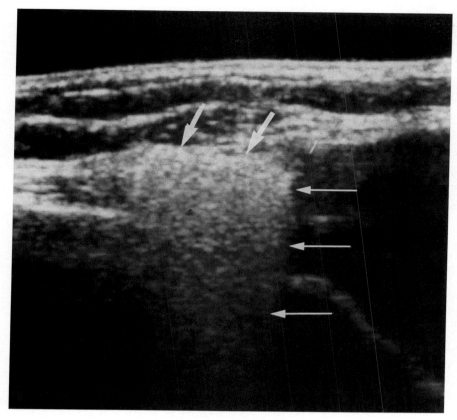

FIG. 10-7 *(Continued)* **E.** *Sonographically, the characteristic echogenic "snowstorm" of free silicone within the tissues overlies the implant edge in this confined leak. Note the well-defined anterior margin (thick arrows). Echogenic "noise" is propagated posteriorly and obliterates all the underlying structures (thin arrows). Note the artifactual "squaring off" of the edge of the implant, which is obscured by the overlying echogenic "noise" that is propagated posteriorly.*

echogenic pattern occurs when silicone microglobules mix with the tissues in a foreign-body granulomatous reaction. Occasionally, larger globules of free silicone will be associated with the smaller microglobules, giving a complex pattern of the echogenic "snowstorm" (microglobules of silicone) and hypoechoic "masses" (macroglobules of confluent silicone) (Fig. 10-7*F*). Rarely, a sonographically hypoechoic "mass" corresponding to a free silicone macroglobule is the only sign and is unassociated with the echogenic pattern. A metal marker placed on the skin over the hypoechoic mass seen at US can help to locate the area mammographically and confirm a corresponding radiopaque silicone granuloma within the breast. MR imaging using pulse sequences specific for silicone can confirm that a sonographically detected isolated hypoechoic "mass" represents a large globule of silicone (Fig. 10-8*D, E*).

Since the sonographically detected characteristic echogenic "snowstorm" is highly specific for free silicone microglobules (an oil) mixed within the tissues (water density), we do not recommend confirmation with MR imaging whenever an extracapsular leak is suspected. These patients are recommended for plastic surgical consultation, based on the characteristic sonographic appearance alone.

Implant-Related Lymphadenopathy

Silicone gel microglobules can enter the lymphatic system and be deposited within nodes of the axilla, infraclavicular area, or beyond. Small deposits of silicone within the nodes are most often asymptomatic, do not require surgery, and do not necessarily indicate the implant has ruptured. Occasionally, microscopic gel bleed can enter the lymphatics after traversing the intact silicone envelope and intact fibrous capsule.

US is sensitive in detecting very small amounts of free silicone within the axillary nodes. Sonographically, free silicone within the nodes has the same echogenic "snowstorm" pattern as does free silicone within the breast (Fig. 10-7*G*).

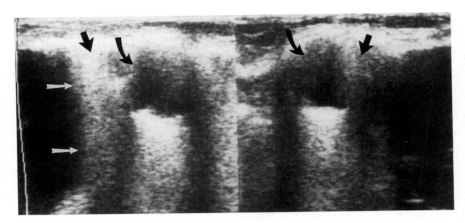

FIG. 10-7 *(Continued)* **F.** *Side-by-side sonographic transverse and sagittal views reveal a hypoechoic "mass" (curved black arrows) within the area of the echogenic "snowstorm" (straight black arrows) in this patient with a silicone implant rupture. The larger confluent collection of silicone that appears as a hypoechoic "mass" transmits sound like a "miniature implant." Smaller microglobules of silicone within the breast tissue appear as a highly echogenic "snowstorm" pattern. The lateral portion of the implant is obscured by the echogenic noise (white arrows).*

Mammographically, the axillary nodes that contain smaller amounts of silicone may not be radiopaque. Occasionally, radiopaque nodes containing larger amounts of silicone (Fig. 10-7H) accompany a ruptured silicone implant.

MR imaging is insensitive in detecting small amounts of silicone in axillary nodes. Larger amounts of silicone are required for MR imaging to detect signal differences between silicone within the tissues, due to partial volume averaging.

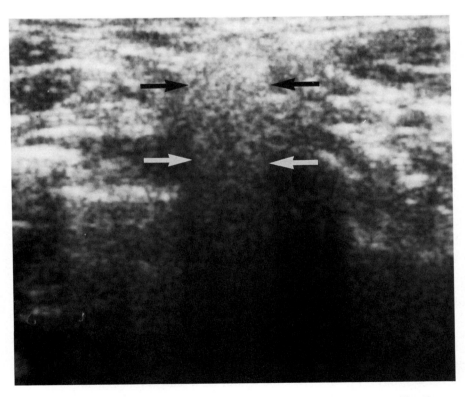

FIG. 10-7 *(Continued)* **G.** *During sonographic evaluation of the axilla, the echogenic "snowstorm" pattern of free silicone (opposing white and black arrows) was serendipitously detected in this asymptomatic patient.*

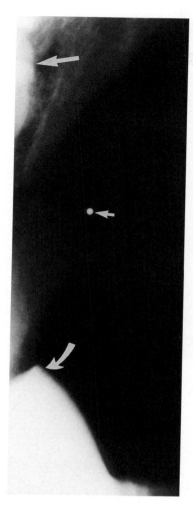

FIG. 10-7 *(Continued)* **H.** *In the same patient as Fig. 10-7G the radiodense axillary nodes containing silicone gel (long straight arrow) are seen in the special mammographic axillary view. At ultrasound the metal marker (short arrow) was placed on the skin over the echogenic area to ensure inclusion of the lymph nodes mammographically. This represented retained silicone within axillary nodes from an old rupture. The superior aspect of the new implant is seen (curved arrow).*

Polyurethane from polyurethane-coated implants can also enter the lymphatics and can present as bilateral axillary adenopathy, having an appearance similar to reactive lymph nodes. Polyurethane is not radiopaque, and the enlarged nodes are not opaque mammographically. In patients with polyurethane-coated silicone implants, the characteristic sonographic "snowstorm" pattern can occasionally be seen within the axillary nodes. In these cases the echogenicity is associated with silicone microglobules as well as with polyurethane shards in the lymph nodes. It has never been demonstrated that polyurethane shards alone cause the snowstorm.[20] Since these nodes are most of-

ten asymptomatic, surgical removal is rarely performed for confirmation or for investigation of the types of material within the nodes.

MAGNETIC RESONANCE IMAGING OF IMPLANTS

The MR pulse sequences are selected to maximize silicone visibility. In addition to using T2-weighted images, "silicone only" images can be obtained[7] using the relative resonance frequency of silicone compared to fat or water and adding chemical suppression techniques. Better detail is obtained by using a dedicated breast coil with the patient prone, imaging each implant separately. Multiplanar images are acquired with a 1.5 Tesla superconducting magnet.

MR imaging and CT have been shown to be more reliable in detecting intracapsular rupture than mammography or US in an animal model.[19] The most reliable sign of intracapsular leak by MR imaging is the "linguine sign" which represents the collapsed silicone envelope (curvilinear lines of low-signal intensity) (Fig. 10-8A) surrounded by the silicone gel which has escaped through tears in the envelope. The silicone gel remains confined by the fibrous capsule in an intracapsular leak. Radial folds within the implant (Fig. 10-8B) or periprosthetic fluid collections are not a sign of implant failure. It is unknown whether isolated water droplets within the implant are related to implant failure (Fig. 10-8B).

The exact anatomic location of free silicone within the breast or chest wall (Figs. 10-8C, D) can be assessed with MR imaging (Fig. 10-8E) using various planes and silicone-selective pulse sequences. When prior US indicates free silicone in sites remote from the breast, customized MR scans for the area of suspected silicone can be obtained. MR imaging can also evaluate the integrity of a new implant in the presence of residual silicone within the adjacent tissues from a previous rupture (Fig. 10-8F).

MR imaging is the only modality capable of detecting excessive gel bleed (silicone gel confined to the space between the fibrous capsule and the outer side of the envelope in the absence of a gross envelope tear or collapse of the envelope). Excessive gel bleed is recognized with MR imaging as the "noose" or "inverted teardrop" signs (Fig. 10-8G). This sign, however, is nonspecific and can also be seen with an intact envelope as well as with a small tear in the envelope without an envelope collapse.[7] Microscopic amounts of gel bleed, which occur in all silicone implants, are *not* a sign of

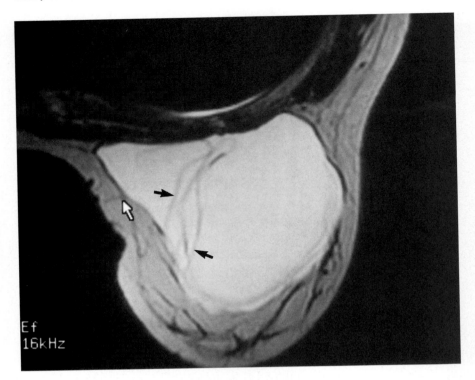

FIG. 10-8   A. *Fast-spin echo T2-weighted axial MR image of a silicone implant reveals curvilinear, thin, low signal intensity lines called the "linguine" sign (black arrows) which represent the collapsed envelope in this intracapsular leak. The low signal line surrounding the implant represents the fibrous capsule, which contains the intracapsular leak. The white arrow is incidental. (Courtesy of Peter Davis, MD.)*

implant failure and cannot be detected by MR imaging but can occasionally be detected with US as the echogenic "snowstorm" within asymptomatic axillary nodes.

EVALUATING THE BREAST AFTER EXPLANTATION

The implant can be removed along with the overlying fibrous capsule (capsulectomy) or through incisions in the fibrous capsule (capsulotomy). With total capsulectomy, the entire overlying fibrous capsule is removed along with the underlying implant. With partial capsulectomy, a portion of the fibrous capsule may be left within the breast. Capsulectomy is a more lengthy and tedious surgical procedure. If new implants are not inserted, a mammopexy procedure to reshape the breasts is usually performed. With capsulotomy, the old implant can be "slipped out" and the new implant inserted within the original fibrous capsule. If new im-

plants are not inserted, the collapsed fibrous capsules remain within the breast.

Mammography and US can evaluate the breast after explantation for residual hematomas or seromas, residual silicone, or residual fibrous capsules. With capsulotomy and explantation without implant replacement, the post-op mammogram can reveal the collapsed fibrous capsules posteriorly.

RECONSTRUCTION

Surgery to reconstruct a "new breast" can be performed immediately at the time of a mastectomy or can be delayed for months or years. In delayed reconstruction, the space for the new implant may be created using a saline-filled tissue expander implant that can be repeatedly injected with saline to achieve the desired size pocket to receive the new implant. Mastopexy or reduction mammoplasty of the contralateral breast is often performed at the time of surgery to achieve bilateral symmetry.

Silicone or saline implants are commonly used for reconstruction. Most often the implant is placed in

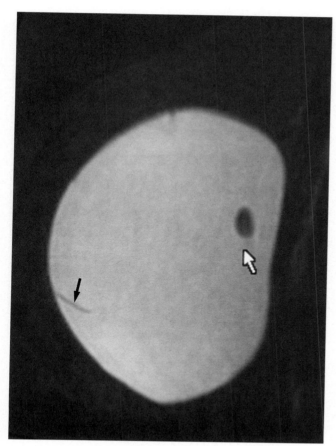

procedure are a more natural-appearing and -feeling breast, and the absence of complications associated with synthetic implants. The disadvantages are a more lengthy surgical procedure, a long postoperative recovery, possible abdominal wall herniation where the rectus muscle was removed (the fascia transversalis constitutes the anterior abdominal wall), and scars over the abdomen and chest.

Complications of fat necrosis can occur in areas of diminished blood supply. Although it is usually unnecessary to image the reconstructed breast,[21] patients with fat necrosis can present with a palpable mass in the reconstructed breast. Areas of fat necrosis have the same appearance mammographically (increased density, dystrophic calcifications, and oil cysts) and sonographically (focal echogenicity) in the reconstructed flap as in breast tissue following trauma. Early calcifications within fat necrosis associated with a pal-

FIG. 10-8 *(Continued)* **B.** *Sagittal MR image of an intact silicone implant reveals a water droplet (white arrow). The significance of water droplets within the implant is unknown. A radial fold (black arrow) extends from the surface but does not cross the entire implant. The radial fold is not, however, a sign of implant failure. This image was obtained with Fast STIR and water suppression to generate a "silicone only" image. (Courtesy of Peter Davis, MD.)*

the retropectoral (submuscular) position. The overlying muscle between the skin and the implant gives a more "natural" appearance and is thought to decrease the likelihood of formation of capsular contracture.

The surgical technique of *musculocutaneous flap transfer* utilizes *autogenous tissue* to move a patient's own tissue from the abdomen (rectus abdominis flap) or back (latissimus dorsi flap) to create a new breast. The more frequent method of autogenous tissue reconstruction is the transverse rectus abdominis musculocutaneous (TRAM) flap technique. An ellipse of lower abdominal fat and skin, along with one or both rectus abdominis muscles, and its intact blood supply are rotated and tunneled subcutaneously to the new breast site and sutured in place to create a breast mound. A nipple and areola can be created with tattooing and/or with skin grafts. The advantages of this

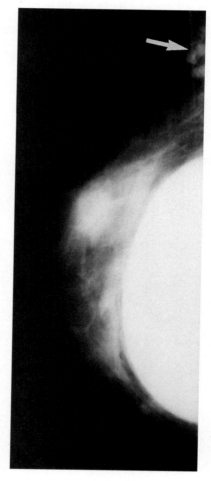

FIG. 10-8 *(Continued)* **C.** *Radiodense nodules (arrow) are seen superiorly on the MLO mammographic view. Silicone granulomas were suspected in this patient with a history of a prior silicone implant rupture and a new silicone implant.*

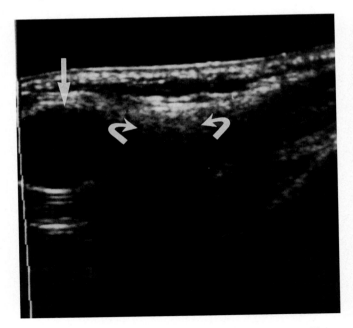

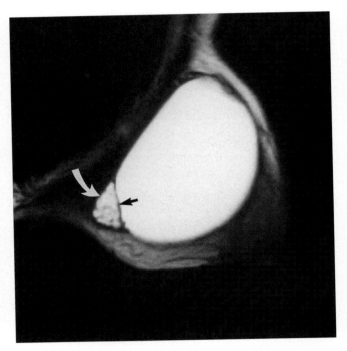

FIG. 10-8 *(Continued)* **D.** *In the same patient as Fig. 10-8C, US reveals a hypoechoic mass (straight arrow) in the vicinity of an ill-defined echogenic area (opposing curved arrows) with loss of detail posteriorly. The hypoechoic mass represented a larger silicone globule at the 12 o'clock position above the right breast.*

FIG. 10-8 *(Continued)* **F.** *Residual silicone (white arrow) from a prior rupture is identified adjacent to an intact silicone implant which was placed subsequent to the original leak. There was a question with US whether the new implant was intact. The MR image confirms the intact implant. A line of demarcation (black arrow) is noted between the intact silicone implant and the residual silicone from the prior rupture.*

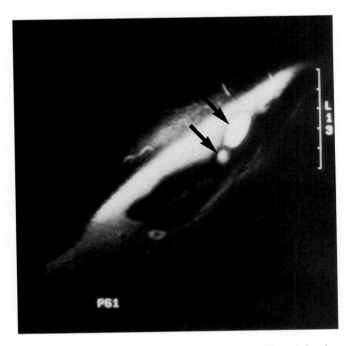

FIG. 10-8 *(Continued)* **E.** *Fast-spin echo T2-weighted axial MR image of the same patient in Figs. 10-8C and 10-8D confirms high-signal-intensity silicone globules (arrows) within the posterosuperior chest wall at the 12 o'clock position. The new implant was intact (not shown).*

pable mass must be differentiated from recurrence of carcinoma. Since the autogenous flap does not contain breast tissue, a recurrence would be situated posteriorly near the chest wall and not within the transplanted tissue. Fat necrosis, however, also occurs posteriorly where the implanted flap is sutured to the chest wall.

SUMMARY

Multiple imaging modalities may be required to fully evaluate patients who have had augmentation or reconstruction mammoplasty. There are advantages and limitations of each imaging modality for detecting implant complications and concomitant breast parenchymal disease. The appropriate intervals for surveillance for implant failure and the choice of the most effective imaging modality or combination of modalities will depend on the experience of the radiologist and the availability of the various imaging techniques. For women at the appropriate age for breast cancer screening, whenever implant failure is suspected, mammography supplemented with sonography is the most cost effec-

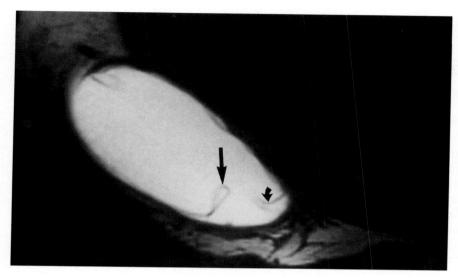

FIG. 10-8 *(Continued) **G.** The "inverted teardrop sign" (long arrow) and "noose sign" (short arrow) represent silicone gel that has entered radial folds. This can be a sign of excessive gel bleed without an implant tear or can result from a small tear without collapse of the envelope.*

tive initial evaluation, followed by MR imaging for equivocal findings of intracapsular leakage or suspected leakage posterior to the implant. The advantages and limitations (Tables 10-1, 10-2, and 10-3) of each modality as well as the reliable and unreliable signs of implant failure (Tables 10-4 and 10-5) are noted in this chapter. Continued assessment of the various imaging modalities will better establish the most accurate and cost-effective methods for detecting free silicone in the tissues and occult tears in the silicone envelope.

REFERENCES

1. Ganott MA, Harris KM, Ilkhanipour ZS, et al. Augmentation mammoplasty: normal and abnormal findings by mammography and ultrasound. RadioGraphics **12:**281–295, 1992.
2. Gerow FJ. Breast implants, in Georgiade NG (ed): *Reconstructive Breast Surgery.* The C.V. Mosby Co, St. Louis, 1976; pp. 31–49.
3. Shestak KC, Ganott MA, Harris KM, et al. Breast masses in the augmentation mammoplasty pa-

TABLE 10-1

ADVANTAGES AND LIMITATIONS OF MAMMOGRAPHY IN THE PATIENT WITH BREAST IMPLANTS

Advantages of mammography
- The single best method for detecting asymptomatic breast cancer
- With double-lumen implants (outer saline and inner silicone implants) mammography can better demonstrate the integrity of the outer saline component than can US.
- Most cost effective
- Reproducible; less operator dependent
- Can detect gross silicone implant leakage

Limitations of mammography
- Difficulty in differentiating a confined leak from a bulge or hernia
- Cannot image all the breast tissue, despite four views of each breast, because of radiopacity of the implant and compaction of the tissues
- Uses ionizing radiation and is therefore not indicated in young patients
- Cannot visualize the posterior wall of the implant
- Cannot compress over the implant
- Radiopaque implant can hide a breast mass or calcifications
- Periprosthetic lesions are displaced out of view on ID images

TABLE 10-2
ADVANTAGES AND LIMITATIONS OF ULTRASOUND IN THE PATIENT WITH BREAST IMPLANTS

Advantages of ultrasound
- Can image all the breast tissue, including the periprosthetic area
- Can image the axilla, infraclavicular area, and superficial areas of the anterior chest and anterior abdominal wall
- The echogenic "snowstorm" is highly specific for free silicone and can identify free silicone even in remote locations
- Very accurately predicts extracapsular leaks
- Can differentiate a confined leak from a bulge or hernia
- Uses no ionizing radiation
- More cost effective than MR imaging
- Can differentiate a cystic or solid breast mass from a silicone granulomatous mass secondary to implant rupture
- Can differentiate pathologic adenopathy associated with disease from silicone lymphadenopathy
- Can better define the extent of the leak into the surrounding tissues than can mammography or clinical examination
- Scan can be performed the same day as the mammogram

Limitations of ultrasound
- Can miss silicone leaks that occur posteriorly because of difficulty in visualizing the posterior implant wall, especially in larger implants within larger breasts
- Cannot be used to evaluate patients who have had percutaneous silicone injections
- In some cases, there may be difficulty in differentiating intracapsular leaks from nonspecific internal echoes produced by folds, wrinkles, proteinaceous material, and reverberation echoes
- Because of obliteration of all detail by the "snowstorm," anatomic detail is lost in the area of free silicone
- Very operator dependent; a learning curve is required to diagnose subtle signs of leakage
- Cannot identify microcalcifications as a sign of breast cancer

TABLE 10-3
ADVANTAGES AND LIMITATIONS OF MAGNETIC RESONANCE IMAGING IN THE PATIENT WITH BREAST IMPLANTS

Advantages of MRI
- More accurately identifies intracapsular leaks by the "linguine" sign
- Detects silicone leaks posterior to the implant, including free silicone in the pectoral muscle and/or chest wall
- Displays the exact anatomic location of free silicone and its relationship to muscle groups, vessels, or nerves
- Can confirm silicone in an isolated "mass" seen with US using silicone-selective pulse sequences
- Can evaluate the integrity of a new implant in the presence of residual silicone from an old rupture
- Can detect excessive gel bleed (free silicone between the implant envelope and the fibrous capsule) without collapse of the envelope
- Can image the outer saline and inner silicone compartments of a double-lumen implant
- Uses no ionizing radiation
- Reproducible

Limitations of MRI
- Cannot detect small amounts of silicone mixed within the tissues, due to partial volume averaging which "dilutes" the silicone-specific signal and also due to limitations in spatial resolution
- Areas outside the breast coil are not routinely imaged; prior knowledge of the location of free silicone in remote locations is needed to customize the MR examination
- Most costly of the three modalities
- Requires a separate appointment
- Is not available in every community
- Does not identify calcifications
- Not intended to identify solid breast masses, since the contrast agent gadolinium is not used

TABLE 10-4
RELIABLE SIGNS OF IMPLANT RUPTURE

Mammography
- Free silicone within the breast tissue or axilla

Ultrasound
- For extracapsular leaks, the "snowstorm" pattern is highly reliable. It may or may not be associated with hypoechoic "masses."
- Signs of intracapsular rupture include short, horizontal double lines ("doublets" or "stepladder" sign), diffuse low-level echoes throughout, bizarre patterns of complicated echoes, and echogenic bands that cross the entire implant.

MRI
- "Linguine" sign of a collapsed envelope
- Silicone outside the implant

TABLE 10-5
UNRELIABLE SIGNS OF IMPLANT RUPTURE

Mammography
- Contour deformities (wrinkles, bulges, or hernias)

Ultrasound
- Contour deformities
- Reverberation echoes
- Radial folds extending from the implant surface but not crossing the implant
- Periprosthetic fluid collections

MRI
- Contour deformities
- Radial folds
- Periprosthetic fluid collections

tient: the role of ultrasound. Plast Reconstr Surg **92:**209–216, 1993.

4. Eklund GA, Busby RC, Miller SH, et al. Improved imaging of the augmented breast. AJR **151:**469–473, 1988.

5. Harris KM, Ganott MA, Shestak K, et al. Silicone implant rupture: detection with US. Radiology **187:**761–768, 1993.

6. Rosculet KA, Ikeda DM, Forrest ME, et al. Ruptured gel-filled silicone breast implants: sonographic findings in 19 cases. AJR **159:**711–716, 1992.

7. Gorczyca DP. MR imaging of breast implants, in Davis PL (ed): *Breast Imaging.* Magnetic Resonance Imaging Clinics of North America; WB Saunders Co, Philadelphia, **2:**659–672, Nov 1994.

8. Middleton MS, McNamara M, Jr. Does silicone gel really bleed? (Abstr RSNA). Radiology **197** (Suppl)**:**370, 1995.

9. Berg WA, Caskey CI, Hamper UM, et al. Single and double-lumen silicone breast implant integrity: prospective evaluation of MR and US criteria. Radiology **197:**45–52, 1995.

10. Robinson OG Jr, Bradley EL, Wilson DS. Analysis of explanted silicone implants: a report of 300 patients. Ann Plast Surg **34:**1–6, 1995.

11. Reynolds HE, Buckwalter KA, Jackson VP, et al. Comparison of mammography, sonography, and magnetic resonance imaging in the detection of silicone gel breast implant rupture. Ann Plast Surg **33:**247–255, 1994.

12. Gorczyca DP, Sinha S, Ahn CY, et al. Silicone breast implants in vivo: MR imaging. Radiology **185:**407–410, 1992.

13. Gorczyca DP, DeBruhl ND, Mund DF, et al. Linguine: Does it represent the collapsed silicone implant shell? Radiology **191:**576–577, 1994.

14. DeBruhl ND, Gorczyca DP, Ahn CY, et al. Silicone breast implants: US evaluation. Radiology **189:**95–98, 1993.

15. Berg WA, Caskey CI, Hamper UM, et al. Diagnosing breast implant rupture with magnetic resonance imaging, ultrasound, and mammography. RadioGraphics **13:**1323–1336, 1993.

16. Caskey CI, Berg WA, Anderson ND, et al. Breast implant rupture: diagnosis with ultrasonography. Radiology **190:**819–823, 1994.

17. Levine RA, Collins TL. Definitive diagnosis of breast implant rupture by ultrasonography. Plast Reconstr Surg **87:**1126–1128, 1991.

18. vanWingerden JJ, vanStaden MM. Ultrasound mammography in prostheses related breast augmentation complications. Ann Plast Surg **22:**32–35, 1989.

19. Gorczyca DP, DeBruhl ND, Ahn CY, et al. Silicone breast implant ruptures in an animal model: Comparison of mammography, MR imaging, US, and CT. Radiology **190:**227–232, 1994.

20. McNamara MP, Jr. Personal communication. Mt. Sinai Medical Center, Cleveland, OH, 1996.

21. Mendelson EB. Evaluation of the postoperative breast, in Bassett LW (ed): *Breast Imaging: Current Status and Future Directions.* The Radiologic Clinics of North America; WB Saunders Co, Philadelphia, **30:**107–138, Jan 1992.

Chapter 11

THE ROLE OF MAMMOGRAPHY IN BREAST CONSERVATION THERAPY

As the size of breast cancer at the time of detection becomes smaller, more women find themselves having the option of choosing between breast conservation therapy (BCT) and more extensive surgery such as mastectomy. Mammography plays an important role in the initial evaluation of patients considering BCT as well as in their follow-up care. The radiologist must be able to recognize the early signs of recurrent cancer in patients electing breast conservation and differentiate them from expected postsurgical and postirradiation changes. He or she must also be able to detect new foci of tumor at sites distant from the original tumor.

EVALUATION OF THE PATIENT FOR BREAST CONSERVATION THERAPY

The primary reason for choosing BCT is based on the expectation that the cosmetic outcome of the treated breast will be acceptable. There is little reason to conserve the breast if, after therapy, there will be a poor cosmetic result. The cosmesis depends upon the size of the tumor, the location of the tumor, and the size of the breast.[1]

Sometimes patients with palpable breast carcinoma have undergone biopsy without ever having had a mammogram. If this is the case, mammography of both breasts should be performed as part of the initial evaluation.

Obtaining a baseline of the contralateral breast is necessary for future follow-up. Of equal importance is that patients may have simultaneous bilateral breast cancer (Fig. 11-1) and the aggressiveness of treatment may be modified if the other breast harbors an occult malignancy. An unsuspected contralateral metastasis may already be present at the time of initial presentation.

There are several purposes for obtaining an immediate baseline of the ipsilateral breast. If an unsuspected separate focus of tumor is present, then there may no longer be the option for BCT. Surgical excision of the second tumor focus may so distort the breast that its resultant appearance will be predictably poor and eliminate any consideration for conservation (Fig. 11-2).

If the woman opts for BCT and no further surgery is necessary because the initial excision contained all of the tumor with surrounding clear margins, the examination serves as a baseline for the future. The practice of obtaining a postsurgical preirradiation baseline in all patients undergoing BCT has been recommended.[2] The rationale is that without this examina-

138

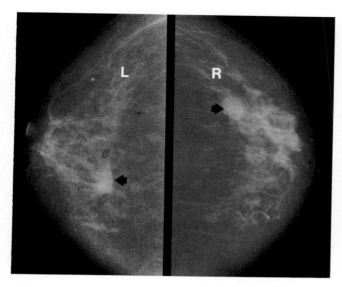

FIG. 11-1 *This patient presented with bilateral simultaneous breast cancer. The malignancy on the left side was palpable but the one on the right was not.*

FIG. 11-2 *(Continued)* **B.** *This patient also has widespread multicentric tumor and has no therapeutic option other than mastectomy.*

tion, the radiologist would face the task of having to compare a postsurgical postirradiation mammogram with a presurgical preirradiation exam, or having no prior mammogram at all for comparison. Despite the difficulty of obtaining adequate compression of the recently biopsied breast, and knowing that there will almost always be postsurgical edema and occasionally a hematoma or seroma, it may be easier to compare this baseline with a follow-up examination. As a general rule, no matter how abnormal the postbiopsy preirradiation baseline looks, within 6 months the lumpectomy site should look no worse, and in fact, most changes should begin to regress. The only changes that

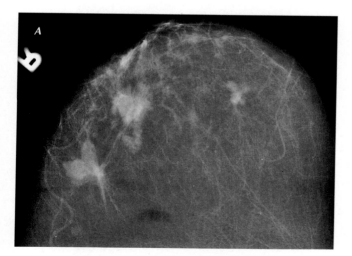

FIG. 11-2 **A.** *This patient presented with multicentric breast cancer and is not a candidate for breast conservation therapy.*

can be expected to appear at 6 months are generalized skin thickening, increased overall breast density, and calcifications, all of which may occur as a result of radiation therapy. It is not a policy at NEMCH to routinely obtain a postsurgical preirradiation mammogram on every patient.

The postsurgical preirradiation baseline mammogram is used by some to aid in the evaluation and management of the patient with possible incomplete tumor excision or inadequate documentation of tumor excision by histopathologic examination. When the postbiopsy mammogram shows evidence of residual tumor at the lumpectomy site either by demonstration of a mass or microcalcification, there is a high probability that residual gross macroscopic tumor is present. A mammogram showing no definite residual tumor implies that either there is no residual tumor or that only residual microscopic disease remains.[3] Unfortunately, a mammogram showing no definite residual tumor is not, by itself, enough to guarantee that there is no residual disease because of the markedly decreased sensitivity of the examination in the surgically disturbed breast. Even a specimen radiograph documenting complete removal of the mammographic abnormality cannot guarantee completeness of tumor removal. Microscopic tumor commonly extends beyond the mammographic abnormality.[4] At NEMCH, documentation of clear margins by histopathology is the only accepted criterion for assessment of the completeness of tumor excision. Mammography and breast palpation are inadequate for making this determination.

Even though all residual tumor should be removed, in certain circumstances the clinician may choose not

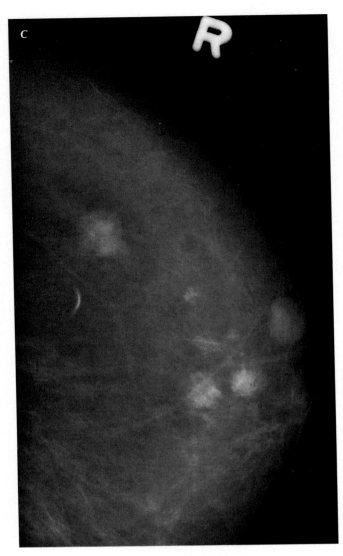

FIG. 11-2 (Continued) C. Every mass in this breast proved to be malignant. BCT is not a possibility with such widespread disease.

to perform a reexcision. In this case, mammography is far more accurate than breast palpation in assessing the extent of residual disease in order to guide radiation to the breast and can be used to map the boost field or iridium implant site.[5]

MAMMOGRAPHY OF THE POSTSURGICAL PREIRRADIATED BREAST

Assuming that all tumor has been removed, the findings on the postbiopsy mammogram are similar to the findings in any breast that has recently undergone

biopsy.[6] Since optimal compression is impossible to achieve because of the recent surgery, the overall density of the breast will often appear increased when compared to the contralateral side. The postoperative findings of localized skin changes including thickening, dimpling, or gross retraction are usually evident. There will almost always be localized increased density at the biopsy site which may be accompanied by postsurgical architectural distortion. On occasion, an actual mass representing hematoma or seroma may be present, obscuring the entire biopsy area (Fig. 11-3).

MAMMOGRAPHY OF THE POSTSURGICAL POSTIRRADIATED BREAST AT SIX MONTHS TO ONE YEAR

The postsurgical changes present on the baseline examination such as increased density and/or architectural distortion will be no worse on this examination and in most cases should be resolving (Fig.11-4). As discussed in Chap. 9, traumatic lipid cysts can develop at the biopsy site (Fig. 11-5). This form of fat necrosis typically has a characteristic evolutionary sequence of

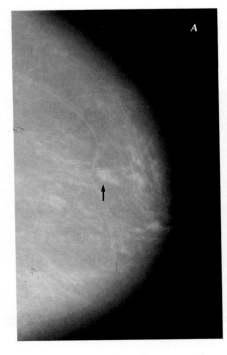

FIG. 11-3 A. A nonpalpable stellate mass (arrow) was detected on routine screening mammography.

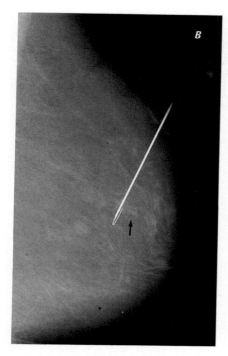

FIG. 11-3 (Continued)   B. It was successfully localized and excised. Histology revealed an 8-mm invasive ductal carcinoma.

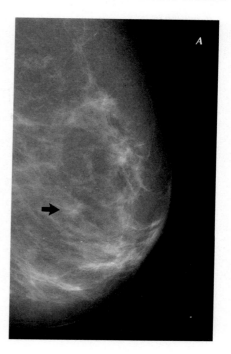

FIG. 11-4   A. A small palpable carcinoma (arrow) was seen on mammography.

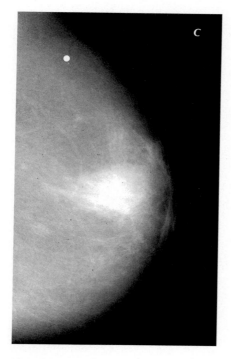

FIG. 11-3 (Continued)   C. This postsurgical preirradiation film demonstrated a hematoma obscuring the biopsy site as well as expected periareolar postsurgical skin thickening.

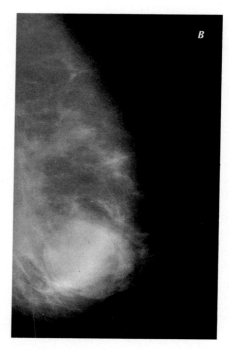

FIG. 11-4 (Continued)   B. A postsurgical preirradiation exam reveals a hematoma or seroma at the lumpectomy site.

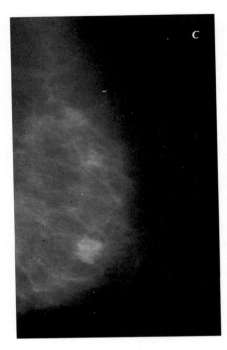

FIG. 11-4 *(Continued)* **C.** *A film taken 9 months later reveals regression of the mass at the lumpectomy site.*

findings. Initially, one or more lucent densities will appear at the biopsy site. This fat density is surrounded by a pseudocapsule. Over time, dense macrocalcifications, some with lucent centers and some with more linear shapes, will appear. Microcalcifications may also

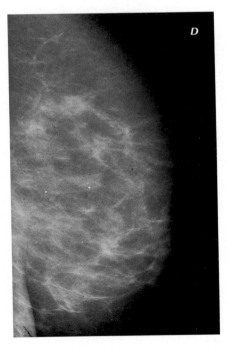

FIG. 11-4 *(Continued)* **D.** *A mammogram obtained 2 years after initial surgery reveals total resolution of all the postsurgical changes.*

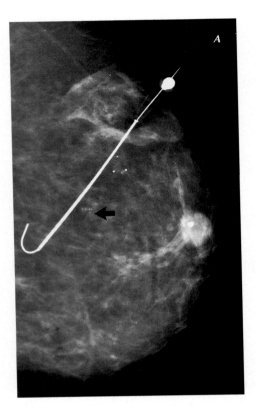

FIG. 11-5 **A.** *A nonpalpable cancer with microcalcifications (arrow) was successfully localized.*

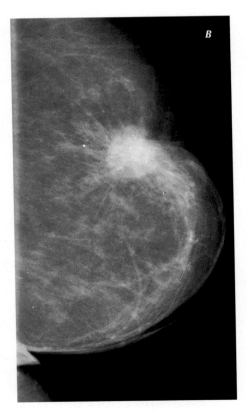

FIG. 11-5 *(Continued)* **B.** *The postsurgical preirradiation film shows a hematoma at the lumpectomy site.*

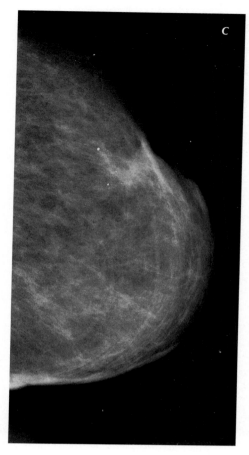

FIG. 11-5 *(Continued)* **C.** *Eight months later the hematoma is resolving.*

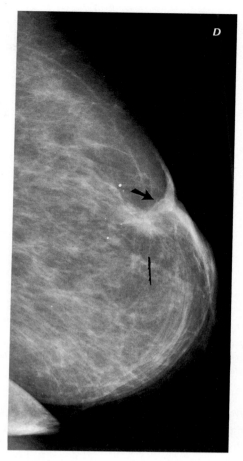

FIG. 11-5 *(Continued)* **D.** *One and one-half years after biopsy, there is further resolution of the hematoma. A traumatic lipid cyst (arrow) has developed at the biopsy site.*

become apparent within the lipid substance or at the margin of the lucent zone. However, they should not be misinterpreted to indicate recurrent tumor, since the early stage of the characteristic benign macrocalcification is the development of microcalcification. As long as the microcalcifications are confined to the area of fat necrosis and do not extend beyond it, we do not recommend biopsy of the area (Fig. 11-6).

Dermal calcifications may also develop at the biopsy site. These will often have the usual clues of dermal location such as polygonal shape, peripheral location, and lucent center. They can be proven to be within the dermis using superficial marker techniques which have been previously described (Fig. 11-7).

Three expected mammographic changes produced after breast irradiation are generalized skin thickening, increased markings throughout the breast, and the production of calcifications. The generalized skin thickening and increased density are the result of radiation dermatitis resulting from the presence of intracellular and extracellular edema.[7] These findings are always evident on the 6-month examination after the beginning of irradiation (Fig. 11-8).

The natural history of postirradiation generalized skin thickening and increased breast density is variable. They are usually maximal at the conclusion of irradiation. In most patients they will decrease over time, and in a majority of patients they will totally resolve. This return to normal may take as long as 4 years. In a minority of patients, postirradiation generalized skin thickening will not totally regress.[8]

The development of postirradiation calcification has been estimated to occur in approximately 25 to 40 percent of patients.[7] It may appear as soon as a few months after the start of irradiation or may be considerably delayed. These postirradiation calcifications assume several appearances, including coarse macrocalcifications with linear shapes, round phlebolith-like macrocalcifications, as well as calcifications of suture material (Fig. 11-9).[9] On occasion, postirradiation calcifications can have the appearance of irregular microcalcification indistinguishable from malignancy,[10] and biopsy to exclude recurrent tumor is usually unavoidable (Fig. 11-10).

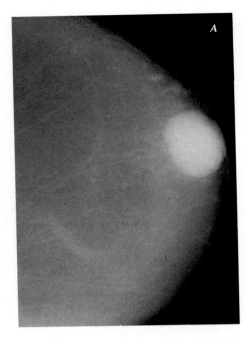

FIG. 11-6 A. *This large subareolar mass proved to be a medullary carcinoma. It was excised and the breast was irradiated.*

When known tumor calcifications are irradiated, they may remain stable, regress, or even totally disappear after radiation therapy. Stability of tumor calcium does not necessarily mean treatment failure, since the residual tumor may be totally sterilized.[11] When a

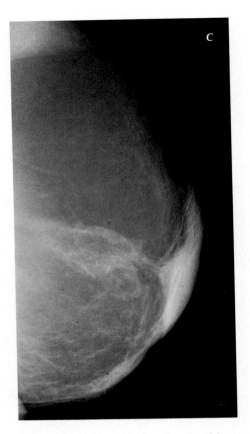

FIG. 11-6 *(Continued)* C. *Two years after biopsy, the lipid cyst has developed internal calcifications.*

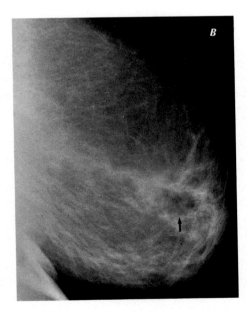

FIG. 11-6 *(Continued)* B. *Nine months after biopsy, the postirradiation change of generalized increased breast density is evident. A large traumatic lipid cyst (arrow) has developed at the biopsy site.*

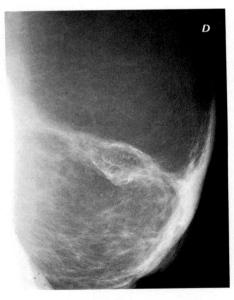

FIG. 11-6 *(Continued)* D. *Two and one-half years after biopsy, the calcification process has continued. Notice that no calcification has developed outside the volume of the lipid cyst. (Courtesy of the Dept. of Radiology, New Rochelle Hospital, New Rochelle, NY.)*

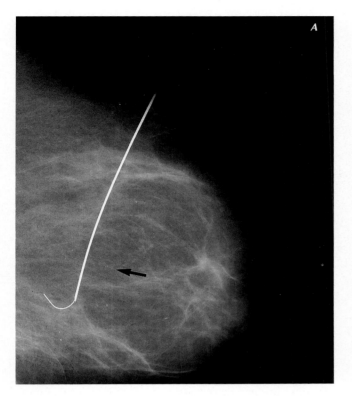

FIG. 11-7 A. *This patient underwent a successful needle localization for a geographic area of microcalcifications (arrow).*

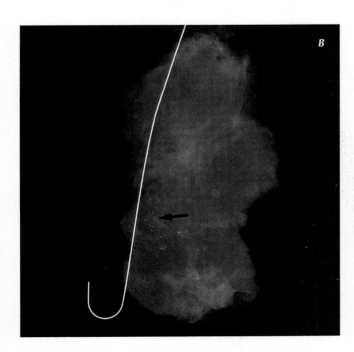

FIG. 11-7 *(Continued)* **B.** *Specimen radiograph confirms excision of the microcalcifications. They are benign.*

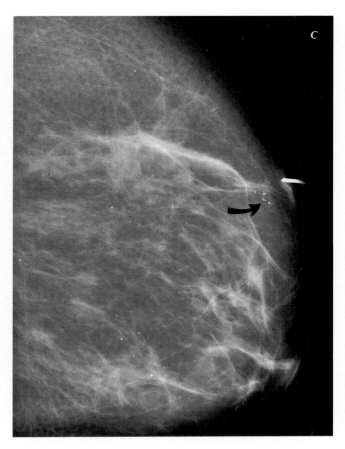

FIG. 11-7 *(Continued)* **C.** *Ten months later dermal calcium (arrow) has developed at the biopsy site. A metallic strip marks the biopsy scar. Notice that there are no obvious postsurgical changes deep in the breast at the site of the excised microcalcifications.*

known residual tumor mass is irradiated, it may not completely regress despite successful sterilization by radiation, but it should show some decrease in size within 6 months.[12]

FOLLOW-UP OF PATIENTS WITH BREAST CONSERVATION THERAPY

A woman who has already had breast cancer is at the highest risk for developing another breast cancer. It has been estimated that the probability of recurrent tumor at the biopsy site is 2 percent every year for the first 14 years after therapy.[13] The radiologist should always be on the alert to detect the development of recurrent tumor at the lumpectomy site or a new focus of tumor in either the ipsilateral breast distant from the

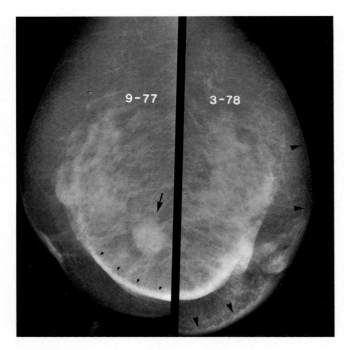

FIG. 11-8 *This patient presented with a palpable carcinoma (arrow) and clinically obvious skin thickening and retraction (small arrowheads). The tumor mass was excised and the patient received breast irradiation. Six months later expected postirradiation generalized skin thickening (large arrowheads) and general increased breast density are apparent.*

biopsy site (Fig. 11-11) or in the contralateral breast.

Metastatic disease to the breast may be impossible to differentiate from a second primary tumor by mammographic criteria, but some features favor the diagnosis of metastatic spread. Since most primary breast cancer occurs in the upper outer quadrant, one or more masses developing in the medial aspect of the contralateral breast or the presentation of contralateral lymphatic obstruction (generalized skin thickening and increased breast density) should suggest the possibility of crossover metastatic disease.

The mammographic features of a new cancer developing in the ipsilateral or contralateral breast do not differ from the usual signs of breast cancer. The radiologist must not automatically assume that changes on follow-up examinations are caused by prior surgery or radiation if they were not evident on the latest previous examination. At NEMCH, all future examinations of the patient with BCT consist of five views—the two standard views of each breast as well as a magnification view of the lumpectomy site. Some advocate that a magnification view of the lumpectomy site should only be done in selected cases.[14]

The optimal follow-up protocol for patients undergoing breast conservation therapy has yet to be established.[15,16] The usual follow-up protocol at NEMCH begins with mammography of the treated breast performed 6 months after completion of radiation therapy. This examination serves as the baseline for all future comparisons. As stated previously, the views obtained of the treated breast include an oblique view, a craniocaudal view, and a magnification view of the lumpectomy site. Ideally all future magnification views should be performed in the same projection to allow for easy comparison. Then bilateral mammography is performed 6 months later (1 year after completion of the

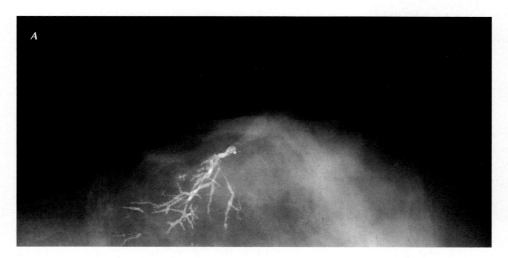

FIG. 11-9 A. *An entire ductal system has calcified after irradiation in this patient.*

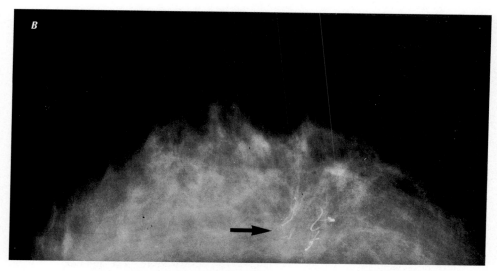

FIG. 11-9 (Continued) **B.** *Calcified suture material (arrow) is present in this postirradiated breast.*

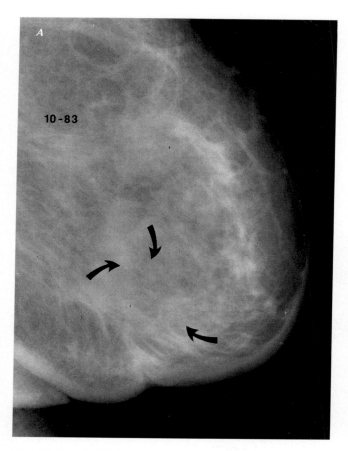

10-83

FIG. 11-10 **A.** *Eight months after excision and irradiation, subtle microcalcifications (arrows) developed at the biopsy site.*

radiation therapy). The patient is subsequently followed by annual mammography.

The follow-up for patients treated by mastectomy is annual mammography of the remaining contralateral breast. The views obtained are the standard oblique and craniocaudal projections. Ancillary views are added only when necessary to resolve a problem. Routine imaging of the mastectomy site[17] or the performance of special axillary views[18] have not proved to be useful in the detection of recurrent breast cancer and are not done at NEMCH.

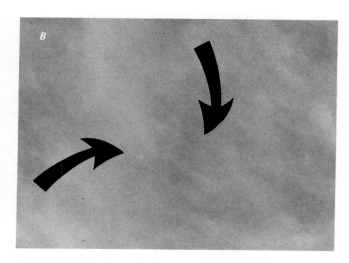

FIG. 11-10 (Continued) **B.** *Close-up view.*

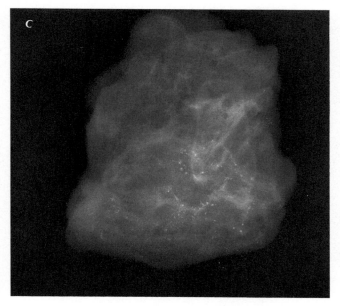

FIG. 11-10 *(Continued)* **C.** *Specimen radiograph confirmed excision of the microcalcifications. Histology revealed atypical lobular changes and microcalcifications most consistent with radiation change. No tumor was present.*

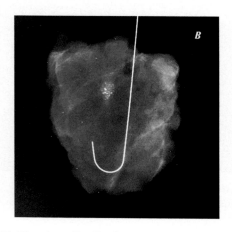

FIG. 11-11 *(Continued)* **B.** *Specimen radiography confirmed its excision. Histology revealed intraductal carcinoma. The margins were clear, and the patient received no further treatment.*

REFERENCES

1. Dershaw DD. Mammography in patients with breast cancer treated by breast conservation (lumpectomy with or without radiation). AJR **164**:309–316, 1995.

2. Mendelson EB. Imaging the post-surgical breast. Semin US, CT, MR **10**:154–170, 1989.

3. Homer MJ, Schmidt-Ullrich R, Safaii H, et al. Residual breast carcinoma after biopsy: role of mammography in evaluation. Radiology **170**:75–77, 1989.

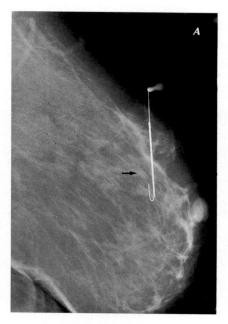

FIG. 11-11 **A.** *A geographic cluster of microcalcifications (arrow) was needle localized in this 52-year-old asymptomatic woman.*

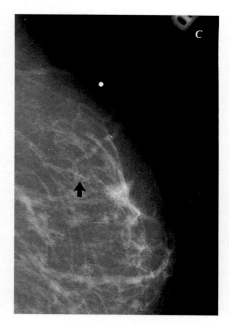

FIG. 11-11 *(Continued)* **C.** *One year later on the annual follow-up mammogram, new microcalcifications (arrow) appeared near the previous biopsy site.*

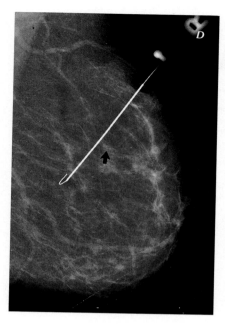

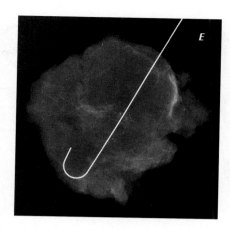

FIG. 11-11 *(Continued)* **E.** *Specimen radiograph confirms their excision. Histology revealed intraductal and invasive ductal carcinoma. The patient underwent a modified radical mastectomy.*

FIG. 11-11 *(Continued)* **D.** *The calcifications were needle localized prior to excision because they were nonpalpable.*

4. Graham RA, Homer MJ, Sigler CJ, et al. The efficacy of specimen radiography in evaluatig the surgical margins of impalpable breast carcinoma. AJR **162**:33–36, 1994.

5. Paulus DD. Conservative treatment of breast cancer: mammography in patient selection and follow-up. AJR **143**:483–487, 1984.

6. Mendelson EB. Evaluation of the postoperative breast. Radiol Clin North Am **30**:107–138, 1992.

7. Dershaw DD, Shank B, Reisinger S. Mammographic findings after breast cancer treatment with local excision and definitive irradiation. Radiology **164**:455–461, 1987.

8. Libshitz HI, Montague ED, Paulus DD. Skin thickness in the therapeutically irradiated breast. AJR **130**:345–347, 1978.

9. Stacey-Clear A, McCarthy KA, Hall DA, et al. Calcified suture material in the breast after radiation therapy. Radiology **183**:207–208, 1992.

10. Rebner M, Pennes DR, Adler DD, et al. Breast microcalcifications after lumpectomy and radiation therapy. Radiology **170**:691–693, 1989.

11. Libshitz HI, Montague ED, Paulus DD. Calcifications and the therapeutically irradiated breast. AJR **128**:1021–1025, 1977.

12. Paulus DD, Libshitz HI, Montague ED. Malignant masses in the therapeutically irradiated breast. AJR **135**:789–795, 1980.

13. Stomper PC, Recht A, Berenberg AL, et al. Mammographic detection of recurrent cancer in the irradiated breast. AJR **148**:39–43, 1987.

14. DiPiro PJ, Meyer JE, Shaffer K. Usefulness of the routine magnification view after breast conservation therapy for carcinoma. Radiology **198**:341–343, 1996.

15. Hassell PR, Olivotto IA, Mueller HA, et al. Early breast cancer: detection of recurrence after conservative surgery and radiation therapy. Radiology **176**:731–735, 1990.

16. Orel SG, Fowble BL, Solin LJ, et al. Breast cancer recurrence after lumpectomy and radiation therapy for early-stage disease: Prognostic significance of detection method. Radiology **188**:189–194, 1993.

17. Fajardo LL, Roberts CC, Hunt KR. Mammographic surveillance of breast cancer patients: Should the mastectomy site be imaged? AJR **161**:953–955, 1993.

18. Propeck PA, Scanlan KA. Utility of axillary views in postmastectomy patients. Radiology **187**:769–771, 1993.

Chapter 12

MAMMOGRAPHY OF MALE BREAST DISEASE

The two primary conditions that affect the male breast are cancer and gynecomastia. Eccentric masses in the male breast almost invariably require excisional biopsy for diagnosis. Gynecomastia can usually be diagnosed clinically. Therefore, male patient management rarely depends on mammography and that is why at NEMCH this examination is infrequently performed.

CANCER

Male breast cancer is much less common than female breast cancer. This malignancy represents less than 1 percent of all cancers in men. Its peak incidence is between the ages of 60 and 70. Clinically it presents as an eccentric, painless, hard mass and its mammographic features are identical to those in the female breast.[1,2]

GYNECOMASTIA

Gynecomastia is a hyperplasia of ducts and connective tissue.[3] Since the only place ductal tissue exists in the male breast is beneath the nipple, by definition, gynecomastia must be subareolar. It may be painless or painful, unilateral or bilateral. It is commonly seen in the young man after puberty, but it also has a second peak incidence after the age of 50.

The most common etiology of gynecomastia is idiopathic. Numerous drugs have been identified which can cause gynecomastia and these include phenoth-

iazines, thiazides, reserpine, cimetidine, estrogen, digitalis, isoniazide, amphetamines, marijuana, vincristine, and busulfan. Gynecomastia may be caused by systemic conditions such as cirrhosis and chronic renal failure. Other causes include neoplasms and hormonal imbalance.

The mammographic appearance of gynecomastia is that of increased ductal tissue (Fig. 12-1). When a man with gynecomastia seeks medical attention, it is either because of a palpable lump beneath the nipple or because the gynecomastia is painful. In either case, excisional biopsy can be both diagnostic and therapeutic. If the etiologic factor can be identified and removed, the process should regress. With idiopathic gynecomastia, the ductal tissue may regress spontaneously. There is an end-organ responsiveness in gynecomastia because unilateral gynecomastia may occur even though the etiology is one that should affect both breasts (Fig. 12-2).

REFERENCES

1. Dershaw DD, Borgen PI, Deutch BM, et al. Mammographic findings in men with breast cancer. AJR **160:**267–270, 1993.
2. Chantra PK, So GJ, Wollman JS, et al. Mammography of the male breast. AJR **164:**853–858, 1995.
3. Cooper RA, Gunter BA, Ramamurthy L. Mammography in men. Radiology **191:**651–656, 1994.

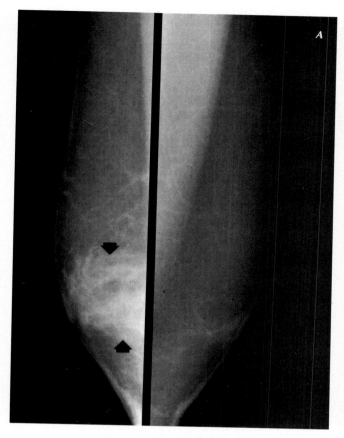

FIG. 12-1 A. *This is an example of painless unilateral gynecomastia (arrows).*

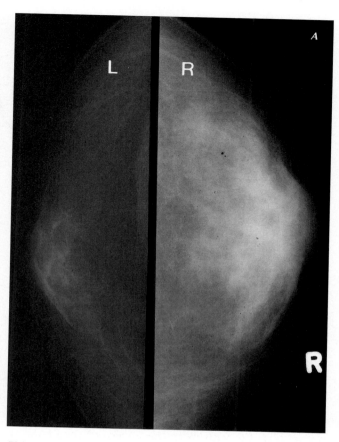

FIG. 12-2 A. *This man is taking estrogen for prostate carcinoma. There is unilateral gynecomastia on the right.*

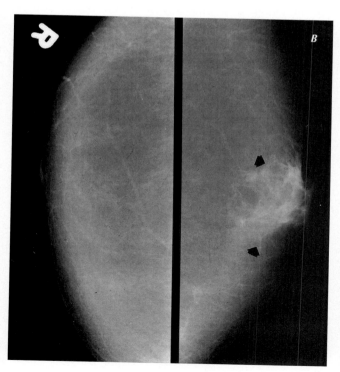

FIG. 12-1 (Continued) B. *This is an example of painful unilateral gynecomastia (arrows).*

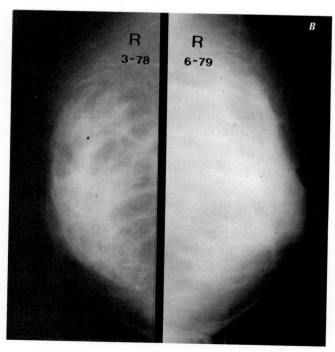

FIG. 12-2 (Continued) B. *Since the patient is continuing his estrogen therapy, the unilateral gynecomastia in his right breast is increasing.*

Chapter 13

BREAST ULTRASOUND

Frederick J. Doherty

Although mammography is the only accepted screening tool for the detection of nonpalpable breast cancer, most mammographic abnormalities are not malignant. Modern ultrasound (US) has proven itself to be a facile, accurate, and reliable diagnostic tool to complement mammography, since it can help reduce the need for unnecessary surgery for benign processes.

An equivocal mammogram may present a specific problem, which can be answered easily with a directed, high-quality US scan. With the increased resolution of modern scanners, along with the increased experience of those operating the scanners, new and sophisticated problems can be handled confidently with breast US.

For those who are relatively new to this modality or to this application, there may be a rational fear of breast US, which is simply due to a relative lack of experience. A comfort level in breast US can only be reached through experience in scanning and in operating the equipment. This chapter is designed to offer assistance in shortening the learning curve in order to become more comfortable with the uses of breast US. Those who are more experienced in breast US will recognize the problems so often encountered in daily scanning, when things do not seem to behave according to the rules.

The only breast US worth performing is one that is of high quality and offers diagnostic significance about the management of a specific problem. The radiologist must be familiar with the objectives and proper uses of breast US, and also must understand both the strengths and limitations of the modality. When the US is done to evaluate a mammographic finding, the radiologist must be confident that the sonographic finding is the exact correlate of the mammographic abnormality. Comfort in breast US comes with an ever-expanding awareness of the normal sonographic anatomy of the breast and its normal anatomic and sonographic variations. While the differentiation between cystic and solid masses represents its most common and basic usage, US will have other roles that will be found, as experience develops.[1] For example, the use of US to guide needles into lesions in the breast is now commonplace.

In this chapter, general concepts about the objectives and proper applications of breast US will be described as outlined in Table 13-1. The strengths and limitations of breast ultrasound will be stressed. The normal sonographic anatomy of the breast, as well as the sonographic appearance of cysts and solid masses, will be covered in detail. Technical and anatomical variability will be emphasized. Other breast abnormalities will be shown, and a discussion of needle intervention in the breast will be presented. This chapter is intended to provide a logical and practical approach to developing confidence in the use of modern breast ultrasound, and it is not meant to be an exhaustive review or an atlas on the topic.

OBJECTIVES AND APPLICATIONS OF BREAST ULTRASOUND

Breast Ultrasound—Yesterday and Today

After an initial flurry of excitement in the late 1970s in an effort to challenge mammography as a screening tool for breast imaging, the results of the early use of breast ultrasound to detect cancer were dismal. Since

TABLE 13-1
THE USES OF ULTRASOUND IN THE BREAST

1. Objectives and applications of breast ultrasound
2. Understanding the strengths and the limitations of breast ultrasound
3. Normal sonographic anatomy of the breast
4. Breast cysts
5. Solid masses
6. Other things that are found in the breast
7. Sonographically guided procedures with needles

mammography could detect about 90 percent of cancers in all categories, versus about 50 percent with ultrasound, the use of ultrasound for the detection of early breast cancer fell into disfavor. It was only able to detect about 10 percent of cancers under 1 cm in size.[2] However, although it was unable to detect breast cancer, ultrasound was easily capable of showing benign cysts in the breast.[3]

While dedicated automated breast scanners were made in the 1980s, a modern generation of high-resolution, all-purpose, real-time scanners simultaneously developed. Equipped with high-frequency probes these new scanners placed the ability to do good breast ultrasound into many more radiologists' hands. The ability to diagnose a cyst, with confidence, became an easily available tool for those radiologists who acquired these new all-purpose scanners. As more experience developed, ultrasound became a valuable diagnostic tool to clarify issues which were raised by equivocal mammographic findings, to answer specific clinical questions, and to place needles easily and accurately into lesions of the breast.[4]

Goals of Breast Ultrasound

The most important goal of breast ultrasound is to avoid unnecessary surgery. This is achieved when the diagnosis of a perfect cyst can be made, and a biopsy avoided. Core biopsy of presumed benign lesions also can reduce the number of surgical biopsies of fibroadenomas or fibrocystic changes. A focal asymmetric density that is shown to be only fibroglandular tissue with ultrasound can be followed with mammography, since follow-up is an option for a high probability benign lesion.

It would be ideal to be able to detect cancers with ultrasound, which cannot be seen by mammography. Though this occasionally happens, ultrasound is not a screening tool and its use as such may lead to unnecessary surgery. It has been shown that incidental masses seen with ultrasound have a very low probability of being malignant.[5] This fact should be seriously considered when there appears to be an ultrasound abnormality in a region of the breast, where the mammogram shows normal adipose tissue. This unsuspected sonographic finding may not even be real. The technical limitations of ultrasound can at times cloud the picture, and scanning artifacts may mimic abnormalities.

At NEMCH ultrasound of the breast is directed at answering a specific clinical or mammographic question and it is not used to search in other areas of the breast for unsuspected abnormalities.

Applications of Breast Ultrasound

The majority of breast ultrasounds performed at our hospital are referred from mammography because of a non-palpable focal abnormality that may be a cyst. Sometimes a focal asymmetric density, seen on mammography, will be evaluated with ultrasound to see if it can be explained by focal and matching normal fibroglandular tissue, without evidence of anything else in the region.[6] This will be discussed later in this chapter. Sometimes a clinician will refer a symptomatic patient for a clinical or palpable abnormality, which cannot be visualized by mammography. Women who have a mammogram, which is highly suspicious for cancer, are not ordinarily sent for ultrasound, since the sonogram adds no further information.

Modern ultrasound images normal breast parenchyma, and it is capable of making the diagnosis of a cyst in the breast with close to 100 percent accuracy.[7] If a mass is solid, it should not be mistaken for a cyst. Ultrasound clearly shows normal breast parenchymal tissue, normal breast adipose tissue, cysts, and solid masses (Fig. 13-1). Normal tissue and simple cysts require no surgery. The nature of solid masses is often indeterminate, and biopsy or follow-up is necessary to manage the problem. Very careful real-time scanning is frequently necessary to resolve equivocal and technically artifactual ultrasound findings.

Ultrasound is also used to guide needles into breast abnormalities. It can be used for cyst aspiration, needle localization for surgical excisional biopsy, or core biopsy.

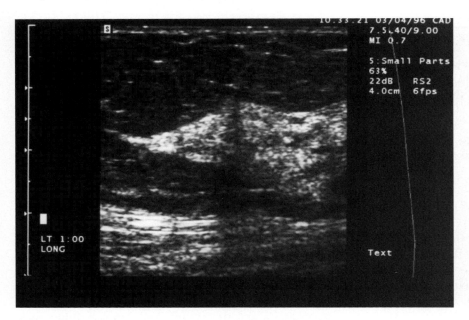

FIG. 13-1 *Typical breast ultrasound findings.* **A.** *Normal breast architecture showing a region of echogenic parenchymal tissue surrounded by hypoechoic fatty breast tissue, lying upon chest wall structures.*

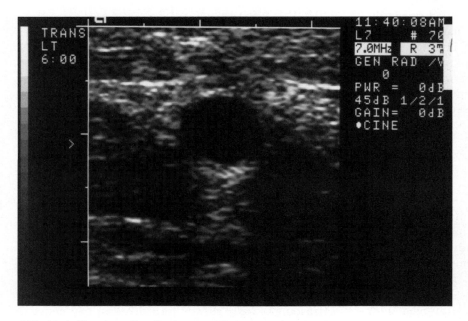

FIG. 13-1 *(Continued)* **B.** *A magnified view of a classic cyst.*

UNDERSTANDING THE STRENGTHS AND LIMITATIONS OF BREAST ULTRASOUND

In order to perform good breast ultrasound, scanning experience is one of the most critical factors, and it is really the only way to develop an appreciation of the strengths and limitations of ultrasound in imaging the breast. Perhaps more than in any other area of medical imaging, the image produced is directly related to the quality of the equipment coupled with the creative and artistic skill and experience of the operator of the scanner. While patient body habitus may often limit scanning, most ultrasound problems are related to scanner operation. This section will discuss the strengths and limitations of ultrasound, and how it affects one's ap-

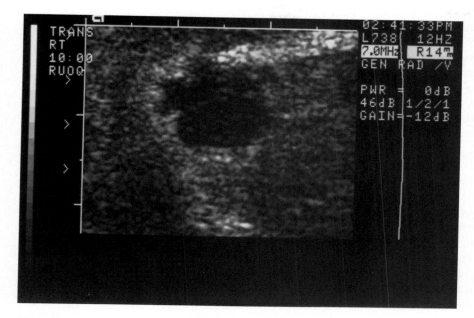

FIG. 13-1 *(Continued)* **C.** *A hypoechoic solid mass proven to be medullary carcinoma.*

proach to breast imaging. Technical factors of ultrasound scanning will be stressed throughout the chapter. The appearance of the different breast tissue characteristics will show how ultrasound images may offer diagnostic confidence or little reliability.

Strengths of Ultrasound

The high-resolution, real-time probes available today offer exquisite spatial and contrast resolution, where fine structures can be imaged with clarity. The most important use of modern ultrasound is its ability to diagnose a perfect cyst with confidence. In good hands, cysts as small as 2 to 3 mm can be commonly found, even in a large fatty breast, if the operator knows where to look and is very carefully searching for them (Fig. 13-2). Finding a cyst usually answers the question and eliminates need for further anxiety. Solid masses require further management.

For the inexperienced, larger cysts are easy to find in small glandular breasts. Experience in breast ultrasound permits the detection of smaller cysts in very large fatty breasts.

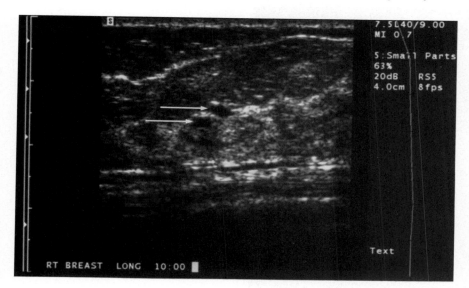

FIG. 13-2 *Two tiny cysts (arrows) in a large fatty breast, where natural tissue contrast is less than optimal. Nevertheless, these two small cysts are clearly seen.*

Modern scanners also allow for accurate evaluation of solid masses. It is possible that very careful analysis of all of the features of a presumably benign solid mass may allow nonsurgical management.

As previously mentioned, real-time ultrasound also provides a quick, easy, and safe route for the very accurate placement of needles into lesions in the breast for various purposes.

Limitations of Ultrasound

It must be stressed that ultrasound imaging has many factors that can limit the quality of the image. These include the equipment, the operator, the patient, and the lesion itself. It is obvious that newer scanners provide far better images than older scanners, and this is a very important factor in image quality and resolution. The equipment's level of resolution is the most critical nonvariable factor in limiting the image. A machine cannot show what it cannot resolve. It is most unusual to see microcalcifications with ultrasound (Fig. 13-3). It is also difficult for it to detect small breast cancers.

Variable factors that also come into play include operator experience, the architecture and size of the breast, and the size, location, and characteristics of the lesion itself. These variables may be present as only individual factors, but there will be times when all of these variables will simultaneously affect the quality of the scan. Increased operator experience helps to tame these variables, and this results in an improvement of the quality of breast ultrasound over time.

The size and tissue makeup of the breast along with the size, tissue characteristics, and mobility of a lesion, can all affect the ability of ultrasound to detect a breast abnormality. Small, mobile, solid masses and cysts are hard to find in a large breast, even for the most experienced sonographers. These lesions can be missed very easily. There just is not enough tissue contrast for these rapidly moving small lesions to be identified. The mobility of both the breast tissue and the lesions themselves compounds the degree of difficulty in trying to detect small abnormalities. A small mobile lesion can quickly slip under the probe, never to be seen again, as it jumps out of the plane of the image. This is a good reason why ultrasound is not a good screening tool for breast cancer detection.

An anechoic cyst is easy to find when it stands out against an echogenic fibroglandular tissue background, whereas a hypoechoic solid mass may be impossible to locate against a background of hypoechoic adipose tissue. Contrary to many people's beliefs that fat is echogenic, it is important here to emphasize the fact that adipose tissue in the breast, similar to its appearance elsewhere in the body, is hypoechoic (Fig. 13-4). It is a myth that adipose tissue is hyperechoic.[8]

Another limitation of ultrasound is in the evaluation of the area deep to the nipple. This area is commonly lost in intense shadowing, and, as a result, imaging is compromised here.

The purpose of doing good breast ultrasound is to provide an answer to a specific question. Inability to find a cyst or answer the question tosses the problem back to mammography for management, and ultrasound becomes non-information. Non-information does not play a role in patient management, since the question was not answered, and the possibility of breast cancer remains in the differential.

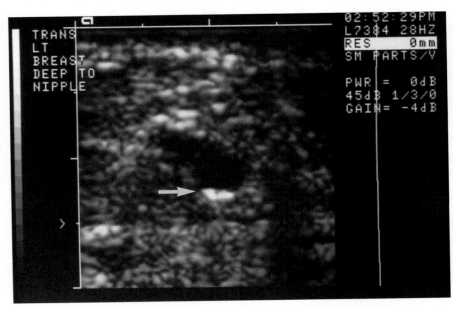

FIG. 13-3 *A rarely seen example of microcalcifications (arrow) layering dependently in a very small cyst in a breast.*

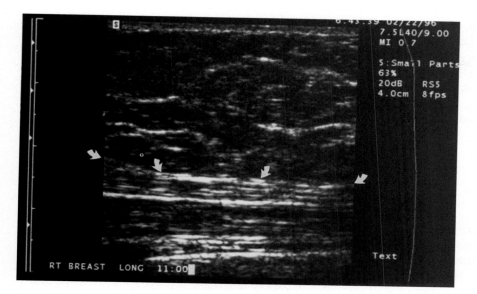

FIG. 13-4 *A totally fatty breast is shown, where no echogenic fibroglandular tissue exists. The horizontally striated pectoral muscles are seen in the chest wall deep to the retromammary fascia (arrows).*

Multiplicity of findings also raises the issue of not answering the specific mammographic question. A specific question requires a specific answer, and ultrasound must be able to locate an area geographically that can be the only answer to the question. When there are multiple abnormalities or findings, it becomes difficult and often impossible to correlate each finding exactly with the mammogram. When multiple asymmetric densities cannot all be matched with multiple areas of fibroglandular tissue, a tumor could easily be missed. Although multiple, rounded densities may all have the identical mammographic appearance, ultrasound may show a solid mass among numerous cysts. Obtaining histology either by core biopsy or needle localization can be performed with ultrasound guidance.

It has long been recognized that ultrasound is not helpful in distinguishing between benign and malignant solid masses in the breast, since there is a significant overlap in the appearance of both benign and malignant tumors.[9] Attempts are being made now to identify probably benign solid masses, where the findings indicate little chance of cancer, and unnecessary surgery can be avoided.

Most modern probes are equipped with color and pulsed Doppler capability. Whether this offers anything significant in breast diagnosis is uncertain.[10] Some claim success in certain specific applications, such as following post-operative treatment of breast cancer patients looking for signs of either healing or tumor recurrence.[11] Experience with the use of microbubble contrast agents for color Doppler evaluation of solid masses may offer help in differentiating benign from malignant lesions in the future.[12]

US Scanners and High-Frequency Real-Time Scanning of the Breast

Modern ultrasound scanners are equipped with high-frequency real-time probes that provide superb images of the breast. These probes have Doppler capabilities, which some people are using in evaluating breast abnormalities.

It is important to use the highest frequency probe available that will penetrate to the depth needed to be imaged. 5-MHz probes are really not acceptable now, except in very rare circumstances, that are most likely size-related. In these rare circumstances, one is looking only for gross abnormalities in a very limited scan. 7-MHz is the lowest frequency that provides good resolution throughout most breasts. 10-MHz probes offer excellent resolution, especially in the very near field close to the skin. It has been our experience to scan most breasts successfully at 7 MHz regardless of size. Compression can thin a large fatty breast to a reasonable thickness for good imaging. There have been only a few instances of complete failure due to breast size.

Because of the small footprint of the probes, it is easy to miss small mobile masses when trying to scan a region of a large breast. The narrow field of view raises the level of difficulty in finding small lesions in a large breast. This is a good reason why breast ultrasound is not a good scanning tool, since it is too easy to miss small lesions. While not a good tool for whole breast evaluation, ultrasound is reliable and easy to use for focused problem solving, where a relatively confined region of interest is generously and carefully evaluated. For small palpable abnormalities, scanning while simultaneously palpating a mass may be helpful in determining if the mass is cystic, solid, or normal breast tissue. An extension of this principle is used in free-handed, sonographically guided, needle placement procedures. Small superficial masses may benefit from the use of a standoff pad, since getting the lesion away from the transducer surface will reduce artifacts. This can improve both contrast and spatial resolution (Fig. 13-5).

Breast Tissue Characteristics Seen with Ultrasound

The breast is an organ which undergoes a change in architecture during life. The normal breast tissue is basically a mix of echogenic fibroglandular parenchymal tissue and hypoechoic adipose tissue. Younger women up to age 30 have more glandular tissue in the central portion of the breast with relatively less amounts of fatty tissue around the periphery. Between 30 and 35 years of age, the echogenic glandular tissue begins to be replaced with adipose tissue.

Breast parenchyma or fibroglandular tissue is very echogenic, and echogenic masses in the breast are not tumors.

Cysts are anechoic lesions that stand out very sharply against a contrasting background of echogenic glandular tissue, but they stand out only moderately well against a hypoechoic fatty background, where there is so much less natural tissue contrast.

Solid masses in the breast are hypoechoic, and while they are easily seen against an echogenic glandular background, they may not be seen if they are very similar in echo texture to the hypoechoic background of a fatty breast. This is why mammography is better than ultrasound at detecting small cancers surrounded by fat. Such small lesions are easily missed with ultrasound.

In a symptomatic woman under age 30 with dense breasts, ultrasound may offer more imaging help than mammography. Ultrasound may also be more helpful than mammography in an older woman with dense breasts.

NORMAL SONOGRAPHIC BREAST ANATOMY

The normal sonographic anatomy of the breast is quite simple as long as the limitations of ultrasound are respected. The skin covered breast tissue is composed of variable amounts of echogenic fibroglandular parenchyma combined with hypoechoic fatty lobules interspersed with thin echogenic fibrous Cooper's ligaments. The breast lies upon the retromammary fascia which is seen as a brightly echogenic line separating the breast tissue from the musculo-skeletal structures of the chest wall (Fig. 13-6).

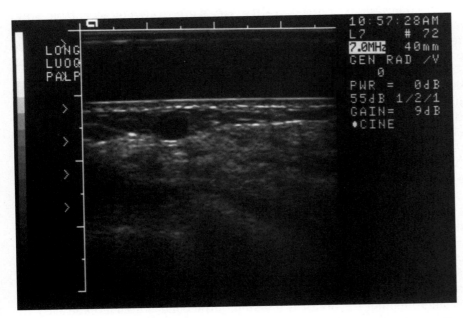

FIG. 13-5 *This is a tiny, superficial cyst in a thin portion of the axillary tail of the breast. This very small cyst located just beneath the skin is better imaged with a standoff pad.*

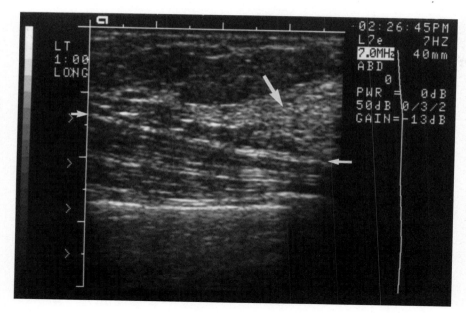

FIG. 13-6 *This is an example of normal sonographic breast architecture. Echogenic fibroglandular tissue (large arrow) is imbedded in hypoechoic adipose tissue. The breast is separated from the structures of the chest wall by the retromammary fascia (small arrows).*

Scanning Position

We scan the breast with the patient either supine or rotated into a posterior oblique position, using a pillow or a sponge wedge, and with the arm held comfortably on the pillow over her head. This tends to stretch and thin the breast, as well as to reduce mobility, and makes ultrasound scanning easier. This position provides natural tissue retraction. This ultrasound position, however, is very different from what appears in mammographic views, and focal regions may be in relatively different areas when comparing the two modalities. Lesions which appear deep to the nipple on a mammogram, may be seen very close to the ultrasound probe, especially when compression is used while scanning. On occasion we scan the patient sitting to find a small palpable lesion, or when we are trying to reproduce the mammographic geometry in search of a lesion.

Normal Breast Tissue

The skin is seen as thinly layered echogenic lines about 2 mm in total thickness. At the areola, the skin appears to thicken slightly as it approaches the nipple. At the nipple, reflective structures such as ducts, are oriented parallel to the ultrasound beam, and this suboptimal imaging situation causes the area deep to the nipple to shadow so intensely that often there is loss of information in this region. Lesions located here can be hidden (Fig. 13-7). Attempts to angle into this area sometimes help.

Under the skin lies hypoechoic adipose tissue divided into lobules by thin echogenic septae. Breast parenchymal tissue is very echogenic and we call it fibroglandular tissue. The echotexture of Cooper's ligaments and glandular tissue is very similar. Glandular tissue tends to be smoothly granular, and it also has some feeling of volume to it, when imaged in biplane fashion. On the other hand, fibrous tissue tends to run in more of a planar or thinner sheetlike fashion. Fibroglandular tissue is distributed throughout the breast in variable and unpredictable ways. Classically it is arranged in a somewhat conical fashion radiating out from the nipple, although this anatomy is rarely perfectly demonstrated. Fibroglandular tissue often is found in patches that are scattered throughout fatty portions of the breast. The lobules of fat tend to be somewhat tubular in shape. They generally are not round nor are they completely surrounded by thin echogenic tissue in a spherical fashion. Ducts and blood vessels are occasionally seen as fluid filled tubular structures (Fig. 13-8). Vessels tend to be straighter and ducts more tortuous.

When scanning with light pressure, Cooper's ligaments tend to be oriented towards the probe. They can serve as strong scatterers of ultrasound, resulting in thin to thick shadows deep to them (Fig. 13-9). This

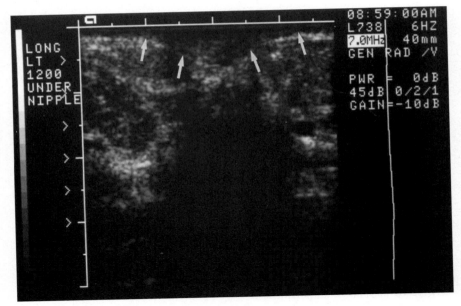

FIG. 13-7 *Shadowing by the nipple is demonstrated here. The skin can be seen to get thicker in the region of the areola (arrows), and the area deep to the nipple is obscured by intense shadowing.*

problem is easily resolved by increased compression and biplane scanning (Fig. 13-10). Thin or thick shadows can disappear in real time as compression is applied. Cooper's ligaments as well as the septae dividing fat lobules become reoriented in a more horizontal fashion to the probe when pressure is applied. This allows good transmission of sound. Firm but gentle compression of a fatty breast definitely improves imaging.

Retromammary Fascia

This is a thin fascial plane covering the chest wall and separating it from the more superficially located breast. The retromammary fascia is clearly seen as a thin strongly echogenic plane which appears as a thin bright line in any one frozen image. It is probably easiest to identify in the axillary region, where it can be seen to

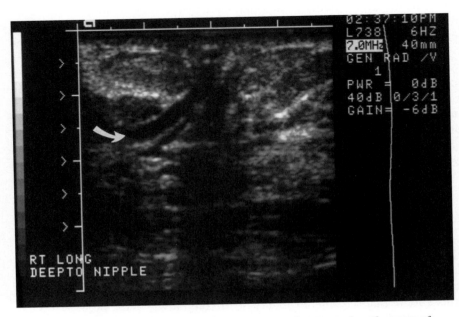

FIG. 13-8 *A portion of a duct (arrow) is seen as it approaches the area of shadowing behind the nipple.*

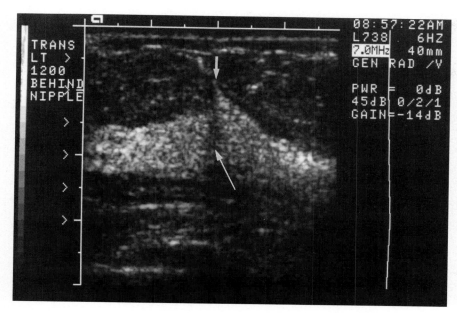

FIG. 13-9 *This is an example of a normally found weak shadow (long arrow) originating form the apex of a prominent area of glandular tissue. This shadow is the result of scattering behind a sharply reflective Cooper's ligament at this site (short arrow). This shadow lacks volume and changes with biplane scanning and compression.*

cover the two pectoral muscles. Once found it can be tracked down into the breast. It is important to identify this structure when scanning, since it is a good marker of the appropriate depth to be scanned (Fig. 13-11).

Chest Wall Structures

Behind the retromammary fascia are chest wall structures that can be identified (Fig. 13-12). The pectoral muscles are easy to see, especially in the axilla. As the pectoral muscles thin, the main structures behind the

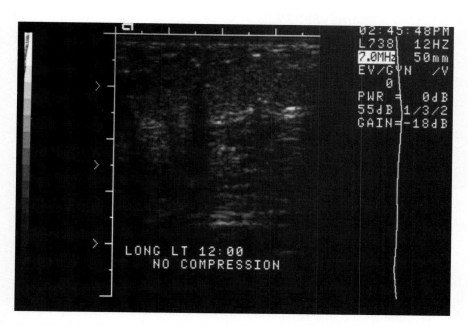

FIG. 13-10 *Deep shadowing reduced by compression.* **A.** *Dense shadowing in the deeper portions of the breast is demonstrated here. The shadowing comes from scattering of ultrasound off sharply angled bright reflectors, such as the apices of Cooper's ligaments and the peaks of fibroglandular tissue.*

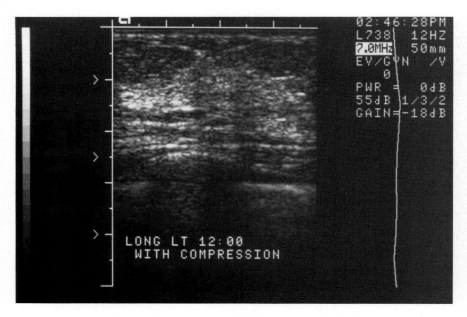

FIG. 13-10 *(Continued)* **B.** *Gentle firm compression reorients these same structures in a direction that is more parallel to the surface of the probe. The shadowing in the deeper portion of the breast disappears.*

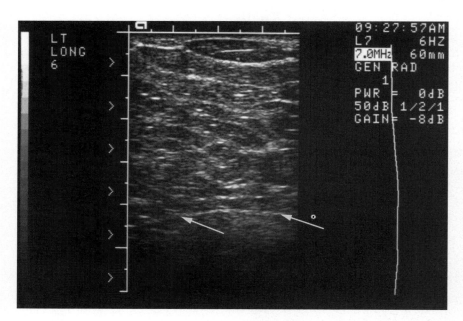

FIG. 13-11 *The retromammary fascia (arrows) is identified in this large fatty breast, offering assurance that the proper depth in the breast is being imaged.*

retromammary fascia are the ribs and intercostal muscles, deep to which lie the pleura and air filled lung. The bony portion of the ribs, and the air-filled lung all cause shadowing. When scanning longitudinally near the sternum, the cartilaginous portions of the ribs are easily imaged (Fig. 13-13). They appear as oval hypoechoic solid structures and should not be mistaken for

small solid masses. Ribs and costal cartilages should be identified as chest wall structures. They begin to shadow in transverse scanning as the transducer overlies the bony portion of the rib. They will also appear to be multiple similar findings in a chain, when scanning along the length of the sternum in a longitudinal fashion.

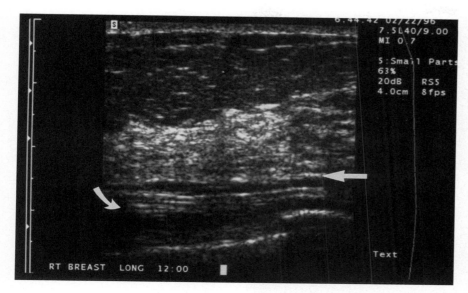

FIG. 13-12 *The retromammary fascia (straight arrow) and pectoral muscles (curved arrow) are clearly shown deep to a fatty breast.*

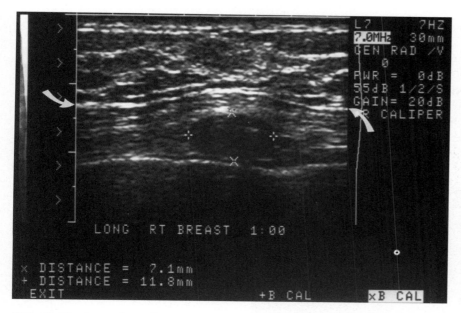

FIG. 13-13 *A costal cartilage in the medial aspect of the right breast is imaged in cross section here. It was mistaken for a solid mass, and its diameters were measured. Biplane scanning would have shown this to be a rib. It should be recognized as being a normal part of the chest wall structure deep to the retromammary fascia (arrow).*

BREAST CYSTS

The classic sonographic appearance of a cyst is a rounded, smooth-walled structure with no internal echoes, a good back wall, posterior acoustic enhancement, and lateral wall shadows. If a classic cyst is found nothing further needs to be done (Fig. 13-14).

The reality in breast ultrasound is that cysts in the breast often do not look classic. It is common for them to be not rounded, to be irregular, to have internal structures, to lack posterior enhancement, and to have internal echoes.[13] These cysts require very careful evaluation. Even though these cysts have unusual imaging characteristics, they nevertheless "talk" cystic to those with experience in breast ultrasound.

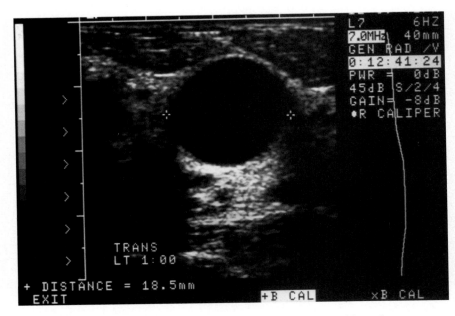

FIG. 13-14 *A perfect cyst is shown here. It is rounded, and has sharp anterior and posterior walls. This cyst has no internal echoes, and it demonstrates posterior acoustic enhancement.*

The most important use of breast ultrasound is its ability to diagnose a cyst with confidence. In the hands of an experienced sonographer, the diagnosis of a simple benign breast cyst should be made with close to 100 percent accuracy. Sometimes these skills are tested in confidently diagnosing a breast cyst.

The Variable Shape of Cysts

Breast cysts are rarely perfectly round, and are commonly ovoid in shape (Fig. 13-15). Pressure on the growing cyst by the weight of the breast exerts a geographical influence on it, causing the cyst to become

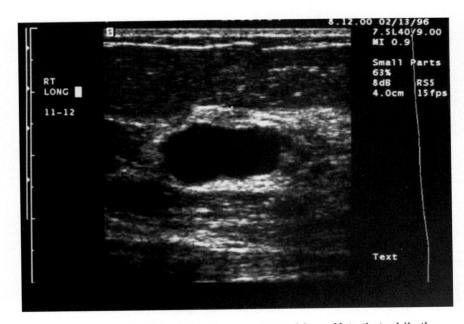

FIG. 13-15 *An ovoid-shaped cyst is demonstrated here. Note that while the walls of the cyst are sharp, their shape is irregular and not smooth. Otherwise this cyst is anechoic with posterior acoustic enhancement.*

compressed and somewhat pancaked in shape. They commonly have a horizontal axis that is greater than their vertical one.

Larger cysts are relatively soft lesions, and, when large enough, their shape can be changed during real-time scanning by applying and removing compression (Fig 13-16). Small cysts, especially in a fatty breast, may not change shape easily when compression is ap-plied. Small cysts are fairly hard lesions, especially in a soft fatty breast.

Large cysts which receive pressure from sur-rounding tough structures such as ligaments or blood vessels appear lobulated (Fig. 13-17). A cluster of cysts can be found, and these can be small or large. Clustered cysts often communicate with each other, and look like a small bunch of grapes. Larger ones, when aspi-

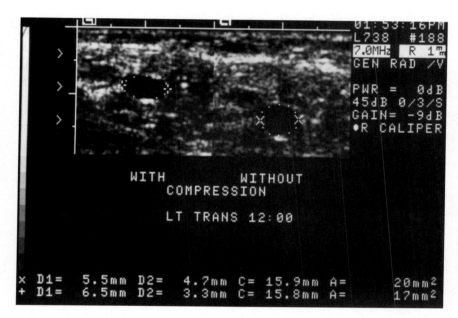

FIG. 13-16 *This is an example of a fairly small cyst changing shape from ovoid to round with compression and without compression.*

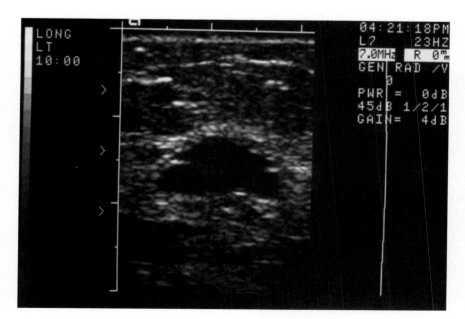

FIG. 13-17 *A cyst with an irregular shape, lobulated borders, and wrinkled walls is shown here. While it is anechoic, posterior acoustic enhancement is weak.*

rated, can completely decompress with one needle stick into only one compartment. These tightly clustered cysts can appear as a lobulated mass on a mammogram.

Cysts with Internal Architectural Structures

Intracystic cancers can be seen with ultrasound. They are cysts which contain a rounded mural nodule or thick irregular septations. The internal architecture is obvious, atypical, and striking (Fig. 13-18).

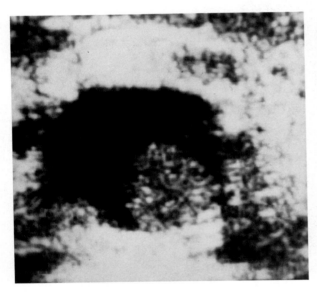

FIG. 13-18 *This is a greatly magnified image of an intracystic carcinoma. While the cyst qualities are straightforward, a large rounded mural nodule is seen here in the lower right quadrant of the cyst.*

However it is common to find fine, thin wrinkles in the wall of an unusually shaped cyst. These are of no significance, and they should be confidently recognized. These membranous internal architectural structures on the edges of cysts are explained by the same forces that change the shape of cysts as previously described. The pronounced wrinkling and tethering effect of a strong structure deforms the cyst to such an extent as to cause a thin internal septation along the cyst wall (Fig. 13-19).

We consider fine, thin-edge wrinkles in a cyst to be a normal and insignificant finding because of the resolution of modern equipment. However when we see cysts with thick septae or rounded solid nodules, we consider these to be malignant until proven otherwise. They require surgical excision. We do not perform diagnostic aspirations of these suspected intracystic carcinomas in order to preserve the target for surgery.

Cysts without Posterior Acoustic Enhancement

While cysts usually have increased through transmission of sound, some do not. A study of 300 sonograms showed absent through transmission in up to 25 percent of breast cysts (Fig. 13-20).[13]

If one looks at the posterior acoustic enhancement area in back of a cyst, it can be seen to be maximal behind the center of the cyst, and to fade off as it gets closer to the edges of the cyst with its lateral wall shadows. The region of increased through transmission of sound has a "comet tail" appearance which is brightest and longest directly in back of the center of

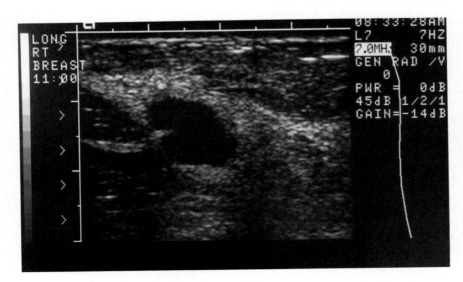

FIG. 13-19 *Thin wall irregularities in a cyst.* **A.** *An image of a large cyst imbedded in echogenic fibroglandular tissue. Note the thin septation at the left side of the cyst.*

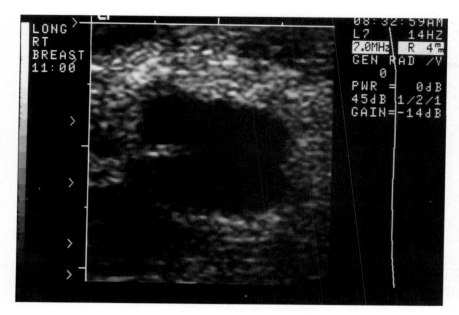

FIG. 13-19 *(Continued)* **B.** *Magnified image of the same cyst. Note the two walls of the thin wrinkle in the edge of the cyst.*

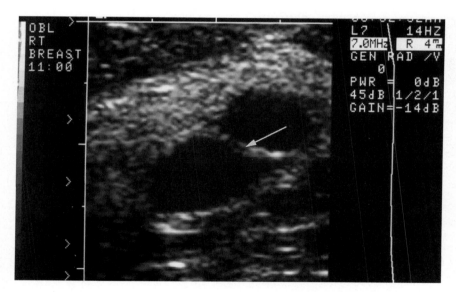

FIG. 13-19 *(Continued)* **C.** *Another view of the same cyst where the invagination along the edge appears as a septum. The hypoechoic channel in the center (arrow) is suggestive of a tiny blood vessel.*

the cyst. As the sides of a cyst are approached, the effects of posterior acoustic enhancement are neutralized by the increased scattering of echoes from the more steeply angled cyst walls. This is why imaging a cyst away from its central axis and at angles approaching tangential can result in absence of through transmission in back of a cyst (Fig. 13-21). The reflective cyst walls, becoming increasingly tangential, start

to scatter ultrasound, and the shorter distance across the cyst fluid closer to the edges helps to cancel the effect of the increased through transmission seen best in the center of a cyst.

Even if there is no increased through transmission in back of an anechoic cyst, it will not cause shadowing, and it will always have a good, sharp wall with good visualization of structures deep to it.

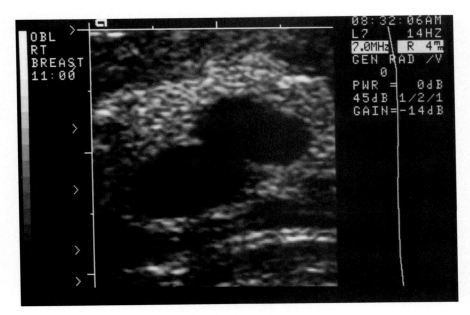

FIG. 13-19 *(Continued)* **D.** *Another view of the same cyst where it appears bilobed. The strong force of an adjacent structure deforming the cyst is shown here.*

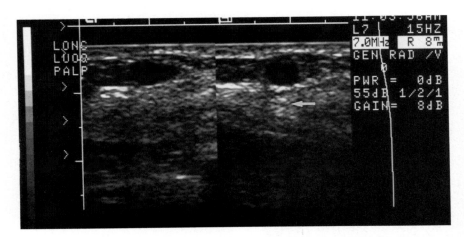

FIG. 13-20 *This is a dual image of the same cyst. On the right side of this dual image, this small and superficial cyst demonstrates obvious posterior acoustic enhancement (arrow). On the left side of this dual image, there is no posterior acoustic enhancement seen.*

Cysts That Have Internal Echoes

There are times when careful scanning technique demonstrates echoes within a breast cyst which will mimic a solid mass. Tiny punctate echoes may be real particles of debris that sometimes may be seen to move. The source of fine particulate debris in a cyst is uncertain but most likely benign. Galactoceles can be filled with moving homogeneous debris giving a false appearance of a solid mass on a frozen image. An incompletely aspirated cyst or a spontaneously or trau-matically decompressed cyst may have the remains of some blood which can be seen.

There may be scanning artifacts from improper gain, dynamic range, or from reverberation of sound. Too much gain can produce internal echoes in a cyst. This is usually obvious since the other tissues in the breast will appear too bright. Adjusting the gain downwards will remove echoes from a cyst before it will remove weak internal echoes from hypoechoic adipose lobules or hypoechoic solid masses. An attempt should

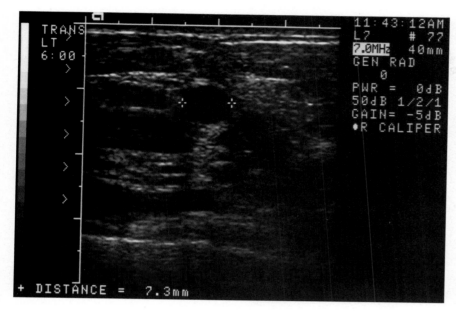

FIG. 13-21 *This is a small perfect cyst with a long tail of posterior acoustic enhancement. Note how the area of increased through transmission has a "comet tail" appearance, where it is brightest directly in back of the center of the cyst, and weakest closer to the edges of the cyst.*

be made to maintain some granularity in the fatty tissue while making a cyst anechoic.

Too high a dynamic range can also place fine echoes in a cyst (Fig. 13-22). In our laboratory we tend to operate at, or slightly higher than, the middle of a scanner's dynamic range. This commonly places streaming low-level echoes in blood vessels in the liver

as well as in scrotal varices, and not infrequently in breast cysts. We have found it helpful to scan the breast at a level just under the middle of the dynamic range, where cysts appear truly anechoic.

Reverberating artifacts are part of working with ultrasound. They are common in large cysts that are close to the skin, near the main bang of the transducer

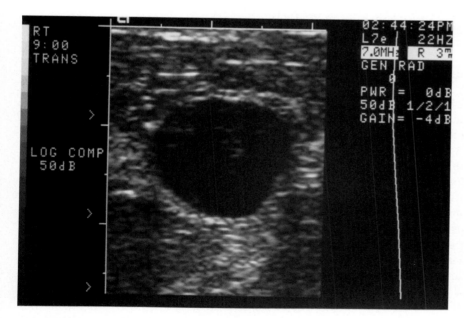

FIG. 13-22 *Reverberation artifact cleared up in a cyst.* **A.** *Irregular low-level echoes placed in a cyst because of reverberation artifact, when this breast cyst was scanned with a dynamic range of 50 dB. The majority of these technically artificial echoes are seen in the more superficial half of the cyst.*

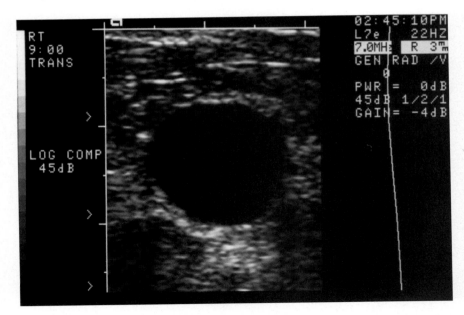

FIG. 13-22 *(Continued)* **B.** *The same cyst is now anechoic when scanned with a dynamic range of 45 dB. No other changes were made in the scanner controls.*

at the skin surface. They should be recognized for what they are. Adjusting the settings or scanning position usually resolves them. They will change position in the cyst with real time maneuvers.

When a lesion "talks" cystic, it probably is, even if it does not satisfy strict cyst criteria. Careful evaluation of scanning technique and readjusting settings may be necessary to diagnose a cyst. If questions persist, then an attempt at aspiration may be necessary.

SOLID MASSES

The approach to solid breast masses is somewhat controversial. In the past an attempt was made to use ultrasound to characterize lesions as benign or malignant. This attempt failed because of a large overlap between the appearances of benign and malignant masses. At our institution we have followed a conservative policy, since we cannot confidently tell whether a solid mass is benign or malignant, and only tissue sampling will positively answer the question.

Now there is renewed interest in evaluating the characteristics of solid lesions, in order to subselect out a group of masses that have no characteristics associated with malignancy, and almost no chance of breast cancer.[14] There is guarded optimism about this approach, and only time will tell whether this differentiation is possible.[15] However there are occasional individual instances when we can feel so strongly that a mass is most likely benign, that follow-up rather than tissue sampling is felt to be acceptable management.

Malignant lesions often have several very obvious worrisome characteristics. A benign lesion, on the other hand, "talks benign," and has an appearance that looks like a heterogeneously filled cyst. In our experience most solid lesions are indeterminate in nature, having a mix of features described with both classically benign and classically malignant characteristics.

Probably Benign Masses

These lesions have a considerable amount of cystic quality to them. While they are rounded or ovoid solid masses with smooth borders, sharp back walls, lateral wall shadows, and posterior acoustic enhancement, they are not anechoic. Instead they are hypoechoic, and filled with heterogeneous internal echoes. They can transmit sound almost as well as a cyst. Most of these lesions are fibroadenomas or fibrocystic changes (Fig. 13-23).

These lesions are slow growing, and like cysts they are under the geographic influence of the weight of the breast, as well as the effect of surrounding strong structures such as Cooper's ligaments. These benign lesions can have a few soft, gentle lobulations in their contour. They also often have a longer horizontal axis, and they are, in fact, somewhat pancaked in shape, and oriented in a plane that is parallel to the chest wall. They also have a thin, echogenic pseudocapsule surrounding them (Fig. 13-24).

We have long followed a conservative and safe "solid or cystic" management approach at our institution. Classic cysts are considered benign and solitary

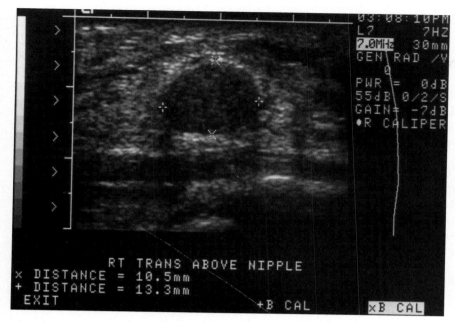

FIG. 13-23 *This is a classic example of a probably benign lesion in the breast. Fibrocystic changes were found at surgery. This rounded-to-ovoid solid mass has smooth borders, a strong back wall, and good sound transmission. An echogenic pseudocapsule is hard to identify against an echogenic fibroglandular background.*

solid masses are biopsied. It must be stressed that ultrasound is only a small portion of the management of breast disease, and that both the mammographic findings and the clinical evaluation of the breast will be the key factors in determining how a breast problem will be handled. Using clinical, mammographic, and sonographic criteria for a probably benign lesion, we have been identifying cases for core biopsy. Others are placing similar cases in follow-up. Developing a comfort level for these criteria depends on experience and the

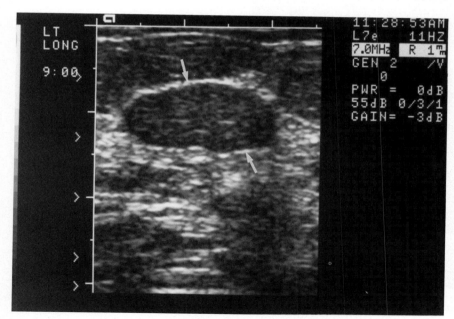

FIG. 13-24 *Another classic "probably benign" lesion. This ovoid fibroadenoma has a horizontal axis greater than its vertical one, and only a couple of very soft and gentle lobulations, at 6 and 10 o'clock. A thin pseudocapsule is also seen (arrows). Except for its ovoid shape, this fibroadenoma is virtually identical in appearance to the fibrocystic changes shown in Fig. 13-23.*

ability to evaluate all walls of a solid mass with complete confidence.

Probably Malignant Masses

Cancers in the breast often have very obvious features that are very different from probably benign masses. Like all masses in the breast, cancers are hypoechoic lesions. However their shape usually is not smooth, but instead they can have sharp multiple lobulations or even sharply angled borders (Fig. 13-25). The lobulations may be either macrolobules or microlobules. They may not have a predominant horizontal axis, and at times can have a vertical axis as long or longer than the horizontal one (Fig. 13-26). These features address the aggressiveness of a cancer where it is not affected by the weight of the breast against the chest wall. It is a lesion that is expanding in all directions and does not respect boundaries.

Cancers also frequently demonstrate some degree of posterior acoustic shadowing. While this is a variable feature, when present it is striking (Fig. 13-27). The entire mass or portions of it can attenuate ultrasound resulting in a focal or diffuse absence of features inside the mass or deep to it. There are times when the back wall of the mass itself cannot be identified.

Microcalcifications ordinarily are not seen with ultrasound. They can be found, on occasion, if scanning is optimal, and if one is searching for them carefully.

Color and pulsed Doppler evaluation of masses may sometimes offer information about a mass. Larger masses can develop tumor vascularity and abnormal flow patterns, but Doppler ultrasound does not seem to offer much help in characterizing smaller lesions in the breast that have not developed enough significant neovascularity to be detected.

Indeterminate Masses

In old clinical studies about 25 percent of lesions that were felt to be classically benign on ultrasound turned out to be cancer. This contributed to the opinion that ultrasound could not reliably be used to differentiate benign from malignant. These studies were done on equipment that was incapable of providing the detail and contrast resolution available today, and now a radiologist has far greater ability to evaluate carefully the contours and features of a mass.

Indeed one can now confidently identify lesions that satisfy the strict ultrasound criteria which suggest a probably benign mass (Fig. 13-28). One can also quite easily identify lesions that are most likely malignant

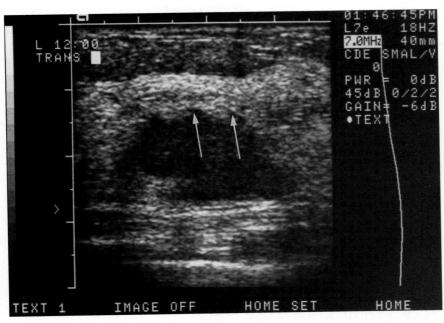

FIG. 13-25 *This is an example of a probably malignant mass. This large, poorly differentiated ductal carcinoma exhibits no attenuation of sound, but its very irregular borders are striking. While all borders of the mass show irregularity, the anterior edge is the most interesting. There is nothing soft and gentle about it. Three sharply angled peaks are seen, and the two on the right appear to end in irregular spiculations (arrows). The borders of this lesion scream "aggressive."*

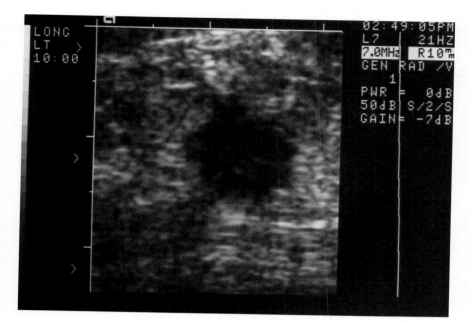

FIG. 13-26 *Infiltrating ductal carcinoma. This hypoechoic mass looks ugly. While it transmits sound well, it has a vertical axis greater than its horizontal axis. It has minimal internal architecture in an otherwise bright image. The borders of this cancer show macrolobulations, microlobulations, and sharply angled edges at contour transitions.*

(Fig. 13-29). Unfortunately, a large number of the solid masses that are seen with ultrasound have an indeterminate appearance, with features suggestive of both benign and malignant disease, and these lesions need biopsy. Future investigation will determine whether the strict ultrasound criteria used to define a benign mass are reliable enough to avoid having to obtain histological confirmation.

Many benign lesions show features that are described with cancer (Fig. 13-30). It is quite common for

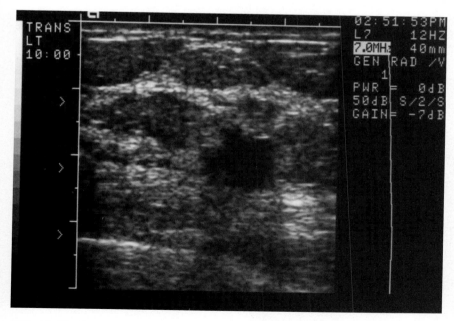

FIG. 13-27 *Infiltrating ductal carcinoma. This hypoechoic cancer shows a paucity of internal echoes in an otherwise bright image. Notice its markedly irregular borders and the moderate attenuation of sound deep to the lesion. While the relative shadowing is not strong, it is obvious, and suggests malignancy.*

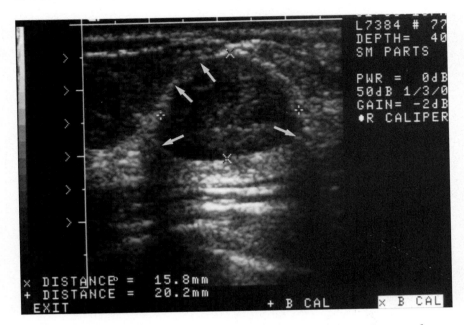

FIG. 13-28 *Classic "probably benign" lesion. This ovoid fibroadenoma shows an elongated horizontal axis, smooth borders, and soft gentle lobulations (arrows) at 4, 8, 10, and 11 o'clock. There is also a sharp back wall, a thin pseudocapsule, and increased through transmission of sound. There are no features suggestive of malignancy.*

fibroadenomas to have lobulated borders and demonstrate posterior acoustic shadowing. Deciding whether lobulated borders are smooth and gentle or sharp and angled is difficult. At either end of the spectrum the contour abnormalities are clear, but the mid range is a gray zone. A prominent bump and dip sign described by some as classic for a fibroadenoma may be perceived by others as a sharply angled lobule (Fig. 13-31). Sharp lobulations are more than just soft gentle bulges of the contour of a mass, and in our practice these lesions are placed into an indeterminate category. A sharp lobulation may be a sign of either a soft benign lesion being distorted by a ligament or a solid malignant tumor being aggressive.

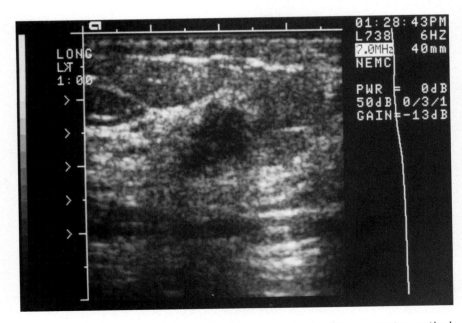

FIG. 13-29 *A breast carcinoma showing aggressive borders, a greater vertical axis, and moderate ultrasonic attenuation.*

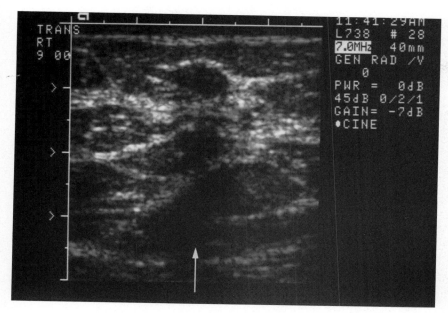

FIG. 13-30 *Four different fibroadenomas, each showing characteristics seen with malignancy.* **A.** *Weak shadowing (arrow) in back of a small lesion.*

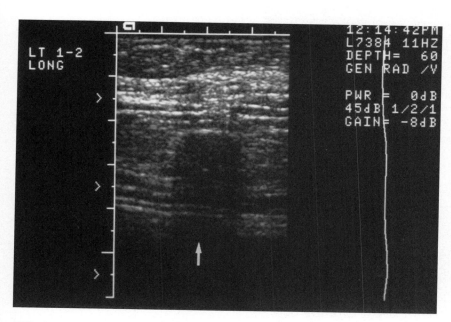

FIG. 13-30 *(Continued)* **B.** *Significant shadowing (arrow) by a larger mass deep in a large fatty breast.*

OTHER THINGS THAT ARE FOUND IN THE BREAST

Focal Asymmetric Densities

A nonpalpable, asymmetric density is an occasional sign of breast cancer. Even after a diagnostic mammographic examination, there are still times when the benign nature of these densities is not certain. When an asymmetric density is focal, we can evaluate it with ultrasound, searching for echogenic fibroglandular tissue that matches the mammographic abnormality in site, size, and shape (Fig. 13-32). Besides cysts, solid masses, and fibroglandular tissue, the only other tissue that is seen in the breast is normal hypoechoic adipose tissue. We are always looking for abnormalities that may be hiding in these mammographic densities.

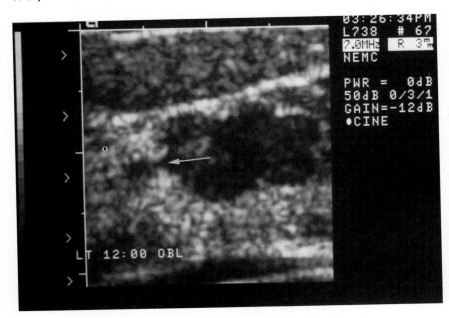

FIG. 13-30 *(Continued)* **C.** *A very sharply lobulated mass with very angular borders on its left side at 9 o'clock (arrow).*

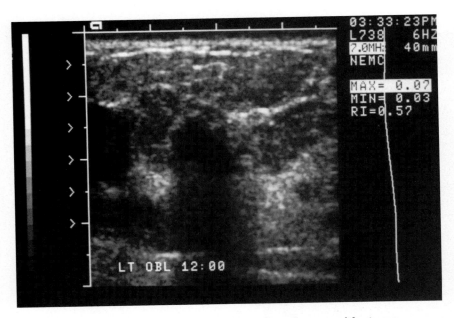

FIG. 13-30 *(Continued)* **D.** *An irregularly shaped mass with strong shadowing.*

When only fibroglandular tissue explains the mammographic finding, these patients are placed into follow-up by mammography, and not by ultrasound. Echogenic fibroglandular tissue is normal breast parenchyma, and breast cancer is not echogenic. The role of ultrasound is finished after it explains the mammographic asymmetric density, and reinforces the mammographic impression of fibroglandular tissue.

We do not evaluate multiple, asymmetric densities since it is impossible to match the ultrasound findings to the mammogram.

Abscesses

Abscesses in the breast are similar to abscesses elsewhere. They have a variable appearance, but usually are seen as a complex cystic mass. They can be filled with internal echoes or have fluid compartments with

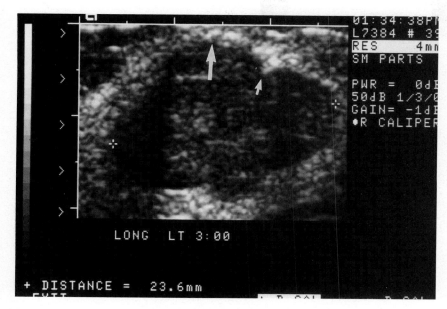

FIG. 13-31 *A very sharply lobulated fibroadenoma. This lesion exhibits a classic bump (long arrow) and dip (short arrow) sign, which can be interpreted as a sharply angled lobulation. While this appearance may be normal in a softer cyst, it is not normal in a solid, and firmer, lesion.*

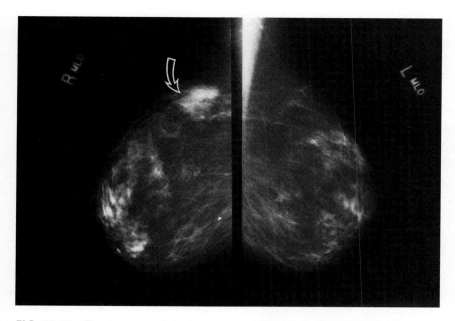

FIG. 13-32 *Focal asymmetric density. **A.** MLO view of mammogram detecting a large area of asymmetry (arrow) in the upper half of the right breast.*

solid-appearing material. At times they can look quite solid and mimic a tumor.

Abscesses are found when a patient has a mastitis which is not responding appropriately to treatment. Thick, echogenic skin may also be seen secondary to the accompanying cellulitis. Acute symptoms, intervention, or follow-up help differentiate these masses from tumors (Fig. 13-33).

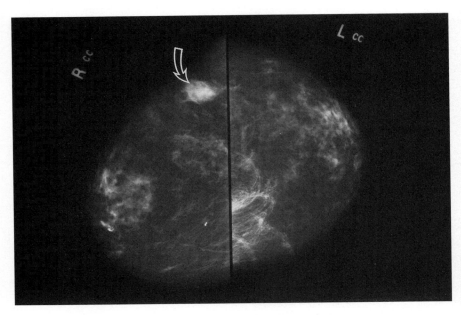

FIG. 13-32 *(Continued)* **B.** *CC view of the same breast localizes the focal abnormality (arrow) in the upper outer quadrant near the axillary tail. This is the ideal patient to evaluate with ultrasound in order to detect normal echogenic parenchymal tissue, which is the most likely explanation of the mammographic finding.*

Galactoceles

Galactoceles can be found in women who are breast feeding. They tend to be large cysts filled with fine particulate and homogeneous debris. At times the debris can be seen to move (Fig. 13-34).

Fat Lobules

There will be times when a hypoechoic fat lobule will be surrounded by echogenic fibroglandular tissue in a single image plane, and look exactly like a solid mass. Employing the old rules of ultrasound and imaging in

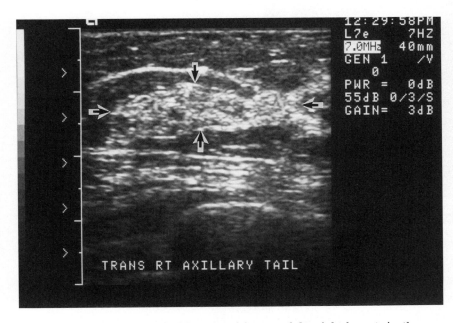

FIG. 13-32 *(Continued)* **C.** *Ultrasound image of the right breast, in the axillary tail, shows a volumetric region of echogenic fibroglandular tissue (arrows), that is similar in size, shape, and site to the mammographic asymmetric density. No other abnormal tissue was found in the entire broad area evaluated, that could explain the mammographic finding.*

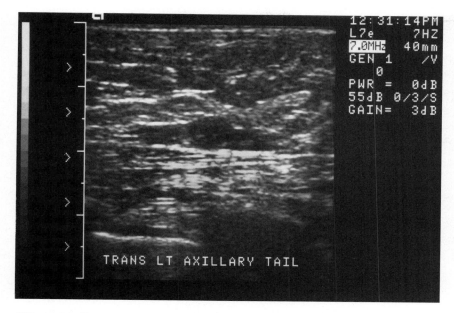

TRANS LT AXILLARY TAIL

FIG. 13-32 *(Continued)* **D.** *Ultrasound image of the contralateral site in the left breast shows only adipose tissue in the region of interest. The ultrasound findings here raise the confidence level that this lesion can be followed safely with mammography.*

a biplane fashion usually resolves the issue. When the probe is rotated around on a fat lobule, the lobule will become elongated and somewhat tubular in shape. It will also blend into the other adipose tissue in the breast (Fig. 13-35). Fat lobules rarely are completely surrounded by thick, echogenic fibroglandular tissue. This is unlike masses which are rounded or ovoid, and often completely surrounded by prominent parenchymal tissue.

Costal Cartilages

Visualization of costal cartilages is often a surprise for those new to breast ultrasound. A costal cartilage can be mistaken for a solid mass. The cartilaginous portions of the rib allow easy transmission of ultrasound, and hence, these structures can be imaged. When imaged in cross section, the costal cartilages appear as smoothly bordered, ovoid, hypoechoic, solid masses.

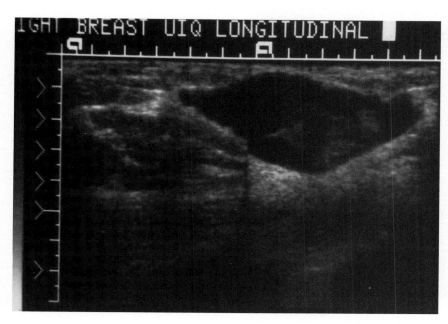

RIGHT BREAST UIQ LONGITUDINAL

FIG. 13-33 *A very large breast abscess is shown here. This complex mass, which is primarily cystic, with internal solid debris, was found in a woman with a severe mastitis that was unresponsive to antibiotics.*

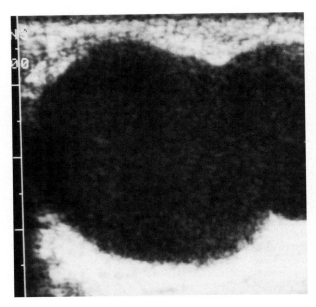

FIG. 13-34 *This is a galactocele in a lactating mother. It is filled with homogeneous internal debris that moved in real time. Note the sharply invaginating walls. Its bilobed appearance is caused by its relatively soft expansion against the stronger and less elastic fibrous structures that are common in the breast.*

They look very similar to a probably benign lesion such as a classic fibroadenoma.

The costal cartilage should not be mistaken for a solid mass. It should be identified as being in the structure of the chest wall, and not in breast tissue. When imaged in biplane fashion, the rib elongates and the bony portion shadows. The costal cartilage is commonly seen when scanning the medial aspect of the breast adjacent to the sternum.

Lymph Nodes

Lymph nodes will be found on occasion, although they are very difficult to identify in a fatty breast. When they are seen, they will be small, smooth, ovoid, hypoechoic masses with a central echogenic hilum. Their appearance is somewhat similar to a miniature kidney (Fig. 13-36).

With careful scanning, an internal blood vessel or two may be found with meticulous color Doppler imaging.

Lipomas

Rarely will one accidentally discover a lipoma in the breast, since the sonographic appearance of the texture of a lipoma is essentially identical to adipose tissue. There may be a subtle lack of internal architecture, such as thin septae. The lipoma has a very thin capsule which usually can be identified with sonography. This capsule can change shape with variable amounts of compression, or with scanning while simultaneously palpating the lipoma (Fig. 13-37).

Phyllodes Tumor

This uncommon tumor is often large and is generally benign. Sonography demonstrates a solid mass with

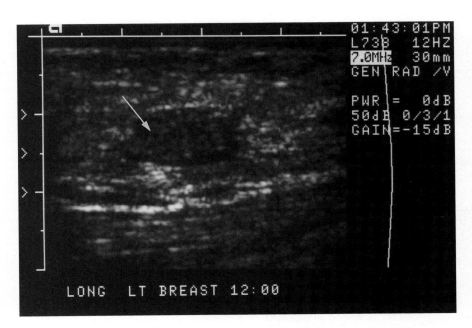

FIG. 13-35 *Fat lobule. **A.** In this longitudinal image, a hypoechoic fat lobule, accentuated by surrounding echogenic fibroglandular tissue, mimics a solid mass (arrow).*

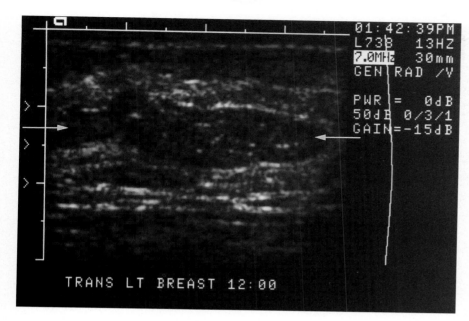

FIG. 13-35 *(Continued)* **B.** *In this transverse image of the same fat lobule, it can be seen to elongate in a tubular fashion, as it blends into the rest of the adipose tissue in the breast (arrows).*

well-defined borders and a variable appearance to its internal architecture. While there are times when the appearance is that of a non-specific solid mass, sometimes it can be seen as a complex mass with pockets of fluid mixed throughout its solid components. Rapid growth of a breast mass in a woman over 30 is suggestive of a phyllodes tumor. The rarely malignant one can only be identified by histology.[16]

Problem Areas

As already mentioned, the technical realities of ultrasound occasionally haunt the user. Breast lesions may not be seen, because either they were geographically missed or they were hidden by normal breast tissue. Cysts can be made to look like solid masses when there is too much receiver gain. Likewise, solid masses can

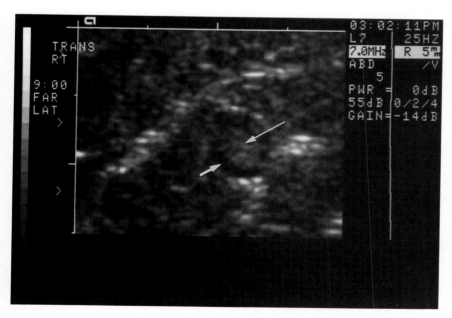

FIG. 13-36 *Normal intramammary lymph node. This small lymph node has a hypoechoic mantle (short arrow) surrounding an echogenic hilar region (long arrow). Note how subtle a finding it is in a fatty breast. It would be very easy to miss this lesion.*

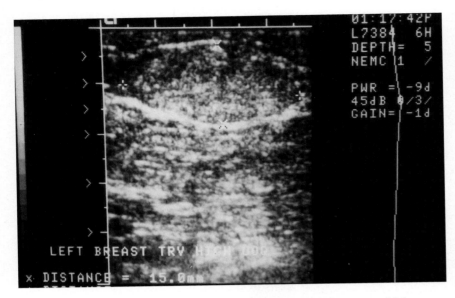

FIG. 13-37 *This encapsulated lipoma is a soft hypoechoic mass which measures 32 mm by 15 mm. It is identical in echo texture to the surrounding adipose tissue. The shape of this lipoma changed easily when compression was applied.*

be made to appear anechoic with too little gain. Visual reference should be made to the sonographic texture of the surrounding, recognizably normal, breast tissue, and technical factors must weigh in the decision.

Even when the low-level echoes in a solid mass are removed because of too little gain, a solid mass should not be mistaken for a cyst, if it is carefully evaluated. If a solid mass is made to appear anechoic, it may not have a good back wall and it may shadow somewhat. A cyst without increased through transmission will at least have neutral sound transmission. A cyst should not shadow. Resolution (or acceptance) of these problems resides in experience with real-time scanning.

SONOGRAPHICALLY GUIDED PROCEDURES WITH NEEDLES

There are many times when ultrasound can provide quick, reliable, and accurate guidance for the placement of needles into the breast for various types of interventional procedures. Cyst aspirations, needle localization of lesions for excisional biopsy, and percutaneous core biopsy of masses are being performed under ultrasound guidance with increasing frequency.

There is no right or wrong way to use ultrasound for needle guidance in the breast, and creative approaches can be taken. The two most critical factors are safety and accuracy. Whatever approach produces positive results with no complications is acceptable.

Creative positioning of the patient can be helpful in the successful placement of needles into breast lesions. We routinely have the patient hold her arm over her head. This compresses and stretches the breast offering firmer tissue for natural retraction in order to suppress mobility. We have found it helpful to use gravity in sticking a lesion, aiming the needle somewhat downwards and toward the floor. Positions where a needle is angled upwards and toward the ceiling, from underneath a lesion is against gravity, and it makes puncture difficult. The lesion tends to bounce around and deflect away from the needle tip, without being hit.

Ultrasound guidance can be done using a "freehand" technique or using a needle bracket. We do not use needle brackets in the breast where they tend to angle the needle towards the chest wall and possible danger. All of our procedures are done freehand with the radiologist performing the puncture by handling the probe with one hand and manipulating the needle with the other. I strive for the best approach that is as parallel as possible to both the chest wall, as well as the probe surface. An assistant operates the scanner controls.

"Homestyle" phantoms using turkey breasts and pimento stuffed olives have been described for a simple way of practicing ultrasound guided needle placement.[17]

Safety

Inserting needles into the breast is a very safe procedure and significant complications are rare. Nevertheless, both minor and major complications exist.

Minor complications relate to bleeding and infection. There is always the real but uncommon chance of a hematoma or sepsis after the insertion of any needle anywhere in the body, but this is usually a minor complication that can be easily treated. For breast cyst aspirations and pre-op needle localizations, the needles that are used are so thin (20 or 21 gauge) that they rarely cause problems. However the larger size of a core biopsy needle (15 gauge) makes bleeding and a hematoma more likely.

Major complications are very rare, but a pneumothorax remains a real possibility during a breast interventional procedure. Care must be taken not to puncture the chest wall deep to the retromammary fascia. Using ultrasound for guidance, this is usually not a problem with cyst aspirations and needle localizations, but it can be a problem with core biopsies. The easiest way to avoid a pneumothorax is to insert the needle parallel to the chest wall.

Skin Preparation

After the site has been scanned, the site selected for needle placement is marked. We also mark the position of the probe on the skin over the lesion for quick reference. We find it helpful to place the lesion about

one-third of the way from the edge of the image, in order to show a region of tissue being traversed by the needle.

The skin is then washed with Betadine and the skin is anesthetized with an intradermal injection of Xylocaine.

While many feel that Xylocaine is unnecessary, we prefer it for the ability to control pain from the beginning. It reduces patient anxiety when there is only one announced tiny needle stick, followed by momentary mild stinging, after which everything else is painless. This allows for repeated attempts after a failed placement. This is very important with core biopsies, where several different samples are taken, and a stab wound is made as well.

Non-sterile gel is applied to the end of the probe, which is then covered with a sterile cover of some sort. Sterile gel is then used for acoustical contact.

Accuracy

Constant visualization of the needle and its tip with ultrasound is the key to accurate placement of needles into the breast. The best way to see the length of the needle is when it is oriented parallel to the face of the probe and perpendicular to the ultrasound scan lines (Fig. 13-38). The more one angles the needle deeper to the face of the probe, the less chance there is of visualizing it (Fig. 13-39). As the needle becomes perpendicular to the chest wall and probe surface it becomes oriented parallel to the scan lines, and it will not be

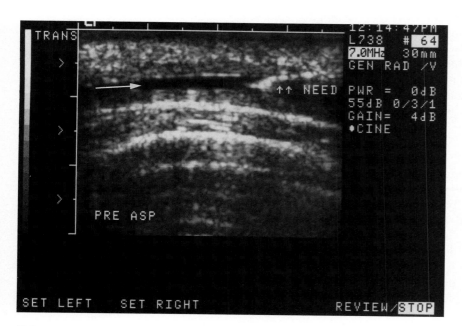

FIG. 13-38 *A thin postoperative seroma (long arrow) is being aspirated here. The needle (short arrows) was positioned as parallel to the face of the probe as possible. This position allowed visualization and accurate placement of the needle tip into this fluid collection that is only a few millimeters thick.*

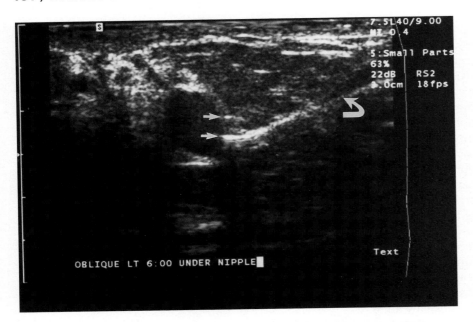

FIG. 13-39 *This is a needle localization prior to biopsy of a noncalcified mass. The needle is placed at an angle approaching 45 degrees to the face of the probe, and while it is identifiable (curved arrow), it is not clearly seen. The curved localizing wire of the Mammalok device is seen imbedded in the surface of the lesion in the region between 3 and 4 o'clock (short arrows). Histology revealed fibrocystic changes.*

seen. Only tissue motion will be seen. This may work in a needle localization, but it is dangerous with a core biopsy.

Keeping the needle parallel to the transducer surface improves safety as well as imaging accuracy (Fig. 13-40). It reduces the chance of pneumothorax, since the needle is more parallel to the chest wall.

Accuracy is important for successful cyst aspiration, especially with small cysts. Extreme accuracy is critical in core biopsies. Needle localizations require less accurate needle placement.

Cyst Aspiration

When aspirating a cyst, we use a 20 gauge needle, 40 mm in length, attached to a 5- or 10-cc syringe. Some people use vacutainers. Most cysts can be safely aspirated without inserting the needle parallel to the chest wall, and most can be reached with a shorter needle and some compression. A more sharply angled needle path into the center of the cyst may be used, with the needle inserted at a site just next to the probe. When a longer path is necessary, a 20 gauge spinal needle is used for its length of 9 cm.

The needle tip can be seen entering the cyst, and if the tip is kept at the center of the cyst, complications will be unlikely. Larger cysts are easy to aspirate, although a cyst often has a layer of very tough tissue sur-

rounding it. Smaller cysts in a fatty breast are more difficult to aspirate, and the needle can stick in the surrounding tissue, pushing the cyst deeper into the fatty breast without puncturing it. The situation is like bobbing for apples.

After we aspirate a cyst in the breast, the mammogram of that breast is repeated to confirm that the cyst has disappeared or is smaller, and also to establish a new baseline. If a hematoma develops, it can be temporally linked to the aspiration procedure and recognized as such. The development of a breast hematoma following cyst aspiration is quite rare.

There have been a couple of instances where we have seen fluid reaccumulate in a cyst, in real time, following a cyst aspiration. An immediate repeat aspiration has produced a similar quantity of fresh blood in the syringe. Manual compression was used afterwards to prevent further reaccumulation before the mammogram. We also have seen the same benign cyst reaccumulate in an interval after the repeat mammogram was taken. When a cyst is barely punctured and develops some bleeding into it, the cyst will become filled with echoes and can mimic a solid mass.

Needle Localization

Most needle localizations at our institution are done under mammographic guidance. However the use of

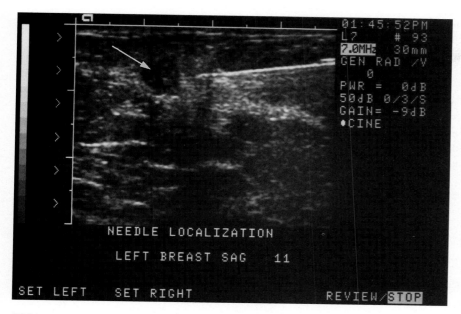

FIG. 13-40 *Needle localization of a small fibroadenoma. The Mammalok needle is very clearly seen since it is positioned so parallel to the surface of the probe. Firm tissue surrounding the lesion prevented closer placement of the needle tip into the lesion (arrow). This firm tissue may also make advancement of the curved end of the wire difficult.*

ultrasound for this purpose is becoming more common. We use whatever length Mammalok needle is appropriate.

The Mammalok is easiest to see when it is parallel to the probe surface. When these needles are placed, accuracy is not as critical as with cyst aspirations or core biopsy, since a volume of tissue surrounding the localizing wire will be surgically excised. Solid masses can be difficult to puncture. If the needle tip is placed into the lesion, it may be difficult to advance the wire. Sometimes the tissue surrounding a solid mass can offer great resistance to advancing the wire. It may be more helpful to try to get close to the lesion without entering it.

When we have localized a solid mass for surgical excision, we draw two simple diagrams of an AP and a lateral view of the breast showing the position of the curved wire and needle tip in relation to the tumor to be removed. This aids the surgeon in planning the approach to the mass. We send this diagram to the operating room with the patient. While presently we do not do specimen ultrasounds, this has been advocated by others.[18]

Core Biopsy

Core biopsies of presumed benign lesions can be performed under ultrasound guidance. Very small and very mobile lesions are difficult to puncture. Superficial lesions are also hard to puncture. Lesions against the chest wall raise the risk of pneumothorax. Masses less than 1 cm in diameter are usually our lower limit for a successful attempt at core biopsy. An automatic biopsy gun is used for core biopsies. At our institution we have been using a 15 gauge, 15-cm-long, Microvasive disposable core biopsy gun (Microvasive "ASAP with Channel Cut" Automatic 15 gauge core biopsy system, Boston Scientific Corporation, Watertown, MA). A shorter length of 10 cm would be adequate. When these automatic core biopsy devices are employed, one must remember that the needle tip will advance almost 2 cm further into the breast after the gun is fired. Here is where a pneumothorax can occur.

Core biopsies are more difficult than cyst aspirations and needle localizations. The patient is scanned, the lesion identified, and a puncture site is chosen and marked. The puncture site is chosen to allow needle placement along a path as parallel to both the chest wall and probe surface as possible. After the skin has been prepared, we make a small stab wound in the skin with a No. 11 scalpel blade. The needle is then advanced through the stab wound into the breast parallel to the chest wall to a site estimated to be close to the lesion, without using ultrasound guidance. Once the needle has been placed into the estimated region of the lesion, ultrasound guidance is then used to see the length of the needle approach the lesion. I will not fire the biopsy gun until I see the needle elongated and I am confident that the needle tip is being imaged. Once the tip is identified at the surface of the lesion, I press the needle gently and firmly into the lesion and fire. This pressure at the end helps to puncture the lesion and assists in preventing the deflection of the lesion away from the needle when it is fired. It is helpful to place the needle tip perpendicular to the tangent of the lesion. This also reduces deflection of the lesion away from the needle.

We try to obtain three good samples from various sites in the lesion. The sample is placed in a sterile jar filled with sterile saline. If the core sinks in the saline, we consider the procedure successful. If it floats, we consider this to be fat and we will repeat the procedure.

REFERENCES

1. Venta LA, Dudiak CM, Salomon CG, et al. Sonographic evaluation of the breast. Radiographics **14**:29–50, 1994.
2. Sickles EA, Filly RA, Callen PW. Breast cancer detection with sonography and mammography: Comparison of state-of-the-art equipment. AJR **140**:843–845, 1982.
3. Jackson VP. The role of US in breast imaging. Radiology **177**:305–311, 1990.
4. Parker SH, Jobe WE, Dennis MA, et al. US-guided automated large-core breast biopsy. Radiology **187**:507–511, 1993.
5. Sickles EA, Filly RA, Callen PW. Benign breast lesions: Ultrasound detection and diagnosis. Radiology **151**:467–470, 1984.
6. Homer MJ, Doherty FJ. Evaluation and management of the solitary asymmetric breast density. Breast Disease **2**:175–186, 1989.
7. Bassett LW, Kimme-Smith C. Breast sonography. AJR **156**:449–455, 1991.
8. Spencer GM, Rubens DJ, Roach DJ. Hypoechoic fat: A sonographic pitfall. AJR **164**:1277–1280, 1995.
9. Fornage BD, Lorigan JG, Andry E. Fibroadenoma of the breast: Sonographic appearance. Radiology **172**:671–675, 1989.
10. Cosgrove DO, Kedar RP, Bamber JC, et al. Breast diseases: Color Doppler US in differential diagnosis. Radiology **189**:99–104, 1993.
11. Kedar RP, Cosgrove DO, Smith IE, et al. Breast carcinoma: Measurement of tumor response to primary medical therapy with color Doppler imaging. Radiology **190**:825–830, 1994.
12. Kedar RP, Cosgrove D, McCready VR, et al. Microbubble contrast agent for color Doppler US: Effect on breast masses. Radiology **198**:679–686, 1996.
13. Hilton SvH, Leopold GR, Olson LK, et al. Real-time breast sonography: Application in 300 consecutive patients. AJR **147**:479–486, 1985.
14. Stavros AT, Thickman D, Rapp CL, et al. Solid breast nodules: Use of sonography to distinguish between benign and malignant lesions. Radiology **196**:123–134, 1995.
15. Jackson VP. Management of solid breast nodules: What is the role of sonography? Radiology **196**:14–15, 1995.
16. Mendelson EB: Breast sonography, in Rumack CM, Wilson SR, Charbonneau JW (eds): *Diagnostic Ultrasound.* Mosby-Year Book, Inc., St. Louis, 1991, pp 541–563.
17. Georgian Smith D, Shiels WE. Freehand interventional sonography in the breast: Basic principles and clinical applications. Radiographics **16**:149–161, 1996.
18. Fornage BD, Ross MI, Singletary SE, et al. Localization of impalpable breast masses: Value of sonography in the operating room and scanning of excised specimens. AJR **163**:569–573, 1994.

Chapter 14

NEEDLE LOCALIZATION: TECHNICAL ASPECTS, NEEDLE CHOICES, AND EXPECTATIONS

TECHNICAL ASPECTS _____

Patient Status

The transformation of excision for a nonpalpable breast lesion from a major surgical procedure to a minor one reflects the confidence that has developed between the radiologist and surgeon. Prior to 1976 at NEMCH, all biopsies for nonpalpable breast lesions were performed on an inpatient basis under general anesthesia. The only guide to direct the surgeon to the lesion was his or her estimation of its distance from the nipple. Since the geometry of the breast on upright compression mammograms bears little resemblance to the supine breast on the operating table, it is understandable why large excisions often were necessary to guarantee removal of the mammographic abnormality. Within 6 years, we converted the procedure to one performed as outpatient surgery under local anesthesia, almost always using a needle-wire localizer system to guide the surgeon to the area of concern.[1] There are some exceptions to our standard method.

We may not perform needle localization for a superficial lesion located within a few millimeters of the skin. Instead the precise location of the lesion is determined preoperatively by radioopaque markers, and this point is marked on the skin.

In certain circumstances, general anesthesia rather than local anesthesia is used. Patients who require general anesthesia fall into one of three categories. The first category reflects surgical preference. When a lesion is deeply located and near the chest wall, especially in a large-breasted patient, the surgeon might prefer the use of general anesthesia, which would provide better control during deep dissection. The second category reflects patient cooperation. Absolute patient cooperation is essential for a breast biopsy performed under local anesthesia, since the woman must remain correctly positioned during the entire operation. The two groups of patients in which this cooperation cannot be guaranteed are foreign-speaking women when a translator is not present and women with mental retardation. The third category reflects patient preference. There are women who absolutely refuse to allow themselves to have a breast biopsy unless they are "sleeping." When the woman demands general anesthesia despite being told how the procedure is routinely performed at our institution under local anesthesia and despite being told about the increased cost and potential morbidity associated with general anesthesia, her preference is respected. The three categories where general rather than local anesthesia is used constitute less than 5 percent of our cases. General anesthesia may be administered on either an inpatient or outpatient basis.

Needle versus Dye Injection

Dye injection localization techniques have never been used at NEMCH and therefore will not be discussed. This does not necessarily reflect the superiority of needle localization over dye injection, since success with dye localization techniques has been reported by others.[2] Perhaps the two most important points for success with dye technique are to avoid overinjection and to minimize the time between injection and surgery, decreasing the potential for dye diffusion.

Surgical Approach

There are two primary surgical approaches to the nonpalpable breast lesion. When the lesion is rather superficially located, some surgeons prefer to cut down directly upon the localizing needle-wire system to the area of concern. The second alternative is making an incision at a site distant from the point of needle entry, tunneling through the breast tissue to approach the localizing guide, and then following the guide down to the lesion. The tissue and localizing wire are removed through the surgical incision. Especially when the lesion is in the subareolar region, an approach via a circumareolar incision should leave the woman with excellent cosmesis. At NEMCH, the surgeon's task is helped by the fact that we leave a 20-gauge palpable needle in place anchored with a curved wire so that the lesion can be easily located. Dissecting toward a nonpalpable breast lesion from a distant site is much more difficult with systems that leave only a thin wire in place to serve as the guide.

Needle Approach

Radiologists have their own personal preferences for the path of needle insertion. Some approach all lesions parallel to the chest wall, while others use a perpendicular path. Some only approach via the shortest distance to the lesion. Many radiologists use a grid localizer device, while others rely on skin markers. What is of paramount importance is not one's bias but the accuracy of the results, specifically the final distance between the localizing device and the lesion. My own practice is to approach all lesions parallel to the chest wall with slight angulation. The needle enters superiorly, inferiorly, or laterally as the case requires, and I use skin markers to determine the point of needle insertion. The technique I use has been described in detail previously.[3,4] I do not necessarily insert the needle via the shortest distance to the lesion if I can achieve greater accuracy by using another path. As a general rule, my goal is for the distance between the lesion and the localizing guide to be no greater than 5 mm. However, in an extremely large breast, a greater distance may be quite acceptable if the resulting cosmesis will be unaffected.

Localization versus Aspiration of Breast Lesions

From the radiologist's point of view, there are distinct differences between a breast localization and aspiration procedure. Perfect accuracy is required for aspiration, since the lesion itself must be sampled. While similar accuracy is desirable for needle localization, this is not mandatory, since the real goal of surgery is not simply to sample the lesion but to excise it along with a margin of normal surrounding tissue. Therefore, the needle must be close to the lesion but does not necessarily have to skewer it. Another important difference between localization and aspiration is defining the success of the procedure. With aspiration, the procedure is over when diagnostic tissue is obtained and the radiologist is a "hero." Even if no diagnosis can be made from the tissue obtained from aspiration, the procedure is still over. However, the end point is much different for a needle localization. Success should not be measured by the accuracy of the needle-wire placement but by whether the lesion has been successfully sampled or removed.

At NEMCH, the team concept in breast disease management also applies to the localization procedure. When the localization fails, everyone fails. In the final analysis, it matters little to the woman whether the localization wire could have been placed closer to the lesion or whether there was an error in surgical technique. The lesion is still within the breast, and the woman must once again return to both the radiologist and surgeon for repeat localization and excision.

NEEDLE CHOICE

Standard Needles

Over the years there has been an evolution in the types of needle-wire systems used for breast localization. Prior to 1976, there were no specialized breast localizing needle-wire systems and only standard needles were available for localization. Standard needles are the most inexpensive type of needle to use, and some radiologists still continue to successfully use them.[5] However, many radiologists experienced the problem of needle movement between the time the woman left the radiology department and the time the biopsy was performed on the operating table. Since the standard needle is not anchored, the relationship between the needle and the lesion depicted by postlocalization mammograms may be different at surgery.

Hooked Needles

In 1976 a breast needle-wire localizer system was created.[6] This hook-wire provided an anchor in the breast so that for the first time the surgeon had a fixed guide to follow (Fig. 14-1). This was a major improvement, and many radiologists, myself included,[7] used this device. As experience was gained with this system, some problems became apparent. First, once the wire was deployed out of the needle, it could not be repositioned. If the placement was inaccurate, a second or even third needle had to be inserted. This proved awkward for the radiologist, patient, and surgeon. Second, since the wire was so thin, it could not be palpated in the breast. This made surgical dissection difficult. Finally, because the wire was so thin, it easily could be inadvertently transected during dissection.[8] If this occurred, not only would the surgeon lose his direction toward the lesion, which could cause him to fail to excise it, but the transected wire fragment might not be successfully retrieved from the breast. This retained fragment can cause serious problems such as migration to areas outside mammary tissue. These hooked fragments have been reported to migrate as far away as the supraclavicular fossa.[9]

In 1980 another needle-wire localizer system was created—the spring-hook wire.[10] The major advantage afforded by this system was the ability to reposition the needle as many times as necessary in order to achieve accurate localization before anchoring the wire in the breast (Fig. 14-2). However, problems became apparent with this system. Since the wire was so thin, it was still nonpalpable, making surgical dissection difficult. This thinness also resulted in the continued pitfall of inadvertent transection. In an attempt to at least partially overcome the possibility of transection, modification of this wire has been created by thickening a portion of the distal end of the wire. Other attempts to eliminate wire transection, such as using a stiffening needle,[11] have been proposed but have not achieved widespread acceptance.

The Curved "J" Wire

In 1985 the "J"-tipped curved-end retractable wire (Homer Mammalok, MD TECH, Gainesville, Florida 32608) was introduced.[12] The three components of this system are a 20-gauge needle, a radiolucent stabilization device, and a memory wire (Fig. 14-3). The wire is

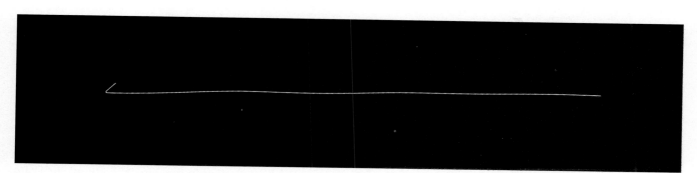

FIG. 14-1 *This is a hook wire created in 1976. The hook remains external to the localizing needle.*

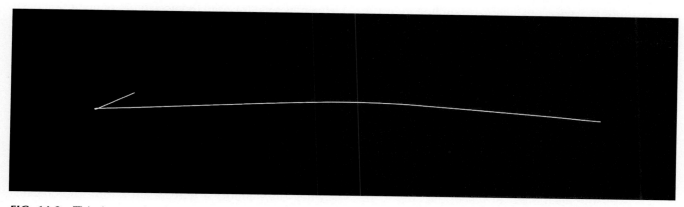

FIG. 14-2 *This is a spring-hook wire. The spring hook is not deployed until the needle is in proper position.*

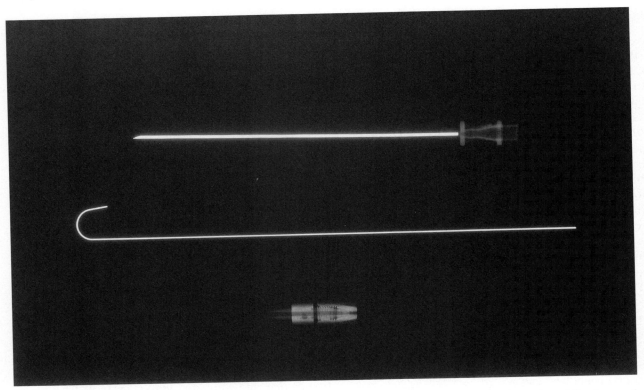

FIG. 14-3 *The three components of the Mammalok system are a 20-gauge needle, a curved memory "J" wire, and a stabilizer.*

made of a nitinol alloy, giving it unique characteristics. The memory J end of the wire allows it to be pushed out and pulled back into the needle as many times as necessary for repositioning. The memory J shape repeatedly reforms (Fig. 14-4). It should be noted that the J end is not floppy but has a significant strength to it, which serves as the anchoring force for the system. Each time the J is out of the needle, the system is anchored in the breast, allowing the technologist to more easily obtain postlocalization films, since she no longer has to worry about accidentally moving an unanchored needle. The radiologist can reposition the system by simply retracting the J wire, redirecting the needle, and pushing the wire out again to anchor it in the breast. For radiologists who need to inject dye, this can also be accomplished through the needle while the J is still anchoring the system in breast parenchyma (Fig. 14-5). Since the J-tipped end of the wire covers the needle bevel, both the needle and wire can be safely left in place. The nitinol alloy is firm and especially with the needle left in place is virtually nontransectable.

Leaving both the needle and wire in place is the recommended way to use the device because it affords distinct advantages to both the radiologist and surgeon.[13] With the needle left in place, the step of removing it has been eliminated so there is no need to

obtain additional films to document the final relationship between the wire and the lesion. Thus the length of the procedure is shortened and there is less radiation to the breast. Additionally, by leaving the 20-gauge needle in place, the surgeon now has a *palpable*, anchored, virtually nontransectable guide to direct him to the nonpalpable mammographic abnormality (Fig. 14-6).

The anchoring strength of the J wire has been reported to be sufficient in the clinical setting. One point to be aware of is that in very fat-replaced breasts, any wire, regardless of the configuration of its tip, may not be anchored firmly in parenchyma and special caution must be paid to avoid the possibility of migration or retraction.[14]

Especially when the surgeon is initially unfamiliar with the Mammalok system, it is prudent to take time to review its features with him. One important piece of information to make the surgeon aware of is that when both the needle and wire are left in place, there is never any need to pull on the system. Surgeons have a habit of pulling on a localizing wire because they are attempting to straighten out the thin, nonpalpable wire in order to avoid accidentally transecting it. Others use a localizing wire as a retractor and pull on it. However, when the memory J wire is left within the 20-gauge needle, it maintains a straight course so that there is

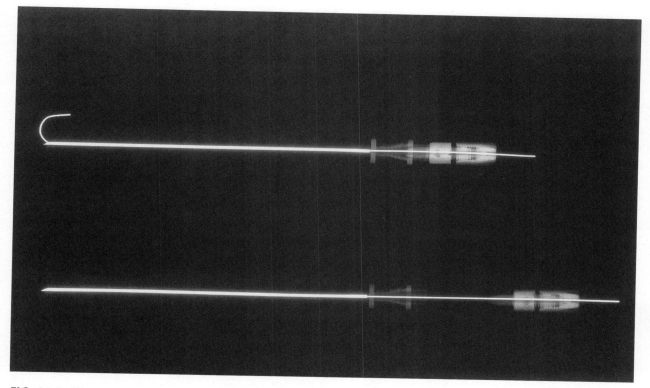

FIG. 14-4 *The top assembly shows the "J" out of the needle in the position that anchors the device in the breast. The bottom assembly shows the "J" wire retracted into the needle in the position for insertion or repositioning.*

never reason to pull on the system. Communicating this important point to the surgeon should eliminate the chance of forcefully pulling the system out of a fat-replaced breast. Sometimes, especially in a dense breast, the surgeon who approaches the system from a distant incision might not be able to palpate the needle

within the breast tissue. The location of the needle can be identified by moving the visible needle hub back and forth. Once again, the important technical point is that there is no reason to ever pull on the system.

A final advantage of leaving both the needle and wire in place is for the radiologist. Since the surgeon

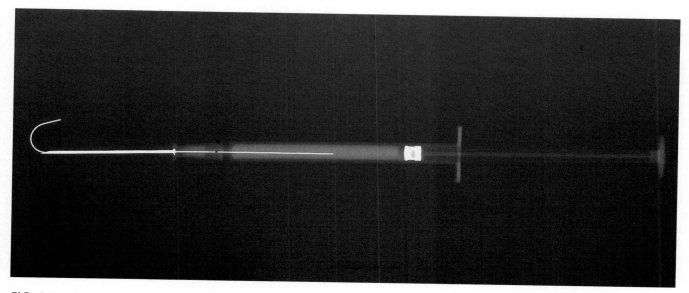

FIG. 14-5 *If the lesion is positioned at the needle tip, dye can be injected to color the site of the mammographic abnormality.*

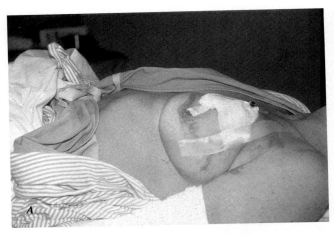

FIG. 14-6   A. *The patient is lying supine on the table in the operating room. The nurse has removed a top covering gauze. The needle hub and stabilizer are visible.*

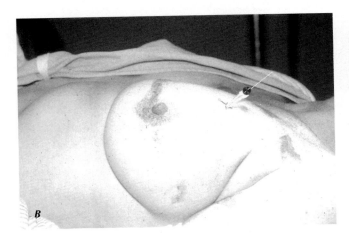

FIG. 14-6 *(Continued)*   **B.** *The bottom gauze has been removed. Notice there is no tape present. Unless the breast is extremely fatty, tape is not used to secure the Mammalok device to the skin. The "J" wire locks the system in place.*

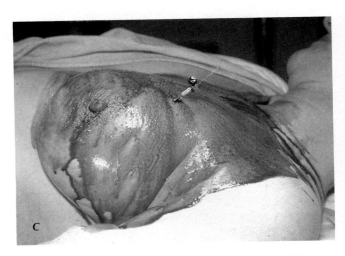

FIG. 14-6 *(Continued)*   **C.** *The skin is cleaned with Betadine prior to surgery.*

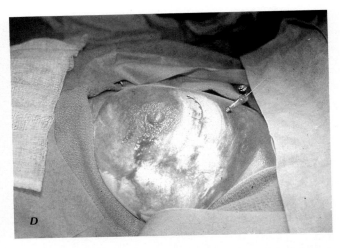

FIG. 14-6 *(Continued)*   **D.** *The surgeon has chosen his site of approach distant from the point of entry of the needle. He will dissect down and intersect the palpable needle.*

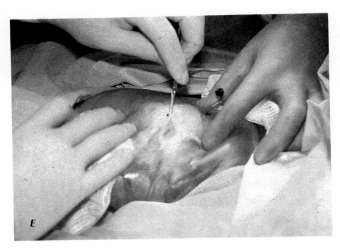

FIG. 14-6 *(Continued)*   **E.** *The surgical incision is made.*

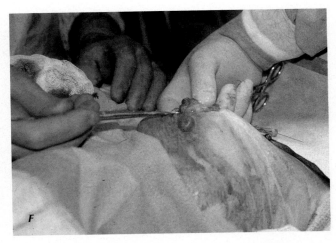

FIG. 14-6 *(Continued)*   **F.** *The breast tissue containing the lesion is being isolated by using the palpable needle as a guide.*

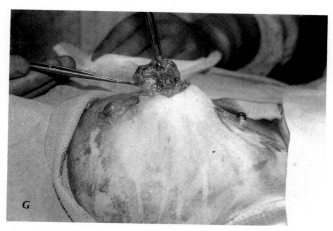

FIG. 14-6 *(Continued)* **G.** *The tissue containing the nonpalpable mammographic abnormality has been isolated and is ready to be excised.*

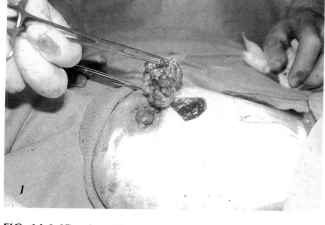

FIG. 14-6 *(Continued)* **J.** *The tissue is then delivered with the "J" wire left in situ.*

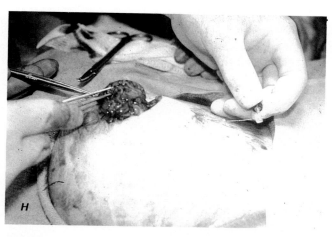

FIG. 14-6 *(Continued)* **H.** *The palpable needle has served its purpose and is no longer required. The stabilizer is unscrewed and discarded.*

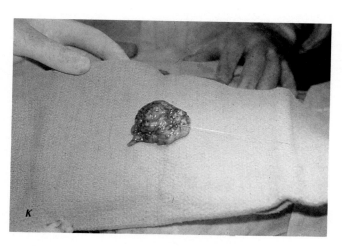

FIG. 14-6 *(Continued)* **K.** *The specimen with the wire left in situ is ready to be brought to radiology for specimen radiography.*

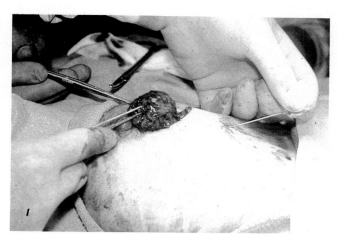

FIG. 14-6 *(Continued)* **I.** *The needle is pulled out of the breast and discarded.*

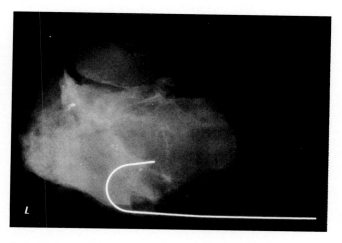

FIG. 14-6 *(Continued)* **L.** *Specimen radiography confirms excision of a solitary cluster of microcalcifications. Histology revealed benign sclerosing adenosis. (Courtesy of Thomas J. Smith, M.D., Boston, MA.)*

has a palpable needle to guide him to the depth of the lesion, there is no need to have the lesion directly at the needle tip. The surgeon can now relate the location of the lesion to its position along the needle length. This makes localization much easier for the radiologist (Fig. 14-7). Of course, if one injects dye, it is still necessary to have the lesion positioned at the needle tip.

I believe that a breast specialty needle should provide a palpable, anchored, nontransectable system that can be repositioned and provide the option of dye injection. The ability to have the device anchored during filming is another feature that eases the technologist's job. My experience with the Mammalok system, using

it in several hundred localizations since 1985, confirms that it possesses all of these characteristics. Undoubtedly, new breast needle designs will be created, and hopefully they will incorporate the characteristics described above.

EXPECTATIONS

Failure Rate

I have published three separate series documenting my failure rate for excising the mammographic abnormality. Using a hooked-wire localizer system, my failure rate was 10 percent.[3] After converting to the Mammalok curved-end retractable wire system, it has decreased to 4 percent[14] and subsequently to 2 percent.[15] In other words, we are now successful in excising or sampling a nonpalpable abnormality in 98 percent of cases.

Very few procedures are perfect. I used to be amazed when I was told that some people have a 100 percent success rate for excising a nonpalpable mammographic abnormality on the first attempt. While my

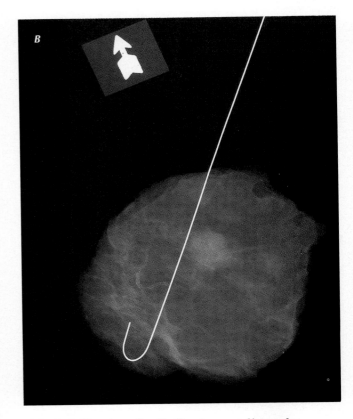

FIG. 14-7 A. A 1-cm nonpalpable noncalcified solid mass was localized by needle prior to surgery. The lesion abuts the distal end of the needle but is not at the tip of the needle.

FIG. 14-7 (Continued) B. Specimen radiography confirms excision. Generous margins were purposefully taken because of the high probability that the lesion would be malignant. Histology revealed intraductal carcinoma extending to the surgical margins. Reexcision was still required.

rate of 98 percent is one that we are proud of at NEMCH, 100 percent is clearly better. However, if one takes the time to view the specimen radiographs, it often becomes clear why someone can have a 100 percent success rate. The specimen radiographs usually show that a huge volume of breast tissue, sometimes approaching the size of a quadrantectomy, needed to be excised. Our success at NEMCH could also be 100 percent if large-volume biopsies were done, but in my institution the volume of excised tissue is kept quite small. However, one cannot judge the accuracy of localization by biopsy volume without relating it to the patient's breast size. While excising a particular volume of breast tissue may be appropriate for a large-breasted woman, leaving her with an excellent cosmetic result, the same size may be very deforming in the small-breasted woman. Since most of the nonpalpable lesions prove to be benign, our goal is not only to excise or sample the lesion but also to leave the woman with an acceptable cosmetic result.

True-Positive Biopsy Rate

In most series the true-positive biopsy rate for excised nonpalpable breast lesions ranges between 15 to 30 percent.[16] This range reflects all lesions biopsied regardless of their mammographic appearance. Data exist establishing the predictive value of lesions with specific mammographic features.[17]

The reported experience in this country with a 15 to 30 percent true-positive rate suggests that if a radiologist has a much lower rate, he is probably being much more aggressive with biopsies, while if one's rate is considerably higher, one is using more stringent criteria for selecting lesions with characteristics giving them a high probability of being malignant. While a 15 to 30 percent true-positive rate is not necessarily the ideal, it is useful for it provides a yardstick for comparison between radiologists. One can easily alter the rate by changing criteria for what triggers a biopsy.

The Biopsy of a Benign Lesion

An important issue verbalized by many radiologists is the guilt, often instigated by the referring clinician, some feel when an asymptomatic woman is subjected to surgery based upon a mammographic finding from a screening mammogram which proves to be benign. Would not the woman have been better off not to have had the mammogram in the first place? Is not the radiologist wrong to have triggered the biopsy? These are important questions that each radiologist doing mammography inevitably confronts and must deal with.

I believe that I am just as wrong for triggering a localization and biopsy for a mammographic abnormality that proves to be benign as is the surgeon who rec-

ommends biopsy for a palpable mass that proves to be benign. A surgeon would reply that he or she is not wrong for performing a biopsy on a woman with a palpable mass, since by surgical criteria he or she had concern that it could be cancer and the mass had to be excised. Why does this differ from what I do if the woman has a mammographic abnormality with radiographic criteria of concern because it could be cancer? In fact, the true-positive rate for finding cancer in palpable masses is virtually identical to the rate for finding cancer in nonpalpable mammographic abnormalities.[18] Radiologists are doing no better and no worse in finding cancer than are our surgical colleagues. Why should we be held to a different standard? Why should mammographic images be required to yield a better true-positive rate than palpating fingers? If a 15 to 30 percent true-positive rate for finding cancer is considered acceptable for the surgeon, it should be considered acceptable for the radiologist. Add this to the fact that as a group, nonpalpable cancers found by mammography are generally discovered at an earlier, smaller stage than are the palpable cancers, giving more favorable odds for survival and increased alternatives to mastectomy such as BCT.

If this problem is one that still exists in your clinical practice, then I suggest that you pay a visit to your pathology department and ask your pathologist to pull the reports for the last 100 consecutive breast biopsies performed for palpable lesions at your hospital. You will discover that the surgical rate for finding cancer is comparable to the mammographic rate. Also, you will probably notice that your surgeon is subjecting very young women (under the age of 30) to biopsy for palpable lesions even though the prevalence of breast cancer at this age is low. No organization would even propose routine mammographic screening of women under the age of 30. Finally, don't be at all surprised if the rate for finding cancer in palpable lesions at your hospital is considerably lower than 15 percent. Armed with these data, you should be able to mount a logical explanation for your position that you are no more wrong than is the surgeon for causing a biopsy for what proves to be a benign mammographic abnormality.

Forcing Biopsies for a Nonpalpable Mammographic Abnormality

One other criticism that radiologists have made me aware of is that they are accused of forcing the surgeon to biopsy a lesion even if it has a low chance of being malignant. In the section devoted to mammographic reporting, I have presented the verbiage of my own "neutral" report, which describes the mammographic abnormality and provides the surgeon with equal options of biopsy or followup. The ultimate choice should not be forced by the radiologist but should rather result from the interaction between the patient and her physician. An analogy with another organ may better illustrate this point. Assume that you have undergone a barium enema for a vague lower abdominal pain of recent onset. You have no other signs or symptoms of disease. Also assume that the pain spontaneously disappears after the barium enema and you feel fine. You then meet with your gastroenterologist, who informs you that the enema is essentially normal except for the incidental finding of a solitary 5-mm smoothly contoured mass on a tiny stalk in your right colon. He proceeds to inform you that based upon its appearance, it has more than a 95 percent chance of being a benign polyp. Nevertheless, a management decision is necessary. Your gastroenterologist tells you that you can have another barium enema within 6 months to document stability of the probable benign polyp, and if it does not grow, it can be followed by periodic barium study. Or you could undergo a colonoscopy. He tells you that a colonoscopy can be a rather uncomfortable procedure and may even fail to reach the area in the right colon. However, if it is successful and the mass can be reached, perhaps it can be snared and excised. With more than 95 percent probability, it should prove to be a benign polyp, but if it is a cancer, then the very biopsy may be curative. I submit that the decision that you make has nothing to do with the radiologist who performed your barium enema. The decision depends upon your anxiety level, your physician's anxiety level, and the general philosophic approach that you have about a "lesion with a high probability of being benign."

The polyp example is analogous to mammography. When I discover a solitary geographic cluster of four punctate microcalcifications without an associated mass density, my experience tells me that there is less than a 5 percent chance of it representing cancer. The two choices that my mammography report offers are excision or follow-up. As the radiologist, I am equally comfortable with each because I know that both are correct management options. In this situation, I do not use my report to force one choice or the other upon the patient or her surgeon. If the referring clinician wants the radiologist to commit to a specific recommendation in every report, I have no problem with this, since recommendations constitute an appropriate component of a consultant's evaluation and the radiologist is a consultant.[19]

Women react to the need for a decision in one of four ways. Some women, without hesitation, will want the biopsy either because it is most important for them to eliminate any possibility of cancer or because their anxiety level cannot tolerate follow-up. Others will opt for follow-up because they understand that it is an acceptable choice and want to avoid a biopsy. Some leave to seek other opinions, and I believe this too is a healthy option. Finally, some women turn to the surgeon and rather than make the choice for themselves prefer to have the choice made for them. In none of these four cases do I as the radiologist enter into the final decision-making process. My role was to find the abnormality, recognize that it could represent an early breast carcinoma, and convey to the clinician through my report a sense of the probability that the specific mammographic characteristics of the abnormality are associated with malignancy. I believe that the radiologist must be sensitive to the wishes of the referring clinician. Ideally, together they should create a report to provide the clinician and patient with the appropriate flexibility necessary in choosing between management options.

REFERENCES

1. Homer MJ, Smith TJ, Marchant DJ. Outpatient needle localization and biopsy for nonpalpable breast lesions. JAMA **252**:2452–2454, 1984.
2. Hermann G, Janus C, Schwartz IS, et al. Nonpalpable breast lesions: accuracy of prebiopsy mammographic diagnosis. Radiology**165**:323–326, 1987.
3. Homer MJ, Localization of nonpalpable breast lesions: technical aspects and analysis of 80 cases. AJR **140**:807–811, 1985.
4. Homer MJ. Preoperative needle localization of lesions in the lower half of the breast: needle entry from below. AJR **149**:43–45, 1987.
5. Feig SA. Localization of clinically occult breast lesions. Radiol Clin North Am **21**:155–171, 1983.
6. Frank HA, Hall FM, Steer ML. Preoperative localization of nonpalpable breast lesions demonstrated by mammography. N Engl J Med **295**:259–260, 1976.
7. Homer MJ. Percutaneous localization of breast lesions: experience with the Frank breast biopsy guide. J Can Assoc Radiol **30**:238–241, 1979.
8. Homer MJ. Transection of the localization hooked wire during breast biopsy. AJR **141**:929–930, 1983.
9. Davis PS, Wechsler RJ, Feig SA, et al. Migration of breast biopsy localization wire. AJR **150**:787–788, 1988.
10. Kopans DB, Deluca SA. A modified needle hook-wire technique to simplify preoperative localization of occult breast lesions. Radiology **134**:781, 1980.
11. Homer MJ, Fisher DM, Sugarman HJ. Postlocalization needle for breast biopsy of nonpalpable lesions. Radiology **140**:241–242, 1981.
12. Homer MJ. Nonpalpable breast lesion localization

using a curved-end retractable wire. Radiology **157**:259–260, 1985.

13. Homer MJ. Localization of nonpalpable breast lesions with the curved-end retractable wire: leaving the needle in vivo. AJR **151**:919–920, 1988.

14. Homer MJ, Pile-Spellman ER. Needle localization of occult breast lesions with a curved-end retractable wire: technique and pitfalls. Radiology **161**:547–548, 1986.

15. Kaelin CM, Smith TJ, Homer MJ, et al. Safety, accuracy, and diagnostic yield of needle localization biopsy of the breast performed using local anesthesia. J Am Coll Surg **179**:267–272, 1994.

16. Homer MJ. Nonpalpable breast abnormalities: a realistic view of the accuracy of mammography in detecting malignancies. Radiology **153**:831–832, 1984.

17. Moskowitz M. Minimal breast cancer redux. Radiol Clin North Am **21**:93–113, 1983.

18. Spivey GH, Percy BW, Clark VA, et al. Predicting the risk of cancer at the time of breast biopsy: variation in the benign-to-malignant ratio. Am Surg **48**:326–332, 1982.

19. Homer MJ. A radiologist's point of view. JAMA **246**:2581–2582, 1981.

Chapter 15

NEEDLE LOCALIZATION: PITFALLS

Except for very superficially located mammographic abnormalities, it is my practice to perform preoperative percutaneous needle localization for all nonpalpable breast lesions. As stated previously, since I have never used dye injection localization techniques, they will not be discussed. Though percutaneous needle localization is a relatively straightforward procedure, several potential pitfalls exist. Five major categories will be discussed (Table 15-1).

LESION SELECTION

The Pseudolesion

Before localizing a lesion, the radiologist should be absolutely certain that the lesion is real and that its location in the breast is clear. If both of these determinations are not certain, localization should not be performed. In order to determine whether a lesion is real or represents a pseudolesion, an overlap of normal breast tissue which makes it appear as a single density, additional views may be required, as was discussed in Chap. 6. Unfortunately, I am no longer surprised that some radiologists perform needle localization of a density even though they are not absolutely certain that it

TABLE 15-1
PITFALLS OF NEEDLE LOCALIZATION

1. Lesion selection
2. Patient problems
3. Wire problems
4. Communication
5. Specimen radiography

is real. Excuses for doing this include, "My partner ordered the localization and I cannot really cancel it" or "The surgeon and operating room are waiting, and it would cause problems to stop the procedure at this time." I feel strongly about something that should be obvious; a patient should not be subjected to surgery unless there is a real indication for it. The primary responsibility for the procedure, with all its consequences, belongs to the radiologist performing the localization and not the one who initially recommended it. If you are not certain where the lesion is located or whether it is real, what will you do when the specimen radiograph is handed to you to determine whether it has been successfully excised? There is a lesson to learn from an examination such as the intraoperative cholangiogram. When the films come from the operating room, the surgeon on the other end of the telephone is not interested in excuses. He simply wants to know if the study is normal or not. Similarly, when the surgeon sends breast tissue from the operating room to determine whether the lesion has been excised, the only question to be answered is, Has the area been excised or not? You had better not answer that you are not certain because you were never convinced that there was anything really there in the first place.

I have two suggestions for avoiding the unenviable situation of having to perform a needle localization for a pseudolesion. First, when an area of concern is seen on a mammogram on only one view but is not positively identified on the other view, the radiologist's report should not recommend biopsy but should recommend additional views to further assess the presence of a significant abnormality and to establish its location. Second, the surgeon must be made aware of your policy (which you should institute) that in order to avoid a potential problem, films must be reviewed in advance with the radiologist who will actually be performing the procedure. Can you imagine any surgeon willing to schedule surgery prior to his own review of a case? Why should we as radiologists allow surgeons to commit us to an interventional procedure without prior review of the case? Not only is this review common courtesy, but it is also appropriate patient care. In the past, I too had been confronted with such problems and have decided that it was important to fight the battle. If you do not choose to fight, and in this case "right" is on your side, then you will deservedly be held accountable for the consequences.

Identifying the Lesion on Only One View

There are techniques for localizing lesions which are seen on only one view[1] using only mammography. I have never localized lesions seen on only one view, and I prefer to resort to ultrasound or CT to localize. However, there is nothing incorrect about localizing a mammographic abnormality seen on only one view as long as the radiologist is absolutely convinced that it is a real lesion.

Mistaking Dermal Calcium for Parenchymal Calcium

The topic of dermal calcium has been thoroughly covered in Chap. 6. The dangers of not recognizing the dermal location of calcium are that the woman will be subjected to needless surgery, and the surgery will fail to excise the calcium unless the surgeon is instructed to remove the dermal layer along with deeper breast tissue (Fig. 15-1).

FIG. 15-1 *The lucent center in some of the calcifications in this cluster is the clue to their dermal location. Once they are proven to be dermal with the appropriate technique, biopsy is unnecessary.*

Decreasing Lesion Size

If a lesion decreases in size with time, localization and biopsy can be deferred, since breast cancer does not spontaneously decrease in size (Fig. 15-2). Probably, such a sequence of events represents a cyst undergoing spontaneous decompression. However, one must be certain that the lesion has not been aspirated between examinations because this may account for the decrease in volume.

Tight compression may rupture a superficially located cyst.[2] If the lesion being localized decreases in volume between compression views, then localization can be deferred. In either situation, it is my policy to obtain a follow-up mammogram within 6 months to document that there has been no regrowth of the lesion.

Ultrasound of a Noncalcified Mass

When simple breast cysts undergo spontaneous decompression, they may develop very irregular borders. It is wise to perform ultrasound on a nonpalpable mass that has any reasonable chance of being a cyst in order to avoid an unnecessary needle localization and excisional biopsy. If one inadvertently localizes a cyst and performs a perfect localization, skewering the mass and causing it to rupture, it may be impossible to document that the mass has been removed by specimen radiography. Even more problematic is that if a nonretractable hook-wire system is used and the cyst is ruptured, the patient may still have to undergo a biopsy just to retrieve the wire. Therefore, another advantage of the Mammalok system is that since the wire can always be retracted, the procedure can be aborted at any time. This fail-safe feature of the system often proves quite useful.

PATIENT PROBLEMS

Consent Form

Sometimes the patient is confused or misinformed about the needle localization and mistakes the procedure for either an aspiration or a biopsy. I always obtain a consent form from the patient to be certain that she has a clear understanding of the procedure and its risks. Fortunately, there are few risks associated with needle localization. The ones that I discuss include fainting, excessive bleeding, allergy to the superficial anesthesia, and failure to excise.

Fainting from a vasovagal reaction is uncommon but may occur during the procedure. The patient is told to let us know immediately if she feels lightheaded

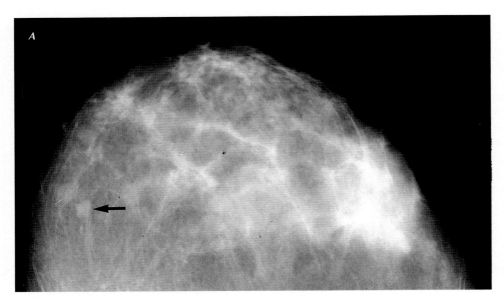

FIG. 15-2   A. *This patient was to undergo needle localization and excision for a nonpalpable mass (arrow) discovered on a routine screening mammogram.*

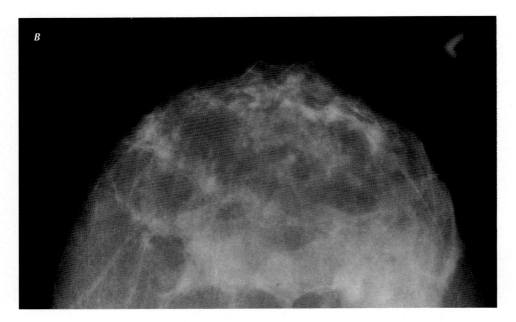

FIG. 15-2 *(Continued)*   **B.** *Two months later the mass is no longer evident.*

so that we can treat her by laying her supine on a stretcher.

The woman is questioned as to whether she has an excessive bleeding tendency or whether she is taking aspirin or other blood thinners. On occasion, a localization has had to be cancelled because the surgeon neglected to ask for this information and we discovered it in our routine questioning prior to the needle localization. The patient is told that normally there is no

bleeding associated with the needle localization. If some minimal bleeding occurs, it can be easily handled with a gauze.

There is a possibility of allergy to lidocaine. Since most women have had dental anesthesia, this is usually not a problem. I routinely use superficial anesthesia during breast localization, not because the localization procedure is painful but because of a theoretical psychologic benefit that some women might have knowing that the breast will be numbed. I fully recognize that anesthesia is not necessary, but it has always been my preference to use it in order to reinforce the concept that the procedure is not painful. This fear of pain, in my experience, is a major source of anxiety that women have about the localization procedure. Rarely, a woman will claim to be allergic to the anesthesia. In this case I tell her that the procedure does not require anesthesia and proceed without it.

The final problem discussed is failure to excise. I tell the woman that there is a chance that the area will not be excised or sampled. In our experience, we have an approximate 2 percent failure rate on the initial localization attempt, which is very low, considering the small volume of breast tissue we typically excise. I explain to the patient that while it is easy to guarantee a 100 percent success rate when one does large breast biopsies, it is our goal to minimize any potential cosmetic deformity because a majority of mammographic abnormalities prove to be benign. It is our philosophy to repeat the localization procedure at a future date rather than to continue excising until the lesion has been removed.

The Mammalok is virtually nontransectable, so I do not discuss the risk of transection. If I used a thin wire that could be transected, I would add this to my consent form.

Excessive Premedication

Since the woman has to be seated upright during the procedure, she cannot be excessively premedicated. Unfortunately, some women are extremely sensitive to even mild medication, and therefore, our rule is that the woman receives no premedication prior to the needle localization. On several occasions we have had the unfortunate experience of having to cancel a localization because the patient was excessively premedicated prior to being brought to the radiology department and was unable to sit upright.

One can eliminate this pitfall with the following procedure. When a localization is scheduled, the person booking the procedure notes whether the biopsy is to be performed on an inpatient or outpatient basis. In our institution there is no premedication of outpatients because they are instructed to report directly to the radiology department. However, if the biopsy is to be performed on an inpatient basis, on the afternoon of admission either the radiologist or technologist briefly explains the procedure to the patient and gives her a letter. The letter states that she must receive no premedication prior to her arrival to the radiology department, since she will be seated upright during the procedure. The letter continues that if there is any problem with her adhering to this, the radiologist must be contacted. The woman is, in effect, told: We do not care if

the chairman of anesthesia comes to your bedside in the morning and threatens you with expulsion from the hospital if he is not allowed to give you premedication. Hand him this letter and tell him to speak to the radiologist. We have had numerous occasions where the woman had to use this letter in order to avoid inadvertent premedication. I know from personal experience that it is not enough to write a note on the patient's chart, speak to the nurse in charge of the patient, or even speak directly to the anesthesiologist.

Vasovagal Reaction

I cannot predict which woman is at risk for having a vasovagal reaction during the procedure. This reaction is by no means rare, and undoubtedly if one performs enough localizations, one will encounter them. It is usual for the anxious, tearful woman to go through a localization procedure easily without incident, while the outwardly assured, calm woman is the one to have the reaction. Therefore, since a vasovagal reaction can occur without warning, I am always prepared for it. There are two absolute rules that I follow. The woman is *never* left alone in the mammography room seated in the upright position, and the localization is *never* performed unless a stretcher is present outside the mammography room.

WIRE PROBLEMS

Wire Migration

There are several pitfalls that are directly related to the specific needle-wire system used. If a wire has a sharp hook and is not firmly stabilized outside the breast, it can migrate deeper into the breast. If this occurs, the final relationship between the end of the wire and the lesion will not be the same as it was on the postlocalization films. This means that the surgeon is being guided by films that no longer depict an accurate relationship between the lesion and the guide. For this reason, even partial movement of the wire into the breast may cause a perfect localization procedure to fail. A secure stabilization device at the skin surface is essential to avoid this. Taping the wire to the breast may not be sufficient to prevent this pitfall.

The radiologist should be especially careful when using wires with short external ends. With a large, pendulous breast, the external end of the wire may become totally enveloped by breast tissue and retracted into it as the woman rises from the chair. Carefully securing the wire with a stabilization device will avoid this complication.[3] The reason the Mammalok localizer system[4] contains a compatible external stabilization device is to eliminate this possibility.

Wires or wire fragments with sharp lead points can migrate through the breast to distant extramammary locations.[5,6] When an entire wire has been retracted into the breast or when wire transection has occurred and the distal end remains in the breast, the radiologist should alert the surgeon to the migration. It would be wise to obtain mammograms to document that the wire is not moving. If the wire is changing position, serious consideration should be given to retrieving it. Since no one has extensive experience with this complication, it has not been established when and how often to obtain follow-up films to document that the wire is stationary.

Wire Transection

The surgeon must be warned if the localization wire used is thin and can be transected.[7] The specimen radiograph should always be scrutinized not only to determine whether the lesion has been excised but also to be certain that the end of the wire is contained within the tissue. If it is not, the surgeon must immediately be informed so that he can decide whether to proceed with further excision in an attempt to retrieve the cut wire end. If the end cannot be retrieved, the woman should be notified. Retrieval at a later date might require another needle localization. Theoretically, leaving the wire in the breast causes no sterility problems, but the possibility of migration must be considered. As stated previously, if I used a wire that could be transected, I would most certainly add this complication to the consent form and discuss it with the patient prior to the start of the localization procedure.

COMMUNICATION

In order for the localization to be successful, there must be communication between all members of the team—the radiologist, the surgeon, transport personnel, nursing personnel, and the pathologist.[8] If there is a break in this chain of communication, significant pitfalls may occur at different points during the localization procedure.

With the Surgeon

An important cause of localization failure is poor communication between the radiologist and surgeon. It is not simple to understand the relationship between the localizing guide and the lesion imaged on two-dimensional upright compression mammograms and correlate this relationship to the noncompressed supine breast in the operating room. After I perform a local-

ization, I sequester the films in my office and release them only to the operating surgeon after I have reviewed the films with him. In this way, I am absolutely certain that the surgeon has a clear understanding of the relationship between the lesion and the localizing guide. I strongly recommend that radiologists do this instead of simply sending the patient and the films to the operating room when the localization procedure is finished. Carefully labeling the films by noting the medial and axillary quadrants and drawing in the nipple should eliminate the possibility of someone hanging the films incorrectly in the operating room. I do not believe, however, that labeling the films can substitute for direct communication between the radiologist and surgeon.

With Nursing Personnel

Nursing personnel must be familiar with the needle localization procedure. We have had the unfortunate experience of a nurse dislodging the wire by forcibly pulling on it because she thought that it was an object caught on the surgical dressing that did not belong there (Fig. 15-3). Any wire, regardless of the configuration of its anchored end, may be forcibly pulled out of the breast.[9] The problem of the wire being pulled out of the breast, or even spontaneously being extruded from a fat-replaced breast, can occur with all wire systems.[10,11]

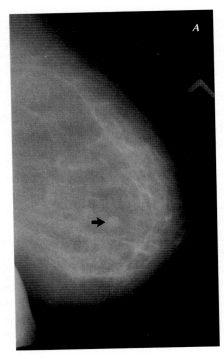

FIG. 15-3 A. *A 1-cm noncalcified mass (arrow) was discovered on a routine screening mammogram. Ultrasound revealed it to be solid.*

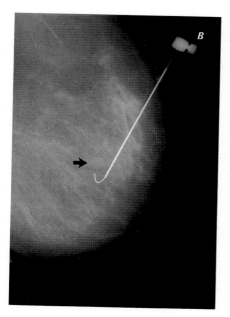

FIG. 15-3 (Continued) **B.** *Since it was nonpalpable, preoperative needle localization was performed.*

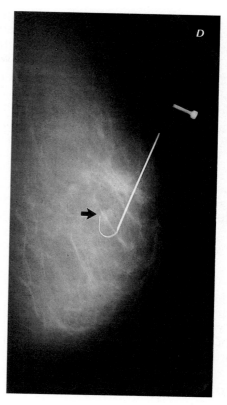

FIG. 15-3 (Continued) **D.** *A repeat localization was performed. The mass (arrow) is at the distal end of the needle.*

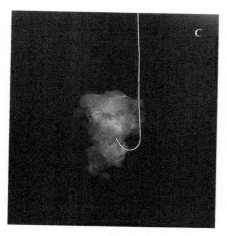

FIG. 15-3 (Continued) **C.** *A nurse who was unfamiliar with the procedure pulled the localization needle-wire system partially out of the breast because she thought it was a needle accidently caught between the covering gauzes. Specimen radiograph shows that the mass was not excised.*

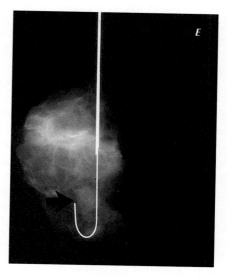

FIG. 15-3 (Continued) **E.** *Specimen radiography confirmed excision of the mass. Notice its angulated borders. Histology revealed a benign fibroadenoma.*

With Transport Personnel

Unless a surgeon can confirm by palpation during his excisional biopsy that the lesion has been removed, it is the routine at NEMCH that the tissue goes directly to the department of radiology for specimen radiography. Since the surgeon is usually unable to confirm this by palpation in most situations, specimen radiography is performed in virtually every case of biopsy of the nonpalpable breast lesion. We attempt to minimize the delay between tissue excision and delivery to pathology. Should estrogen receptor analysis be required, time is important because as time elapses, the estrogen receptor analysis becomes less reliable. Our instruction to transport personnel consists of two important directives. They are told to bring the breast tissue directly to radiology and not to pathology, which is their usual destination, and they are warned not to tarry on their way to the radiology department.

At NEMCH, specimen radiography is performed in the radiology department. In our setting, this is the most efficient way to guarantee that the radiologist, who knows the appearance of the mammographic abnormality, can assume responsibility for determining whether the area has been successfully sampled. However, there is no reason that specimen radiography cannot be performed in another place such as the pathology department, as long as someone who is familiar with the mammographic appearance of the nonpalpable breast lesion assumes responsibility for declaring whether the area has been successfully sampled.

In order to further minimize any delay, a telephone call can be made from the operating room to the radiology department to alert the radiologist that the tissue is on its way. This gives a woman who might be in the middle of having a routine mammogram a chance to temporarily step outside the room.

With Pathology

All too often, although there has been careful documentation that the lesion has been successfully excised, the pathologist has not positively identified the abnormality for histologic evaluation. Especially with large breast biopsy specimens, random sectioning of tissue may not be sufficient to guarantee that the area of concern has been sampled. Just as there should be positive confirmation that the lesion has been removed, there should be positive confirmation that the lesion has been isolated for histologic analysis. This can be achieved when the tissue is sliced and a mass is directly visualized by the pathologist or when definite grittiness is felt as slices are made through an area of microcalcification. However, if the pathologist cannot positively identify the mammographic abnormality, and this is almost always the case with microcalcifications and often the case with asymmetric densities, repeat radiography of the sliced tissue is performed in order to isolate the lesion for the pathologist. This final step of isolation is performed not because of academic purism, but in order to guarantee the correct diagnosis. If this last step of the localization procedure is not performed, what is the proof that the lesion for which the woman has undergone surgery has in fact been placed under the microscope for evaluation?

Convincing the pathologist to work with the radiologist during this last step is not always easily accomplished. If the pathologist does not have enough experience with nonpalpable breast carcinoma, he may be of the opinion that all breast cancer can be found by palpation of the sliced tissue. This is not true. The mammographic examination is so exquisitely sensitive that intraductal and invasive ductal carcinoma may elude detection by palpation of sectioned tissue. I strongly urge the radiologist, with direct support from the surgeon, to open channels of communication with the pathologist in order to work closely during this final step. If the pathologist cannot or will not work with the radiologist, then the next best alternative is to have the radiologist insert needles into the tissue and obtain views in order to direct the pathologist to the precise area in question.[12]

SPECIMEN RADIOGRAPHY

General Technique

We handle all breast specimens in the same fashion; they are compressed in air during filming. Since there is little scatter radiation to deteriorate the image, grids are not necessary for specimen radiography. In fact, the exposure is often so fast that even if one uses a moving grid, grid lines may be seen and may serve to decrease resolution.

The Calcified Lesion

Microcalcifications should be easily evident on specimen radiography and usually appear clearer and more numerous than on the original mammogram. If the mammographic target contained microcalcifications, it is our policy that the pathology report specifically mentions that the mammographic calcifications have been identified on the slides. Close cooperation is necessary between the radiologist and pathologist in this situation because the presence of microcalcifications on the slide does not guarantee that they represent the mammographic calcifications.

A problem occurs when the specimen radiograph unequivocally confirms that the mammographic calcifications have been sucessfully removed but the pathologist is unable to locate them. There are several possibilities in this situation. One possibility is that the calcifications were calcium oxalate crystals. Since these crystals are not easily seen with a hematoxylin-eosin stain but are seen with polarized light, the pathologist should be told to review the slides using polarized light.[13] If calcifications are still not identified on the slides, another possibility is that they are contained within the paraffin blocks so the blocks should be radiographed.[14] The final possibility is that the calcifications were lost during processing of the breast specimen. This occurrence is thought to be unusual but has been reported.[15]

The Noncalcified Lesion

The identification of a noncalcified lesion on specimen radiography is more challenging than identification of microcalcifications. In most situations there should be no difficulty in confirming that a noncalcified lesion has been removed if the lesion is real. On occasion though, there may still be a question even after specimen radiography as to whether the noncalcified area was excised. We instruct the surgeon to leave the localization wire in situ to help us orient both the specimen and wire relative to the noncalcified density. Sometimes two views of the specimen taken at a 90 degree angle to each other will help identify the density.[16]

Whenever there is uncertainty as to whether a noncalcified lesion has been excised, the surgeon is instructed to obtain a follow-up mammogram in the near future. Naturally, this examination is difficult to perform because maximum compression cannot be applied since the woman has a fresh incision. Also, it is difficult to interpret because of the usual postoperative edema or hemorrhage at the biopsy site. However, one of three things will be observed on this mammogram. It will either be evident that the noncalcified lesion has not been excised, that the noncalcified lesion has been excised, or that there is still question as to whether the area has been successfully sampled. In this last situation, another follow-up mammogram must be obtained until the issue is resolved. It is hard to understand the rationale for obtaining specimen radiography only for calcified lesions. The woman is being subjected to a biopsy because there is a concern that she has occult breast cancer, whether or not the area contains calcifications. The same effort should be required to document that the area has been removed whether or not calcifications are present. Specimen radiography of real noncalcified lesions can successfully determine whether the area has been excised.[17]

As previously stated, our surgeons are urged to leave the wire in the specimen. This accomplishes two things. It helps to identify the noncalcified mammographic abnormality by its position relative to the wire. The wire serves another purpose if the lesion is not contained within the specimen. In this case it is not sufficient to call the surgeon in the operating room and tell him to excise more tissue because the surgeon does not know whether to excise more tissue superiorly, inferiorly, medially, laterally, or deeper in the surgical wound closer to the chest wall. He needs direction, and often the orientation of the specimen with the wire can provide this direction.[18] This is another important reason why the radiologist should remain involved during specimen radiography. At best, the pathologist may be able to tell the surgeon whether the mammographic area of concern has been excised. However, only the radiologist is in the position to guide the surgeon to another area for biopsy if the lesion is not contained within the initial excised tissue (Fig. 15-4). It is our practice that if the lesion is not excised after one or two small repeat biopsies, the wound is closed and a follow-up mammogram is obtained as described above.

The final sentence of my dictated radiology report for the needle localization procedure contains a statement as to whether the lesion has been sampled. If the lesion has not been removed, the report has a clear recommendation that a repeat mammogram be obtained and an additional statement to the effect that the surgeon was notified of this by telephone. In this way, total documentation is present in the record. Documenting that the radiologist has carried out his role to the best of his ability is important from a medical-legal point of view.

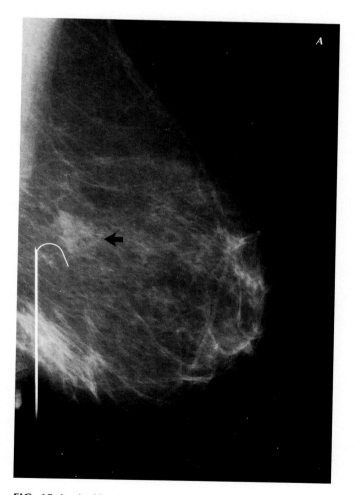

FIG. 15-4 A. *Needle localization via an inferior approach was performed on a noncalcified asymmetric density (arrow).*

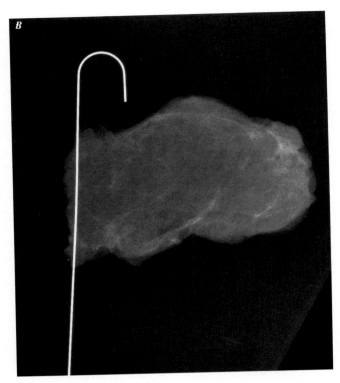

FIG. 15-4 (Continued) B. The asymmetric density is not present on the specimen radiograph. Judging by the position of the wire left in situ, the surgeon was advised to take one more small biopsy slightly more cephalad.

Incisional versus Excisional Biopsy

It is our goal to totally excise a nonpalpable mammographic abnormality with a surrounding margin of tissue. However, on occasion only some of the mammographic abnormality is excised and, in effect, we have performed an incisional biopsy. This is often the case with microcalcifications. If the tissue proves to be benign, we assume that the remainder of the lesion within the breast is benign. However, we always place the patient in our usual follow-up protocol, which means obtaining a repeat mammogram within 6 months and then following the area for a minimum of $2\frac{1}{2}$ to 3 years (Fig. 15-5). In the unlikely event that the tissue sampled does not reflect the entire lesion and that there is an adjacent cancer, we will be able to detect it on follow-up mammography.[19]

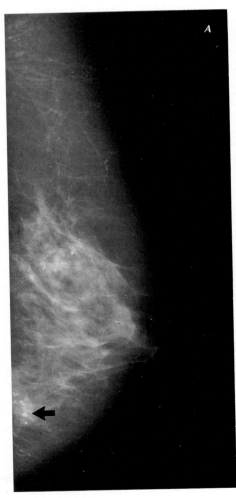

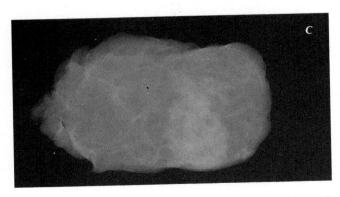

FIG. 15-4 (Continued) C. The next specimen radiograph confirmed excision of the lesion. Histology revealed benign focal fibrosis.

FIG. 15-5 A. A nonpalpable geographic cluster of microcalcifications (arrow) was discovered on a routine screening mammogram.

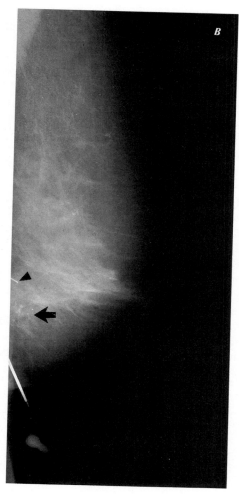

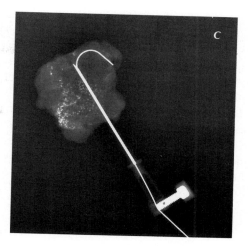

FIG. 15-5 (Continued)   C. Specimen radiograph confirmed excision of numerous microcalcifications extending to the margin of the specimen. It was assumed that the entire lesion had not been removed. Histology revealed focal sclerosing adenosis with extensive microcalcification. The patient was placed into follow-up protocol.

FIG. 15-5 (Continued)   B. An inferior approach was used. The lesion was so close to the chest wall that the distal end of the needle could never be imaged. Since the tip of the "J" wire was clearly seen (arrowhead), the sharp needle tip was being protected by the curved wire so there was no concern that the needle might later penetrate the pleural space. The lesion (arrow) is ventral to the midportion of the needle.

REFERENCES

1. Kopans DB, Waitzkin ED, Linetsky L, et al. Localization of breast lesions identified on only one mammographic view. AJR **149**:39–41, 1987.
2. Pennes DR, Homer MJ. Disappearing breast masses caused by compression during mammography. Radiology **165**:327–328, 1987.
3. Homer MJ. Percutaneous localization of breast lesions. Experience with the Frank breast biopsy guide. J Can Assoc Radiol **30**:238–241, 1979.
4. Homer MJ. Nonpalpable breast lesion localization using a curved-end retractable wire. Radiology **157**:259–260, 1985.

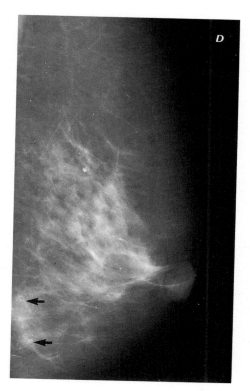

FIG. 15-5 (Continued)   D. A mammogram 6 months later confirms that residual microcalcifications (arrows) remain in the breast. The microcalcifications remained stable throughout the follow-up period and repeat needle localization and biopsy were not required.

5. Davis PS, Wechsler RJ, Feig SA, et al. Migration of breast biopsy localization wire. AJR **150**:787–788, 1988.

6. Bristol JB, Jones PA. Transgression of localizing wire into the pleural cavity prior to mammography. Br J Radiol **54**:139–140, 1981.

7. Homer MJ. Transection of the localization hooked wire during breast biopsy. AJR **141**:929–930, 1983.

8. Homer MJ, Smith TJ, Safall H. Prebiopsy needle localization: methods, problems, and expected results. Radiol Clin North Am **30**:139–153, 1992.

9. Homer MJ. Localization of nonpalpable breast lesions: technical aspects and analysis of 80 cases. AJR **140**:807–811, 1983.

10. Gisvold JJ, Martin JK. Prebiopsy localization of nonpalpable breast lesions. AJR **143**:477–481, 1984.

11. Homer MJ, Pile-Spellman ER. Needle localization of occult breast lesions with a curved-end retractable wire: technique and pitfalls. Radiology **161**:547–548, 1986.

12. D'Orsi CJ. Management of the breast specimen. Radiology **194**:297–302, 1995.

13. Surratt JT, Monsees BS, Mazoujian G. Calcium oxalate microcalcifications in the breast. Radiology **181**:141–142, 1991.

14. Cardenosa G, Eklund GW. Paraffin block radiography following breast biopsies: Use of orthogonal views. Radiology **180**:873–874, 1991.

15. D'Orsi CJ, Reale FR, Davis MA, et al. Breast specimen microcalcifications: Radiographic validation and pathologic-radiologic correlation. Radiology **180**:397–401, 1991.

16. Rebner M, Pennes DR, Baker DE, et al. Two-view specimen radiography in surgical biopsy of nonpalpable breast masses. AJR **149**:283–285, 1987.

17. Stomper PC, Davis SP, Sonnenfeld MR, et al. Efficacy of specimen radiography of clinically occult noncalcified breast lesions. AJR **151**:43–47, 1988.

18. Homer MJ, Rangel DM, Miller HH. Pre- and transoperative localizations of nonpalpable breast lesions. Am J Surg **139**:888–891, 1980.

19. Homer MJ. Nonpalpable breast microcalcifications: Frequency, management and results of incisional biopsy. Radiology **185**:411–413, 1992.

Chapter 16

MALPRACTICE AND MAMMOGRAPHY

The interpretation of mammograms is made more challenging by the numerous medicolegal issues which pertain to this imaging study. As mammographic utilization increases, so does the involvement of radiologists in litigation claiming delay of diagnosis of breast cancer. This growing problem is reflected by the increasing number of articles appearing in the radiology literature addressing issues of medical malpractice in general as well as it relates specifically to mammography. Part of the growing malpractice can be attributed to an incorrect perception on the part of many patients who believe that a normal mammogram means that there can be no cancer within the breast. Given this false perception about the infallibility of mammography, it is easy to understand why many women who have breast cancer diagnosed within 1 or 2 years of a normal mammogram believe that it must have been present on the mammogram and missed. When the message went out to women about the ability of mammography to detect small, curable, nonpalpable breast cancer, it should have been coupled with information about its false-negative rate of approximately 10 percent. The public should have been educated about the significant limitations of mammography such as the possibility that breast cancer can be obscured by dense breast tissue or the possibility that when breast cancer does not form a mass or make microcalcifications, it can have an appearance indistinguishable from normal adjacent breast tissue.

DISCLAIMERS

At the outset it is necessary for me to make several disclaimers regarding the material in this chapter as well as of the other material contained within this book. There are many practices or suggestions proposed in this book which are not meant to be taken as standard of care. This textbook does not define standard of care.

In fact many suggestions in this book are above standard of care.

I am not a lawyer and it is not my intention to give legal advice. My anecdotal observations expressed in this chapter are based on conversations with plaintiff and defense attorneys, reading articles which address medicolegal aspects of breast imaging, reviewing the depositions of others, and personally giving depositions and testimony in court. Different lawyers have different philosophies and different states have different rules. For example, while experts are almost always deposed in some states, they are rarely deposed in other states. While some lawyers maintain a low-key demeanor during depositions, others are very formal, while still others are quite confrontational.

In the legal sense, I am not an authority and nothing I write is authoritarian. In fact, in my opinion, no physician is an authority and no medical textbook is authoritarian. What is contained in the medical literature are the opinions, practices, and results of those writing the article or textbook at that point in time. Since medicine is not static, ideas are commonly changed over time as new discoveries are made or new concepts advanced. There may be a potential pitfall for a physician involved in a malpractice suit to state that a particular physician is an authority or that a particular article or book is authoritarian. If anything that authority does or anything contained in an authoritarian text is not followed, one can question whether the practicing physician has fallen below standard of care. So unless you agree with *everything* someone teaches or writes, perhaps you share my opinion that no physician is an authority and no article or book is authoritarian.

Past performance is no guarantee of future results. This disclaimer or a reasonable facsimile appears in virtually every mutual fund prospectus. Unfortunately this is also true in our legal system. A physician can do everything according to the letter and still be sued and even lose a malpractice case. The reasons for this are fairly obvious. Every case is unique and no two cases have precisely the same set of facts. In every case there is a different combination of judges, attorneys, and jurors. Therefore what proved to be successful in one case may not succeed in another.

PRACTICE MAKES PERFECT

This truism applies to almost everything we do. Unfortunately this also applies to malpractice suits. The more lawsuits in which you are involved, the more depositions you give, the more attorneys who advise you, and the more you understand the rules of our legal system, the more you know what to expect, and the more you feel at ease answering questions posed to you. The obvious problem is that no one wants to develop expertise in this area by being sued a lot! None of us want to be able to say to ourselves "The next time an attorney asks me that question, I'll be better prepared to answer it." A physician involved in a malpractice case hopes there will never be a next time. The purpose of this chapter is to familiarize the reader with some of the medicolegal problems as they relate to mammography, define specific areas of risk, and offer suggestions which may help to minimize the risk.

MAGNITUDE OF THE PROBLEM

On occasion I have been asked whether the legal issues surrounding mammography are being blown out of proportion. The implication of this question is that possibly the problem is not so prevalent and a disproportionate amount of time and worry is being devoted to this topic. The latest information from the Physicians Insurers Association of America (PIAA) breast cancer study clearly defines the magnitude of the problem.[1] Their information is based on 117,000 claims and suits gathered from 21 companies which insure more than 90,000 physicians. Their June 1995 study indicates that the delay of diagnosis of breast cancer continues to be a frequent cause for malpractice claims. In fact breast cancer is the condition for which the patient most frequently files a medical malpractice claim. It is the second most expensive condition regarding indemnity payments which are made in 44 percent of all claims. The study states "Thus it is apparent that breast cancer

claims remain a significant source of concern for the medical malpractice insurance industry," and "Radiologists are the specialists most frequently claimed against in this study."

When one compares the PIAA 1995 study to its 1990 study, the problem is actually getting worse. In 1995 the indemnity payment was 36 percent higher than in 1990, radiologists were named as defendants in 24 percent of cases versus 11 percent, a mammogram was performed in 83.5 percent of cases versus 72.9 percent, and a mammogram was reported as negative or equivocal in 80 percent of cases versus 69.2 percent. It is clear that the medical malpractice issue as it relates to radiologists interpreting mammography is not being blown out of proportion.

THE PROFILE OF THE PATIENT MOST LIKELY TO SUE

One would think that the patient most likely to sue is the patient with a high risk for developing breast cancer who develops a subtle nonpalpable mass or microcalcifications. In fact the PIAA study shows just the opposite. Although the incidence of breast cancer increases with age, claims are more prevalent in younger age groups. More than 60 percent of patients who brought suit were under age 50 and more than 30 percent were under age 40. Furthermore, family history was not a significant factor regarding claims frequency. In addition, despite the fact that the patient herself found the lesion in 60 percent of cases, there was still a delay in diagnosis. Pain or tenderness, symptoms which are more frequently attributed to benign causes, was present in more than 25 percent of cases. In other words, the profile of a patient most likely to sue is that of a younger woman under age 50, with no family history of breast cancer, complaining of a palpable mass which may be painful, and who has undergone a mammogram which was interpreted as negative or equivocal.

From a radiologist's perspective, it appears that we are exposed to malpractice problems in those patients where we least expect it. Although it is true that a mammogram is not even necessary to diagnose a palpable breast cancer, and although we may believe that the purpose of the mammogram in the patient with a palpable mass is really to look for occult disease in the ipsilateral or contralateral breast,[2] in fact a typical case in which the radiologist becomes involved as a defendant is an alleged delay of diagnosis of a palpable mass. In my opinion, at least two important messages are clear. A woman old enough to have a mammogram is old enough to have a breast cancer, and concern for the possibility of the presence of breast cancer must remain high even for the patient judged to be at low risk for developing breast cancer.

AREAS OF POTENTIAL RISK

Since most malpractice claims never come to court because they are eventually either dropped or settled, it may be difficult for the radiologist to get a true overview of the actual facts and situations which represent common causes of malpractice suits from reviewing court cases. Common areas in which radiologists can potentially become involved with medical malpractice claims dealing with a delay of diagnosis of breast cancer can be divided into six general categories. These categories are (1) equipment and technique, (2) the patient-initiated examination, (3) the technologist, (4) interpretation of the mammogram, (5) the mammography report, and (6) needle localization. Potential malpractice risks in each of these categories will now be defined, and strategies which may minimize these risks will be suggested. For every idea proposed regarding aspects of the legal system, the radiologist should ultimately seek guidance from attorneys or risk management personnel who are most familiar with aspects of a particular issue as they relate to a specific practice setting.

Equipment, Technique, and Positioning

The mandatory accreditation of mammography facilities and equipment has been a significant factor in improving the overall quality of mammography equipment and images. Undoubtedly this is the primary explanation for the decrease in the incidence of claims alleging that mammographic images are technically inadequate for diagnosis because they were produced on substandard equipment. Lawsuits based on the fact that mammograms were produced on nondedicated equipment, or that no grid was used, or that a xerogram was performed rather than a film-screen study, have virtually disappeared. Needless to say, mammograms should be performed on equipment which has been approved for use.

However there are still malpractice suits which claim that there has been a delay of diagnosis because of poor technique or positioning. The themes of most of these suits are predictable. The plaintiff's expert is of the opinion that had the breast been pulled harder, or had the film not been so underexposed, or had more of the axillary tail been imaged, the cancer would have been detected. The opinion of the expert is based on his or her personal experience reading mammograms, or articles from the radiology literature discussing technique and positioning.

There are some mammograms which are below standard of care because of improper technique or poor positioning. Yet we all recognize that while we carefully select and submit perfectly positioned mammograms with perfect technique for the accreditation process, in fact many (most?) mammograms produced in our daily clinical practice fall below the ideal standard required for accreditation. Nevertheless we do not judge them all to be substandard for diagnostic purposes. While we strive for perfection in our daily practice, we rarely achieve it consistently. All radiologists recognize that for the accreditation process we submit the best examples of our work and so it should be pretty obvious to any radiologist involved in the daily practice of mammographic interpretation that while not all of our films are judged to be perfect for the accreditation process, this does not mean that they are of inadequate diagnostic quality. The radiologist must make a judgment for every mammogram as to whether the films are of diagnostic quality.

In a recent audit of the positioning quality of mammograms performed at an academic center, it was found that the criteria of the pectoral muscle extending to the nipple or below on the OBL view, and the depth of the tissue on the CC view measuring no less than 1 cm than on the OBL view, were not met in all four views in 64 percent of patients.[3] Does that mean that only 36 percent of all mammograms performed at that institution were standard of care? Of course not! To quote the authors, "These criteria are goals that we should try to attain, but it is understood that they will not be met in all four views in all patients." I would love to audit the practice of any "expert" radiologist who claims that it is below standard of care not to repeat mammograms if they fall short of the standards used for selection of films for accreditation purposes. I would love to audit the practice of any "expert" radiologist who says that a technologist should have pulled harder to image more breast tissue. We all know that since the breast is attached to the chest wall and can never be fully pulled out onto the film, in virtually every case when the technologist is sent back to pull harder, more breast tissue will almost always be able to be imaged on the repeat film. In the screening setting our technologists are constantly making judgements for each patient as to how much pulling and compression can be tolerated. The well-trained, caring technologist is constantly factoring into her work the patient's ability to cooperate and the degree of compression that can be tolerated. It is only with this understanding that judgment of a film's technical quality should be made.

The Patient-Initiated Examination

When the mammogram is initiated by the patient, or in other words, when the patient is self-referred for a mammogram, the radiologist assumes additional responsibilities that fall beyond the usual practices of the radiologist as a consultant. In effect, the radiologist becomes responsible for the care of the patient as it relates to the breast. The only physician receiving the mammography report, whether it is normal or abnormal, is the radiologist. There is nothing wrong with offering patient-initiated mammograms as long as the radiologist is prepared for the additional costs and labor required to handle the added responsibilities in this practice setting.

There are some obvious questions that a radiologist who elects to operate in this setting must have asked and answered. Since screening for breast cancer requires both palpation and mammography, who is responsible for performance of the breast palpation? If there are findings on the mammogram that merit immediate action such as additional views, ultrasound, or establishing a histologic diagnosis, what mechanism is in place to guarantee that it is done? If there are findings that require follow-up mammography, what mechanism is in place to guarantee that the patient returns? If the radiologist converts the patient from a self-referred to a referred patient is the mechanism for this conversion reliable? For instance is it adequate for the radiologist merely to have the patient select the name of a clinician from a listing, or is the radiologist also responsible for being certain that the patient actually sees the clinician? Is there adequate documentation of this? Many of these questions have been addressed by others.[4–6] The prudent radiologist operating a patient-initiated practice should have addressed all of these issues.

The Technologist

Whether or not the technologist is an employee of the hospital, her professional duties fall under the direct responsibility of the radiologist. Often in screening settings, the technologist is the only one the patient sees. The reliance of the radiologist on the technologist is perhaps nowhere so evident as in mammography. In most practice settings the technologist has numerous responsibilities including obtaining history, being the first, and sometimes the only one, to know whether the appropriate views are being performed, and making judgments as to the degree of compression exerted, the technique used, and the image quality.

The importance of the history form has already been covered in Chap. 3. To emphasize a point made previously, if a question is important enough to be asked on the history form, it is important enough to be answered. For optimal efficiency, the patient history form should be periodically reviewed to be certain that it is streamlined and contains the necessary questions. My technologists are taught that *every* question must be answered. Any question left blank permits speculation as to whether it was asked of the patient. I never cease to be amazed when I see a patient history form that has no response for what is probably the most important question asked of the woman prior to the performance of her mammogram "Why are you having this examination?"

The radiologist cannot assume that the cadre of technologists who perform mammography know what is expected of them unless periodic meetings are held with the supervising radiologist. Such meetings can provide valuable teaching opportunities and can also be used for feedback from our technologists who are ultimately the ones on the front line. It should not be surprising that technologist insights and suggestions often provide the radiologist with valuable ideas and suggestions for making a practice more efficient.

The specific responsibilities of my technologists are detailed in Chap. 3. Some of these responsibilities were established as a direct result of the PIAA breast cancer studies of 1990 and 1995 which both indicated that in a majority of malpractice suits, the patient herself was able to palpate the cancer. My technologists are trained to react specially when a patient claims that she has a palpable mass. Extra views of the area containing the alleged palpable abnormality are obtained, and the location is carefully marked on the diagram. In addition, I specifically indicate in my report that I have knowledge that there is an alleged palpable abnormality, describe the special views added to evaluate the area, and comment as to whether any abnormality is evident in the area of concern.

Interpretation of the Mammogram

Since this text, except for this chapter, is devoted to the interpretation of the mammogram, there are no specific points about aspects of interpretation that I intend to make at this time. However there are some general observations about mammographic interpretation that deserve comment. There is a great variability between radiologists regarding mammographic interpretations and recommendations for management.[7]

It is sometimes the case that something was present on a mammogram performed 1 or 2 years earlier (and sometimes even earlier still!) in the area a cancer developed. The question that "experts" must ask themselves when evaluating whether an interpretation is below standard of care in the screening setting is *not* whether there was a finding on an earlier mammogram, but whether it was reasonable for the average radiologist to have interpreted the examination as being within the range of what we accept as "normal" given the wide range of what a "normal" mammogram can look like, given the fact that unless a breast is totally replaced by fat or is totally dense, no two breasts look the same, given the fact that it is common for breasts not to be perfectly symmetrical in their fat-fibroglandular distribution, and given the fact that the radiologist had no knowledge that eventually a cancer would appear.

In an excellent award-winning paper, the difference between a retrospective and blinded interpretation was investigated.[8] This study indicated that nonpalpable breast cancer is frequently evident in retrospect on previous mammograms and failure to detect a retrospectively visible abnormality is not necessarily negligent. In addition, retrospective reviews do not necessarily reflect the everyday practice of screening mammography. While our legal colleagues are fully aware of the reality that often there is a retrospective abnormality present, a malpractice action is rarely brought without a radiologist willing to testify that an interpretation was below standard of care. Therefore the radiologist-expert bears the primary responsibility for the instigation of a medical malpractice suit and this responsibility should be taken seriously because of all of the emotional suffering brought about by a claim without valid basis. An expert has the obligation to judge things fairly. The standards which an expert applies to a colleague should also apply to every radiologist in practice, including the expert himself. No one practices perfect medicine all of the time and standard of care does not require perfection. Earning a medical degree, does not confer omniscience on the recipient. The law does not require that everything the physician did was correct, but rather it requires that the physician exercised "ordinary skill and care that would be applied by other physicians in similar situations."[9] All experts making judgments about the conduct of a physician should understand this.

The Mammography Report

One recurrent legal pitfall that is common to any imaging examination, including mammography, is that the report is either ambiguous or it did not make its way to the eyes of the referring clinician. The added danger regarding mammography is that since in the majority of cases it is a screening study performed on a healthy patient without any signs or symptoms of breast cancer, the referring physician may not have an adequate system to track all reports. Since the woman has no problems, she may not call to learn of her results. To compound the problem further, many patients believe that not hearing mammogram results from the physician means that the test was normal. Various legal aspects of the mammography report have been covered in Chap. 5. Failure to communicate is a recurrent theme in malpractice cases.[10,11] The responsible radiologist should address these issues and seek advice from one's risk management advisors as to the recommended standards expected in one's specific clinical practice. This issue of communication becomes more important in our current changing healthcare environment where the primary care person receiving the report may not even be a physician.

Needle Localization

When a woman undergoes preoperative needle localization for a nonpalpable breast lesion, she has the expectation that the area of concern will be sampled (incisional biopsy) or completely removed (excisional biopsy) and that it undergoes histologic evaluation. The radiologist is an integral part of the procedure. This involvement does not end when adequate needle placement is achieved. To avoid the most common malpractice pitfalls in this area, two questions should always be asked and answered—Is there confirmation that the mammographic lesion has been sampled or removed, and is there confirmation that the mammographic lesion has been put on a slide for analysis by the pathologist?

Not infrequently the surgeon dissects down upon the localizing needle or wire towards a nonpalpable mammographic abnormality and eventually palpates something. The assumption that what is being palpated represents the mammographic abnormality is not necessarily correct. Specimen radiography can provide absolute confirmation that the mammographic target has either been sampled or removed. Although a radiologist might recommend that the surgeon perform specimen radiography in every case, ultimately the surgeon is in charge and cannot be forced to send the breast tissue for radiography. In this situation the radiologist can be factual in his report of the procedure and add that although specimen radiography was offered, the surgeon elected to send the tissue to the pathology department. By doing this the radiologist has documented that specimen radiography was available but the surgeon elected not to to use it.

The smaller the mammographic lesion, the more the pathologist needs help in identification of the mammographic target. Random sampling of excised breast tissue, especially for mammographic targets only millimeters in greatest diameter, provides no guarantee that the mammographic target is on a slide. The radiologist and pathologist should establish a mechanism to be certain that the location of the nonpalpable breast lesion has been identified and isolated for histologic analysis. As noted in Chap. 15, with small mammographic targets, the lesion may be imbedded so deeply within the paraffin block that it may not be contained on any slide for histologic evaluation.

REFERENCES

1. Physicians Insurers Association of America: Breast Cancer Study. Physicians Insurers Association of America, Washington, D.C. 1995.
2. Kopans DB. Breast imaging and the standard of care for the symptomatic patient. Radiology **187**:608–611, 1993.
3. Bassett LW, Hirbawi IA, DeBruhl N, Hayes MK. Mammographic positioning: Evaluation from the viewbox. Radiology **188**:803–806, 1993.
4. Monsees B, Destouet JM, Evens RG. The self-referred mammography patient: A new responsibility for radiologists. Radiology **166**:69–70, 1988.
5. Sickles EA. Mammography screening and the self-referred woman. Radiology **166**:271–273, 1988.
6. Brenner RJ. Medicolegal aspects of breast imaging: Variable standards of care relating to different types of practice. AJR **156**:719–723, 1991.
7. Elmore JG, Wells CK, Lee CH, et al. Variability in radiologists interpretation of mammograms. N Engl J Med **331**:1493–1499, 1994.
8. Harvey JA, Fajardo LL, Innis CA. Previous mammograms in patients with impalpable breast carcinoma: Retrospective vs. blinded interpretation. AJR **161**:1167–1172, 1993.
9. Brenner RJ. Mammography and malpractice litigation: Current status, lessons, and admonitions. AJR **161**:931–935, 1993.
10. Potchen EJ, Bisesi MA, Sierra AE, Potchen JE. Mammography and malpractice. AJR **156**:475–480, 1991.
11. Kline TJ, Kline TS. Radiologists, communication, and resolution 5: A medicolegal issue. Radiology **184**:131–134, 1992.

TEST CASES

This section consists of cases which illustrate principles of mammographic interpretation presented in the first part of this text. The cases are representative of the spectrum of material that will be encountered in an active mammography practice. The exercises are structured so that the reader is able to first evaluate the clinical history and mammograms in order to formulate an opinion about the findings and their significance. Based upon this, the reader should be able to offer recommendations regarding patient management. Then for each case the mammographic findings and recommendations are presented, followed by a discussion of the pertinent teaching points.

HISTORY

This mammogram was performed on a 53-year-old woman with multiple bilateral palpable breast masses.

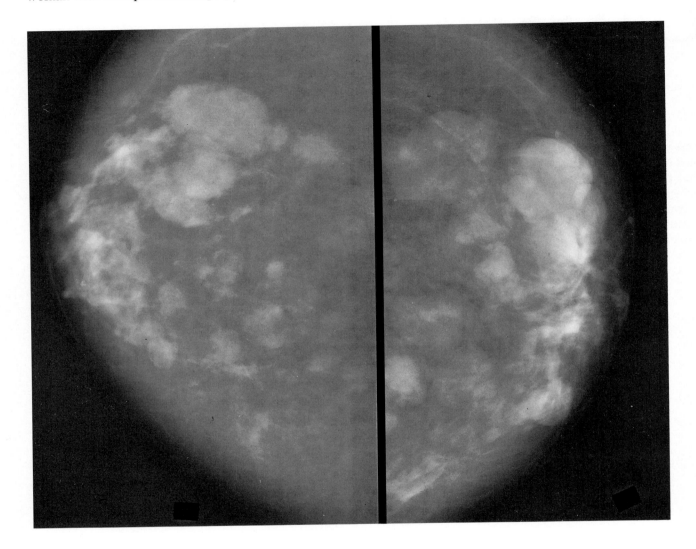

MAMMOGRAPHIC FINDINGS AND RECOMMENDATION

A CC view of each breast reveals numerous bilateral noncalcified moderately well-defined masses. There is no dominant mass. There are no suspicious microcalcifications in either breast.

Place the patient into a follow-up protocol to assess stability of the masses over time. If there is a dominant mass by palpation, its management must be based upon clinical grounds.

DISCUSSION

This is a case of bilaterality and multiplicity. All of the masses have a mammographic appearance that is more likely to be associated with benign disease. Ultrasound would never be recommended unless there were a dominant mass by either mammography or by palpation.

HISTORY

Routine screening mammogram in a 64-year-old woman with known lymphoma.

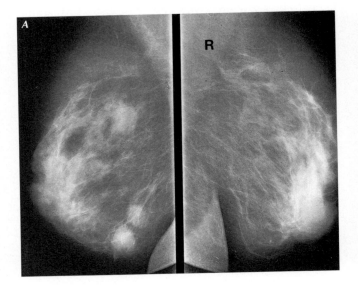

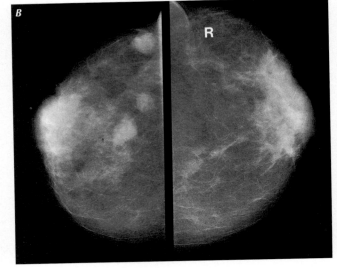

MAMMOGRAPHIC FINDINGS AND RECOMMENDATION

OBL (*A*) and CC (*B*) views reveal multiple noncalcified masses in the left breast with poorly defined margins.

Perform ultrasound to determine whether any or all of the masses are solid.

They all are solid.

One or several of the solid masses should be excised to establish their histology. Although multifocal breast carcinoma is in the differential diagnosis in this patient, lymphoma of the breast is the leading diagnosis.

DISCUSSION

This is an example of multiplicity without bilaterality. This type of pattern should weigh heavily toward obtaining tissue rather than follow-up. Histology revealed lymphomatous involvement of the left breast.

Case 3

HISTORY

These are four different patients who had routine screening mammography. In every case, the breasts were repalpated after the mammogram was interpreted. The breast palpation remained normal.

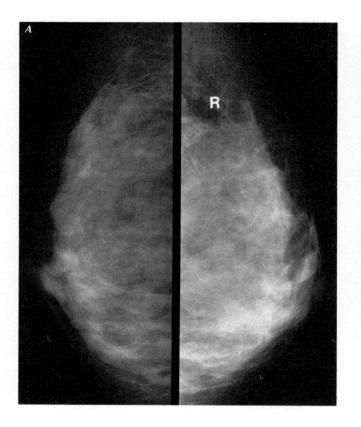

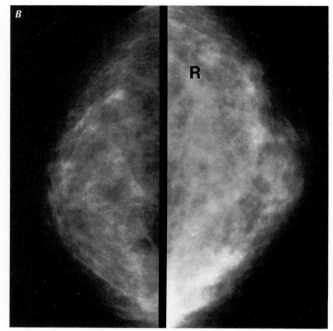

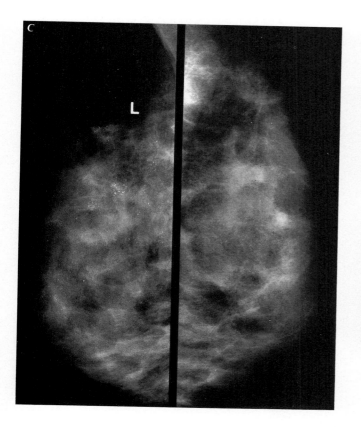

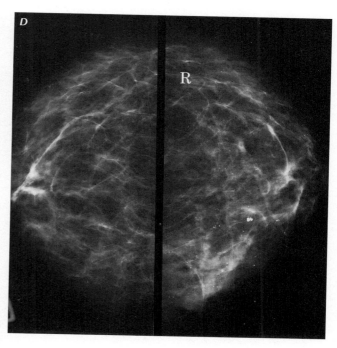

MAMMOGRAPHIC FINDINGS AND RECOMMENDATION

The findings in all four cases are essentially identical. In the right breast of patient #1 (**A**), in the right breast of patient #2 (**B**), in the left breast of patient #3 (**C**), and in the right breast of patient #4 (**D**) there are multiple clusters of microcalcifications. The subtle microcalcifications may be seen better with a magnifying glass! There are no calcifications in the contralateral breasts.

To require excision of all the calcifications would require extensive surgery. An incisional biopsy should be performed to obtain some tissue with microcalcifications to establish the nature of the process. If the histology is benign, place the patient into follow-up to reassess the remaining calcifications over time. Since the process could be benign, tissue should be obtained from an area that will yield the best cosmetic result.

DISCUSSION

All cases are similar in that each represents the situation of multiplicity without bilaterality. In each of these cases, biopsy revealed intraductal carcinoma with a few foci of invasion. Due to the extensive nature of the process, the only therapeutic option was mastectomy.

To believe that an extensive process must be benign because the breast palpation is normal is an incorrect assumption. To assume that the process must represent benign sclerosing adenosis is incorrect because sclerosing adenosis in its diffuse form is usually bilateral. In each case, prompt biopsy should be considered even if the calcifications appear more round and punctate rather than linear and branching. The recognition that these cases represent multiplicity without bilaterality should raise the level of concern that the process is malignant.

HISTORY

Routine screening mammogram on a 79-year-old woman with nodular breasts.

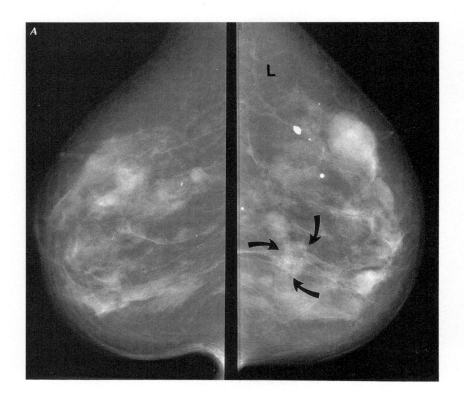

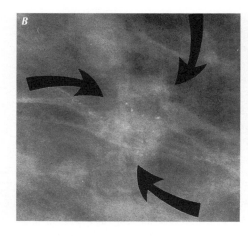

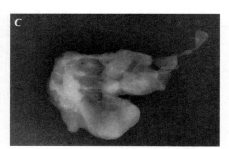

MAMMOGRAPHIC FINDINGS AND RECOMMENDATION

LAT views (**A**) of each breast show multiple bilateral noncalcified masses, more on the left side. In addition, there is a solitary geographic cluster of microcalcifications (*arrows*) on the left side. A closeup view (**B**) shows the cluster to better advantage.

Place the patient into a follow-up protocol for the masses but perform a needle localization and biopsy now to establish the histology of the microcalcifications.

DISCUSSION

Specimen radiograph (**C**) confirms excision of the microcalcifications. Histology revealed an infiltrating ductal carcinoma. The concept of multiplicity and bilaterality must be clearly understood to be used correctly. The two abnormalities on the mammogram were masses and microcalcifications. While there was multiplicity and bilaterality of the masses, allowing the recommendation of follow-up, the microcalcifications were a solitary geographic abnormality. This is why immediate biopsy was performed. In a breast with several abnormalities of differing appearances, each must be evaluated independently for multiplicity and bilaterality.

Routine screening mammograms performed on a 66-year-old woman in 1986 and then two years later, in 1988.

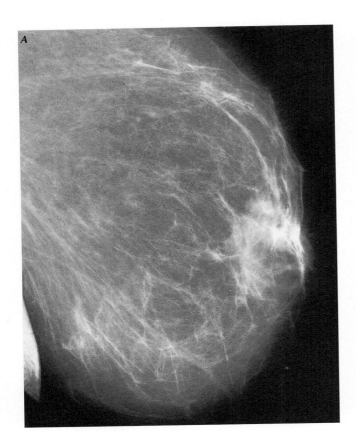

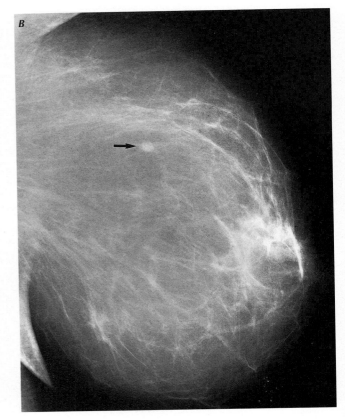

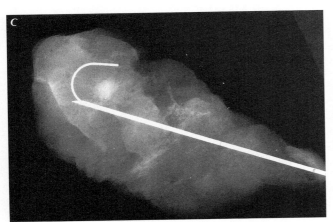

MAMMOGRAPHIC FINDINGS AND RECOMMENDATION ___

Within this two-year interval, OBL views (**A** and **B**) show that a 4-mm noncalcified density (*arrow*) has developed. It has sharp margins.

Perform needle localization and excision to establish the histology of the lesion.

DISCUSSION

Specimen radiography (*C*) confirmed excision of the lesion. Histology revealed an invasive ductal carcinoma. Perhaps nowhere is obtaining old films as important as it is in mammography. Without old films, the characteristics of the mass make it a highly probable benign lesion, and placing it into a follow-up protocol would have been a reasonable option. With a mass this small, it is not the usual practice at NEMCH to perform an ultrasound examination because the mass is beyond the limits of ultrasound to unequivocally declare it a simple cyst even if that is what it really is. Finally, this case clearly shows how mammography should not be used to predict histology. No matter how "benign" the mass appears by mammographic criteria, the only choice the radiologist should have is biopsy versus follow-up when a neodensity is identified.

HISTORY

A routine screening mammogram was performed on a 64-year-old woman in 1983 and in 1987.

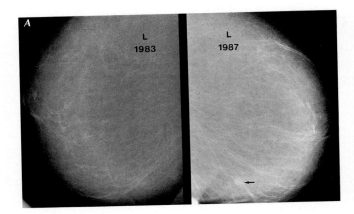

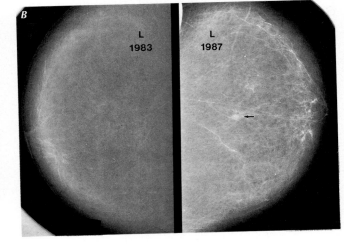

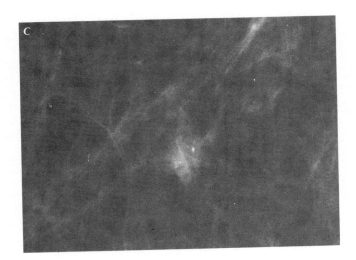

MAMMOGRAPHIC FINDINGS AND RECOMMENDATION

In this four-year interval LAT (*A*) and CC (*B*) views reveal that a neodensity has developed in the left breast. Magnification view (*C*) shows that the density contains microcalcifications. An ultrasound examination was not ordered because the microcalcifications indicate that this can't be a simple cyst.

Perform needle localization and excision to establish the histology of the lesion.

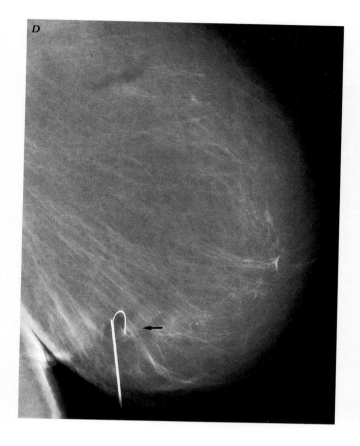

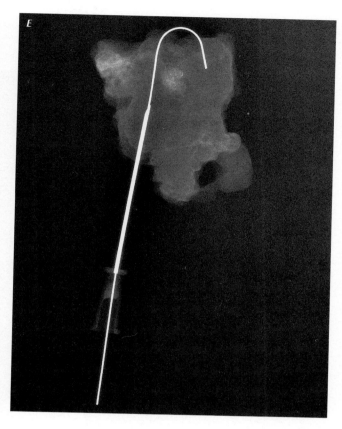

DISCUSSION

An inferior needle localization approach was used (**D**), and specimen radiography (**E**) confirmed excision of the lesion. Histology revealed a 6-mm invasive ductal carcinoma.

This case illustrates two points. This is a neodensity and not an asymmetric density. None of the rules for evaluating an asymmetric density applies in this sit-uation. As a general rule, a moderately well-defined density that has any chance of representing a cyst should probably undergo ultrasound. The presence of microcalcifications on the magnification view eliminated the possibility that this could be a simple cyst. Usually the only calcifications that are associated with a simple cyst are milk of calcium, layering punctate granular calcifications, and rarely rim calcium.

HISTORY

Routine screening mammogram on a 61-year-old woman.

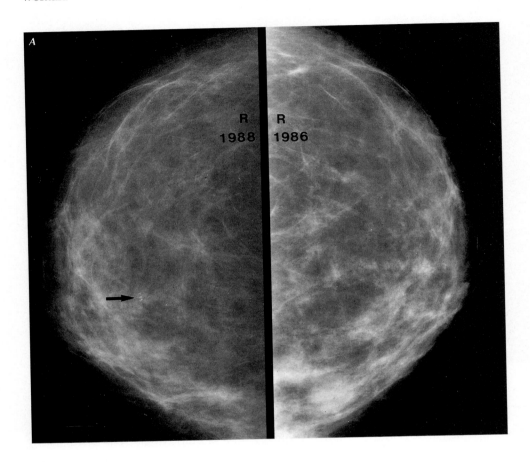

R 1988   R 1986

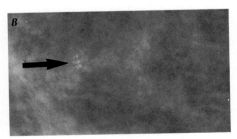

MAMMOGRAPHIC FINDINGS AND RECOMMENDATION

Comparison of CC views (*A*) of the right breast in 1986 and 1988 shows that a new solitary geographic cluster of microcalcifications (*arrow*) has appeared. Closeup view (*B*) shows that there are more than four microcalcifications.

The area should be needle localized and excised to establish the histology of the microcalcifications.

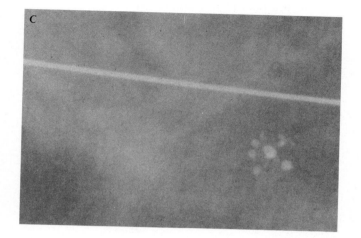

DISCUSSION

The area was excised, and specimen radiography (*C*) confirmed excision of the microcalcifications. They are unassociated with a mass. Histology revealed invasive ductal carcinoma. When one makes the observation that a solitary new cluster of microcalcifications has appeared, the only two options are follow-up or excision. By my criteria, biopsy was recommended, but certainly follow-up is an acceptable alternative. If follow-up is chosen, the clinician must understand that while the radiologist believes the process is most likely benign, the follow-up is necessary because of the possibility of malignancy. Finally, the fact that a small cluster of microcalcifications is unassociated with a density in no way indicates that the process must be benign.

HISTORY

This 62-year-old woman presented with a palpable 1-cm mass in the 3 o'clock position. Based upon palpation, the decision was made to excise the mass. A mammogram was ordered primarily to look for occult disease in the ipsilateral and contralateral breast. There was none. Two weeks later a needle localization was scheduled. Upon questioning the clinician why a localization was necessary for a palpable mass, he said the mass was no longer palpable. It was recommended that another mammogram be obtained prior to scheduling the localization.

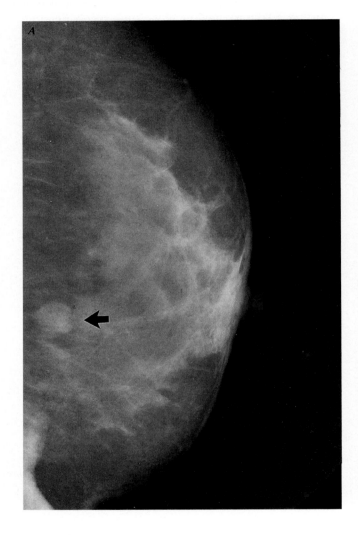

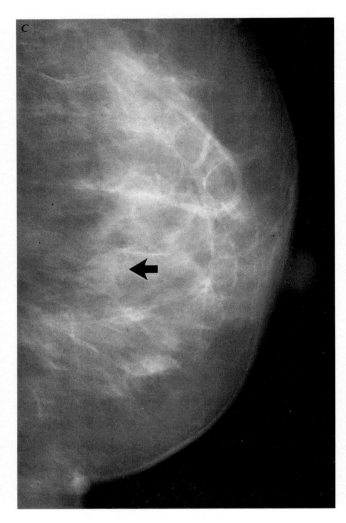

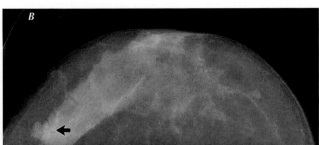

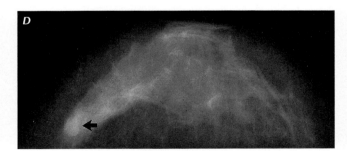

MAMMOGRAPHIC FINDINGS AND RECOMMENDATION

LAT (**A**) and CC (**B**) views show that the palpable mass is noncalcified and has irregular, lobulated margins. Repeat views in LAT (**C**) and CC (**D**) projections two weeks later demonstrate that the mass has decreased in size. This explains why it is no longer palpable.

Assuming that the mass had gotten smaller spontaneously (no aspiration was performed), the localization need not be performed and the patient should return within six months for repeat views of the left breast only to document that the mass does not reappear. Of course, if the mass becomes palpable again in the interval, it can be excised or aspirated based upon clinical grounds.

DISCUSSION

Cancers do not spontaneously grow smaller. By both palpation and mammography, this mass did. It is very important for the radiologist to be absolutely certain that the mass had not been aspirated because that could be the explanation for its decrease in volume. Even if the mass does not totally disappear, spontaneous decrease in size is strong evidence of a benign etiology. We always get a follow-up of the ipsilateral breast within six months just to be certain that the mass does not recur. If it does, then a decision must be made about whether it should be excised.

HISTORY ─────────────────

In 1984 a 76-year-old woman presented for evaluation of left nipple retraction and a palpable mass deep to the nipple. The mass was excised and proved to be an invasive ductal carcinoma. A modified radical mastectomy was performed. The woman returns yearly for mammography of her contralateral breast. In 1988 a nonpalpable mass was detected. It was needle localized.

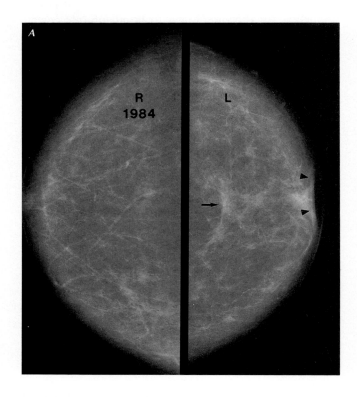

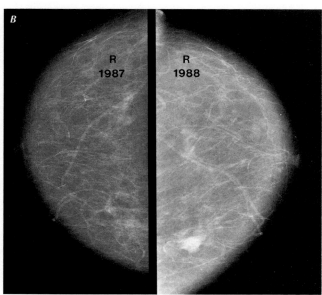

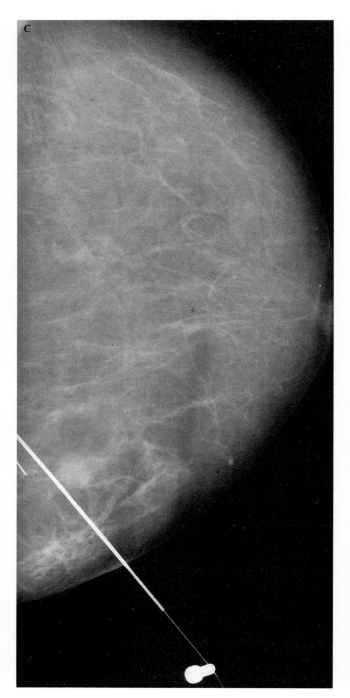

MAMMOGRAPHIC FINDINGS AND RECOMMENDATION

CC views (*A*) of the right and left breasts in 1984 showed left nipple retraction (*arrowheads*) and an irregular mass (*arrow*) located 4 cm deep to the nipple. CC views of the right breast (*B*) show that a 1-cm mass has appeared between annual screens. The mass remained nonpalpable on directed breast repalpation, and needle localization (*C*) was required prior to biopsy. Histology revealed an invasive carcinoma. She underwent a modified radical mastectomy.

DISCUSSION

Probably the highest risk known for the development of breast cancer is a personal history of breast cancer. Women with known breast cancer should undergo annual mammography. If this is not a standard policy where a radiologist practices, then the radiologist would be doing a great service to cause this policy to be adopted. Notice that even in retrospect the cancer was not diagnosable in 1987. Also note that despite its rather superficial location in a very fatty breast, it was nonpalpable.

HISTORY

Routine screening mammogram in a 59-year-old woman.

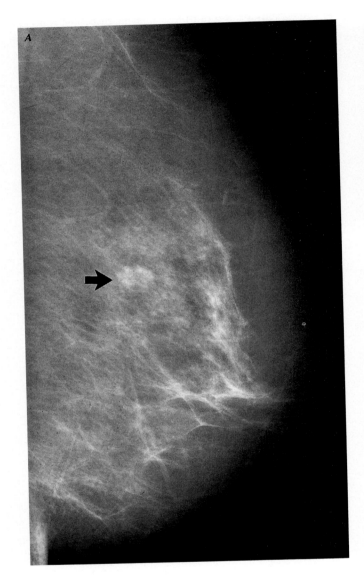

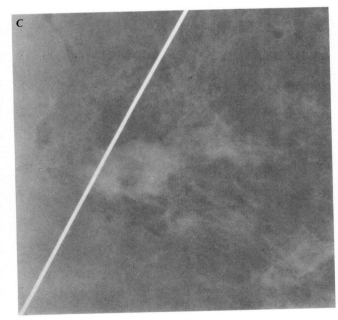

MAMMOGRAPHIC FINDINGS AND RECOMMENDATION

The LAT view (**A**) reveals a 1-cm mass with irregular margins (*arrow*). There is the suggestion that it has a lucent center. Magnification view (**B**) confirms that the lesion has a lucent center.

Perform a needle localization and biopsy of the mass.

Magnification specimen radiograph (**C**) confirms excision of the mass. Notice its lucent center. Histology revealed a 0.7-cm invasive and in-situ lobular carcinoma.

DISCUSSION

This case illustrates that concluding that a mass must be benign just based upon the presence of central fat is incorrect. All aspects of the lesion must be analyzed. When a lesion has some mammographic characteristics that weigh probability toward a benign diagnosis and others that suggest a malignancy, the management should be guided by the "worst" features of the lesion.

HISTORY

This 71-year-old female presented for the evaluation of a hard, painless, fixed palpable mass in the right upper outer quadrant. It measured approximately 3 cm by palpation. Fine needle aspiration was positive for malignancy. A preoperative mammogram was performed.

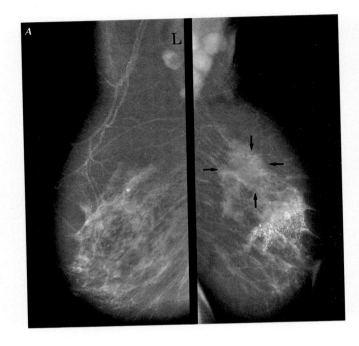

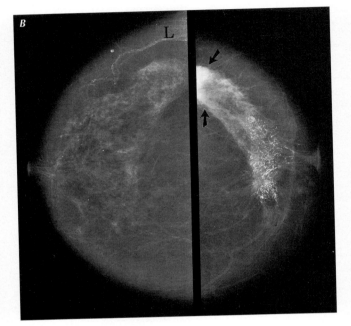

MAMMOGRAPHIC FINDINGS AND RECOMMENDATION

OBL (*A*) and CC (*B*) views of both breasts reveal no dominant mass or suspicious calcifications in the left breast. The palpable mass on the right (*arrows*) is identified. An unsuspected finding was the presence of a large geographic area of linear, branching, pleomorphic calcifications in the right breast above the nipple in the 12 o'clock position.

In addition to performing a biopsy for the palpable mass, the area of calcifications must also be sampled. If it is malignant, then consideration for breast conservation therapy is not an option. Histology of the palpable mass revealed invasive ductal carcinoma, and histology of the microcalcifications revealed extensive intraductal carcinoma with a few foci of invasion.

DISCUSSION

The purpose of the preoperative mammogram had nothing to do with the palpable malignancy diagnosed by fine needle aspiration. It was to evaluate for occult ipsilateral and contralateral tumor. Patient management options will obviously be different with the discovery of occult disease.

HISTORY

Routine screening mammogram in a 65-year-old woman.

MAMMOGRAPHIC FINDINGS AND RECOMMENDATION

OBL (*A*) and CC (*B*) views of the right breast performed on 4/25/88 reveal a 1-cm poorly defined non-calcified mass located 11 cm behind the nipple. The left breast was entirely replaced by fat and had no mass or suspicious calcifications.

Perform ultrasound to rule out the possibility that the mass represents a simple cyst (although this is highly unlikely). If the mass is not a simple cyst, then it should be excised. This patient was managed at another hospital and was followed, instead of undergoing ultrasound.

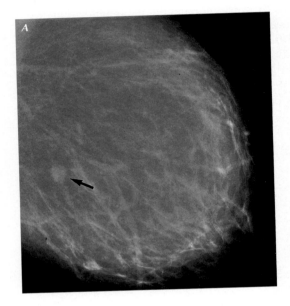

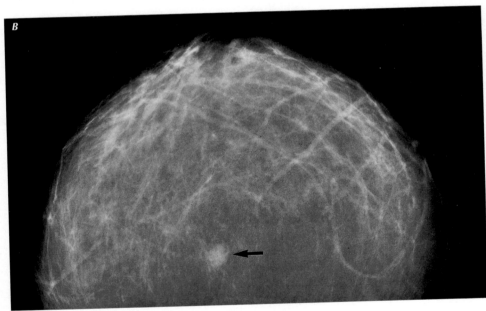

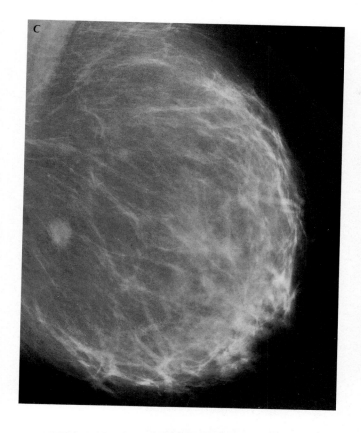

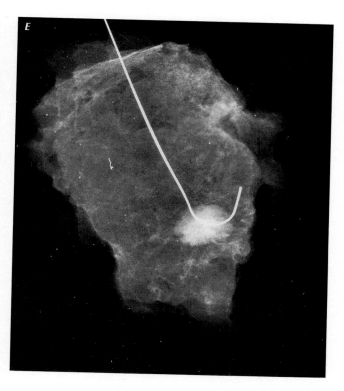

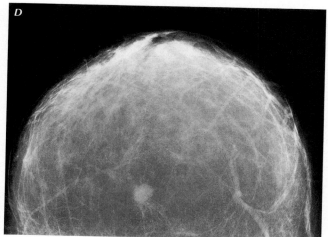

DISCUSSION

A follow-up mammogram was performed on 12/6/88. OBL (**C**) and CC (**D**) views reveal that the mass now measures 1.5 cm in greatest diameter. Since it was still nonpalpable, it was needle localized. Specimen radiograph (**E**) confirmed its excision. Histology revealed invasive ductal carcinoma. This case demonstrates how carcinoma can change within several months. A magnification view performed at the time of the initial examination would have shown the irregular borders to better advantage and should have caused the localization to have been strongly recommended at that time.

HISTORY

Routine screening mammogram on a 59-year-old woman.

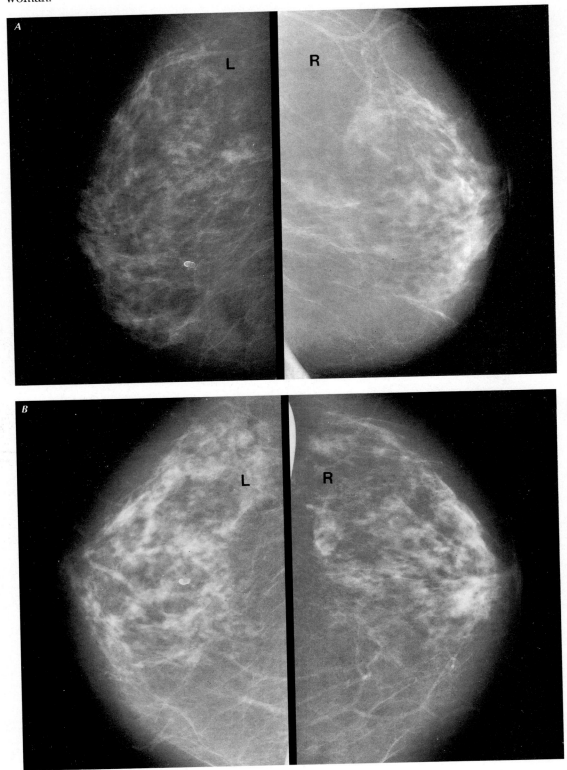

MAMMOGRAPHIC FINDINGS AND RECOMMENDATION

LAT (**A**) and CC (**B**) views demonstrate multiple bilateral asymmetric densities. There is no one area more suspicious to merit biopsy at this time.

Place the patient into a follow-up protocol. The patient refused to return for follow-up mammography. However, she returned two years later for evaluation of a hard palpable mass in the left upper outer quadrant.

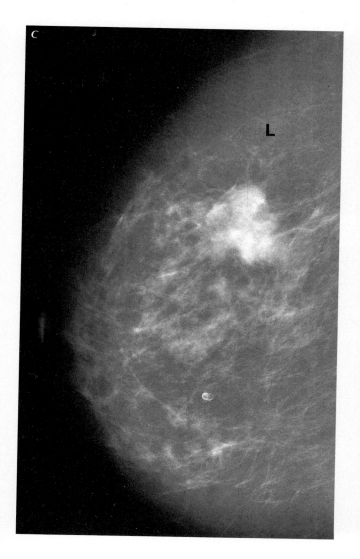

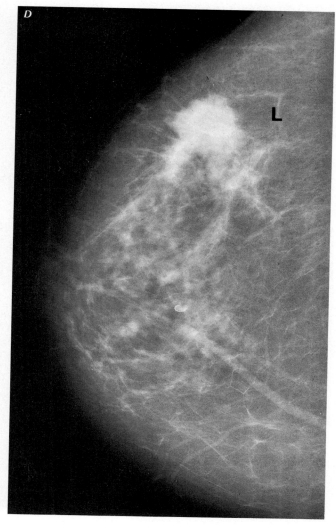

DISCUSSION

LAT (**C**) and CC (**D**) views of the left breast demonstrate a typical carcinoma. Biopsy revealed invasive ductal carcinoma. This carcinoma would have been recognized earlier in the follow-up protocol. In this case, there was clear documentation by the clinician that the patient refused to return for follow-up mammography. It is prudent to be certain that there is appropriate documentation if the patient refuses to return for follow-up.

HISTORY

This 42-year-old woman was referred after an unsuccessful needle localization and biopsy failed to excise a solitary cluster of microcalcifications.

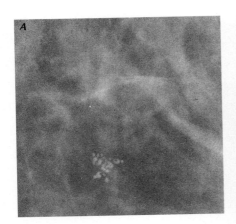

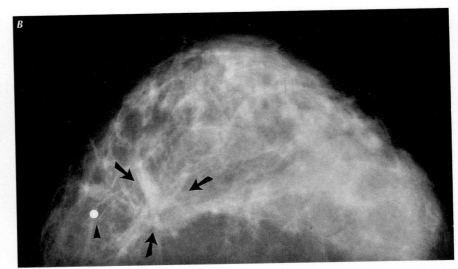

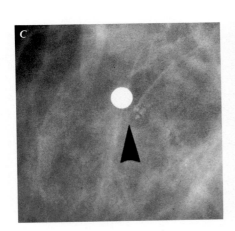

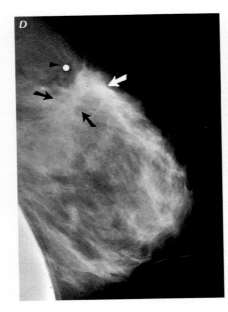

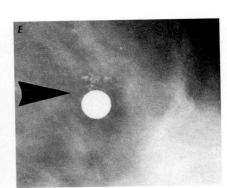

MAMMOGRAPHIC FINDINGS AND RECOMMENDATION

A magnification view of the cluster (*A*) showed that several calcifications had lucent centers. The metallic marker technique was used to determine whether the calcifications were dermal in location. A CC view (*B*) shows the area of architectural distortion caused by the previous biopsy (*arrows*). The metallic marker is directly over the microcalcifications (*arrowhead*). Closeup view (*C*) shows the relationship of the calcifications to the metallic marker. A LAT view (*D*) again shows the postbiopsy architectural distortion (*arrows*). The microcalcifications (*arrowhead*) do not change their relationship to the superficial metallic marker. Closeup view (*E*) demonstrates that the calcifications move with the marker.

The microcalcifications are dermal in location, and no surgery is necessary.

DISCUSSION

This case illustrates how important it is for the radiologist to be certain that microcalcifications are not dermal in location. If their true location is not recognized, then not only will the woman be subjected to needless surgery, but if the surgeon does not take skin with the biopsy (which is not usually done) the microcalcifications will not be excised.

HISTORY _____

This is a routine screening mammogram on a 52-year-old woman. Twenty five years ago she had a biopsy in the right upper outer quadrant for something which proved to be benign. The biopsy scar is easily seen.

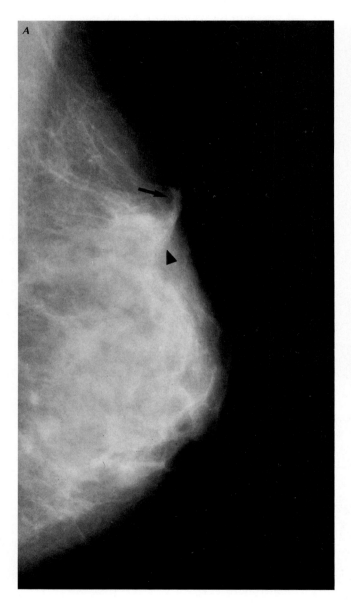

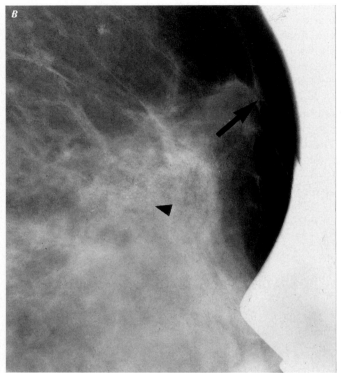

MAMMOGRAPHIC FINDINGS AND RECOMMENDATION _____

A LAT view (*A*) of the right breast shows the biopsy site (*arrow*). Nearby is a solitary cluster of microcalcifications (*arrowhead*). A LAT magnification view (*B*) shows the relationship of the biopsy scar (*arrow*) to the microcalcifications (*arrowhead*). The microcalcifications are generally punctate, but they are too numerous to count and many calcifications are not perfectly punctate. The microcalcifications vary in size.

Have the patient return to determine whether the calcifications are dermal in location.

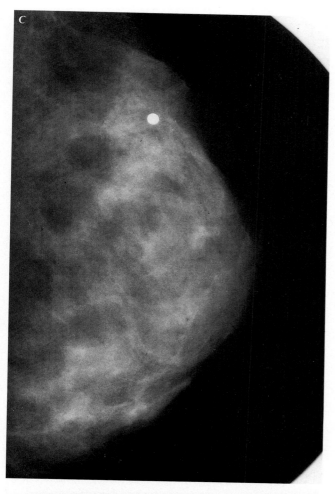

MAMMOGRAPHIC FINDINGS AND RECOMMENDATION

Using the superficial metallic marker technique, many of the calcifications do not separate from the metallic marker either on the LAT (*C*) or CC (*D*) views. Most, if not all, are dermal in location.

Place the patient into a follow-up protocol.

DISCUSSION

Whenever calcifications are near a biopsy site, the possibility of postbiopsy dermal calcifications must be considered. In this case, none of the calcifications had any clues to suspect their dermal location. It is important to remember that just because calcifications are located near a biopsy site for previous benign disease, one can't assume that the calcifications are benign. The patient was placed into a follow-up protocol because these views could not prove that all of the calcifications were dermal. The calcifications have remained stable for nine years.

If the decision were to be made to excise the calcifications to establish their histology, needle localization would not be required. The surgeon should be made aware of their very superficial location.

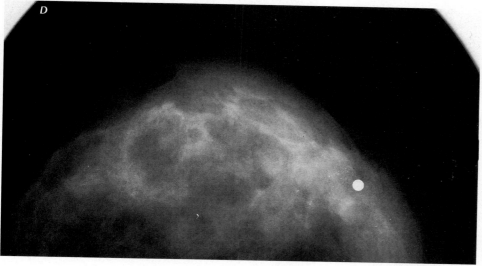

HISTORY

Routine screening mammogram on a 44-year-old woman.

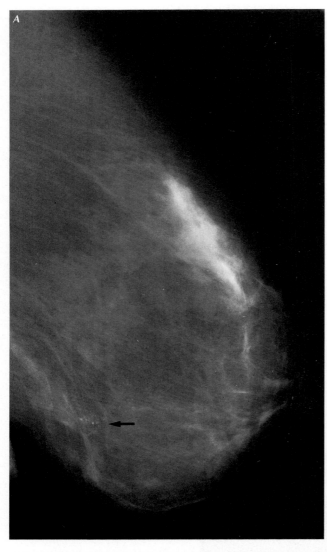

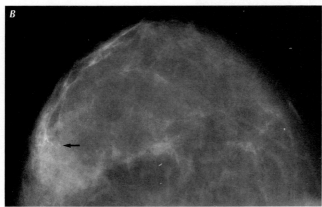

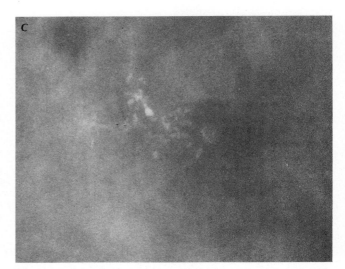

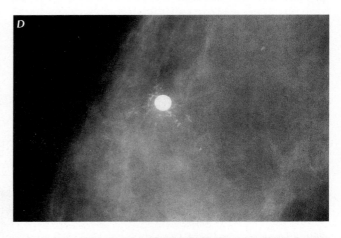

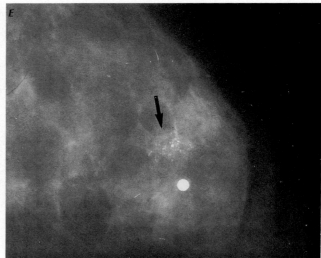

MAMMOGRAPHIC FINDINGS AND RECOMMENDATION

LAT (*A*) and CC (*B*) views demonstrate a solitary geographic cluster of microcalcifications in the right lower outer quadrant. There was no associated mass. Close-up (*C*) shows the microcalcifications to better advantage. The left breast had no dominant mass or suspicious calcifications. Since the calcifications were located very peripherally, the possibility of a dermal location was considered. Before the patient left the department, a metallic marker was used to establish the location of the microcalcifications. On the CC view (*D*) the marker is directly over the calcifications. However, there is separation between the marker and the calcifications on the LAT view (*E*).

Prompt excision was advised to establish the nature of the microcalcifications. Since they were proved to be very superficially located, a needle localization was not required. On the day of surgery the patient returned to the Radiology Department, and the site of the microcalcifications was marked.

DISCUSSION

Specimen radiograph (*F*) revealed excision of many of the microcalcifications. Histology revealed intraductal comedocarcinoma. However, the tumor extended to the margins and reexcision was necessary. On reexcision, areas of invasion were found. An axillary dissection was then performed, and all nodes were free of disease. The patient opted for breast conservation therapy.

The peripheral location of microcalcifications should always raise the possibility of a dermal location. Even though these microcalcifications were not dermal, proof of their superficial location obviated the need for a needle localization procedure. This case illustrates how necessary it is to be certain that all the tumor is removed. Though the initial biopsy only showed intraductal tumor, in fact reexcision demonstrated that there was already invasion, and this changed management, since an axillary dissection was necessary.

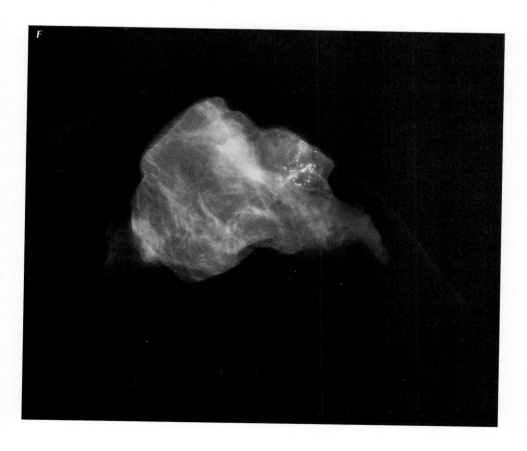

HISTORY

Routine screening mammogram on a 69-year-old woman.

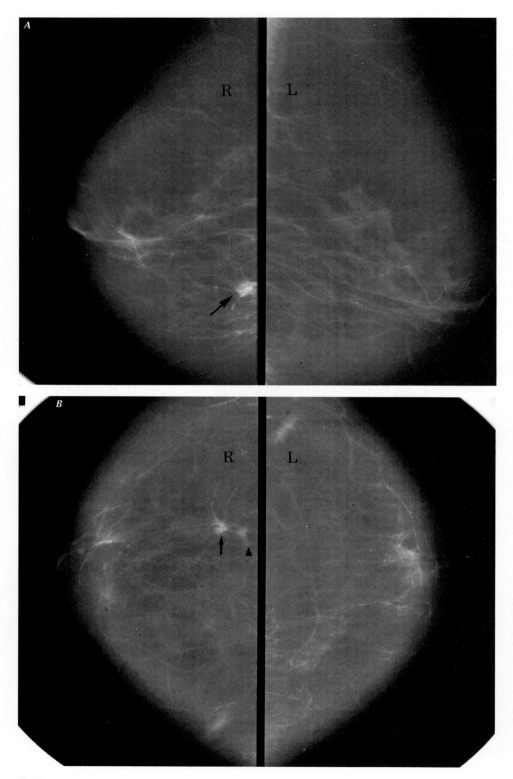

MAMMOGRAPHIC FINDINGS AND RECOMMENDATION

On the OBL views (**A**) and CC views (**B**) there is a 5-mm stellate mass (*arrow*) in the 6 o'clock position of the right breast. On the CC view, a deeper mass (*arrowhead*) is present just posterior to the stellate mass.

Repalpate the patient with special attention to the 6 o'clock region of the right breast. If a mass is palpable, it should be excised. If nothing is palpable in retrospect, the area should be needle localized prior to excisional biopsy.

DISCUSSION

The mass was palpable on redirected palpation. Needle localization was not necessary. Histology revealed invasive ductal carcinoma with an adjacent focus of tumor resulting from direct spread.

Although this mammogram was performed as a routine screening study after a normal breast palpation, indeed the palpation was abnormal when it was directed to the area of concern detected by mammography. The information that a breast palpation is normal must be critically viewed in the context of the examination. A normal breast palpation performed by an experienced person and directed toward an area of suspicion clearly has an advantage over a normal breast palpation performed by a less experienced person without any direction. Ideally if there is a nonpalpable abnormality on the mammogram, the breast palpation should be performed as the person doing the palpation is looking at the mammogram.

HISTORY

A routine screening mammogram was performed on a 78-year-old woman. There are two nonpalpable masses in the right breast. One is calcified, and the other is noncalcified. Assuming that only the OBL and LAT views are available for review, can you predict which lesion is medial and which is lateral without the CC view?

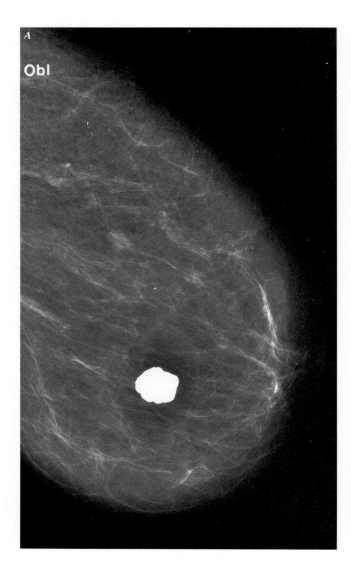

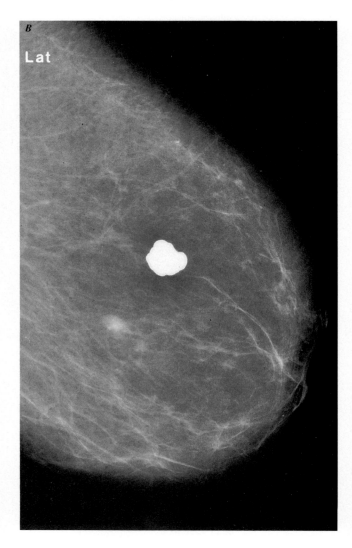

MAMMOGRAPHIC FINDINGS

Compared to the OBL (*A*) view, on the LAT (*B*) view the calcified mass moves up and the noncalcified mass moves down.

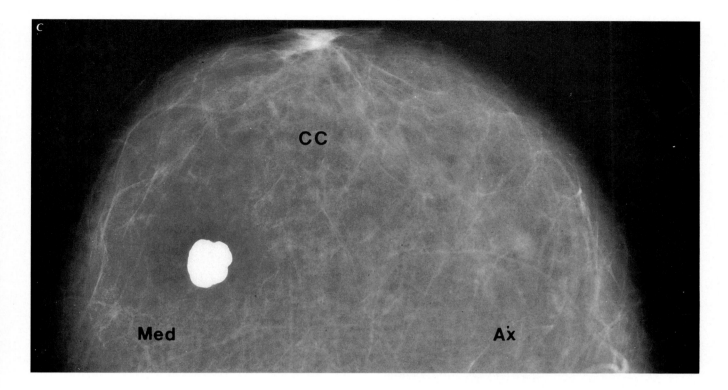

DISCUSSION

The calcified lesion is medially located, and the smaller noncalcified lesion is in the lateral portion of the breast. One of the recurrent mammographic problems is seeing a mammographic abnormality on one view but not on the other. With the aid of additional views, the location of the abnormality can be determined. One of the best articles describing how to do this has been written by Sickles and should be read by every radiologist interpreting mammograms (*Sickles EA: Practical solutions to common mammographic problems. Tailoring the examination. AJR 151:31–39, 1988*). The CC view (*C*) above shows the location of the two lesions.

HISTORY _____

Routine screening mammogram on a 47-year-old woman.

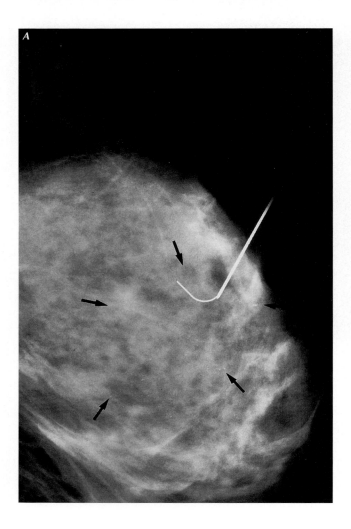

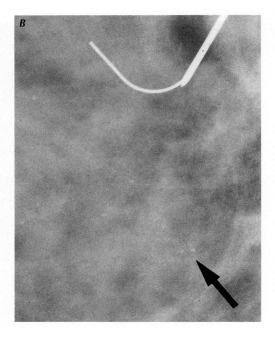

MAMMOGRAPHIC FINDINGS AND RECOMMENDATION _____

There is a large solitary geographic area of microcalcifications in the upper outer quadrant of the right breast. LAT view from a needle localization (*A*) reveals the extensive area involved (*arrows*).

Closeup view (*B*) shows the microcalcifications to better advantage.

Perform a needle localization of the area and sample the lesion. To excise all the microcalcifications would cause unacceptable cosmesis should the process prove to be benign. If the lesion proves benign, place the patient into a follow-up protocol to reassess the residual microcalcifications.

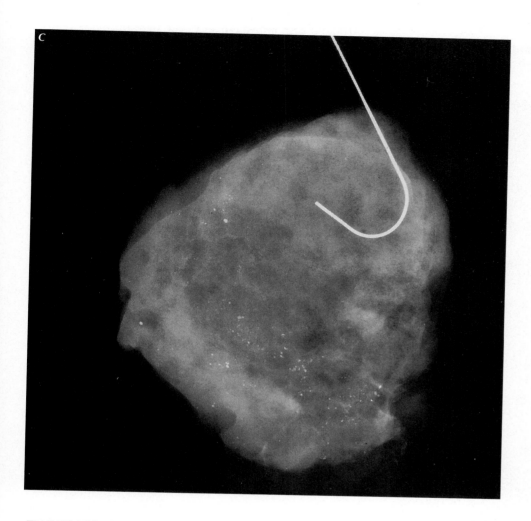

DISCUSSION

Magnification specimen radiograph (*C*) reveals that numerous microcalcifications were excised. Histology revealed fibrocystic disease with focal intraductal hyperplasia and lobular hyperplasia with microcalcifications. Although ideally an excisional biopsy should be performed for all mammographic abnormalities, sometimes all the lesion is not excised, and other times, as in this case, an incisional biopsy is purposefully performed. The patient is placed into follow-up because of the possibility that since the entire lesion was not excised, theoretically a malignancy could have been missed.

HISTORY

A 70-year-old woman presented for evaluation of localized skin dimpling in the *left* upper outer quadrant.

She had known breast carcinoma on the *right* side treated with breast conservation therapy and radiation. There was no palpable mass under the area of the skin dimpling.

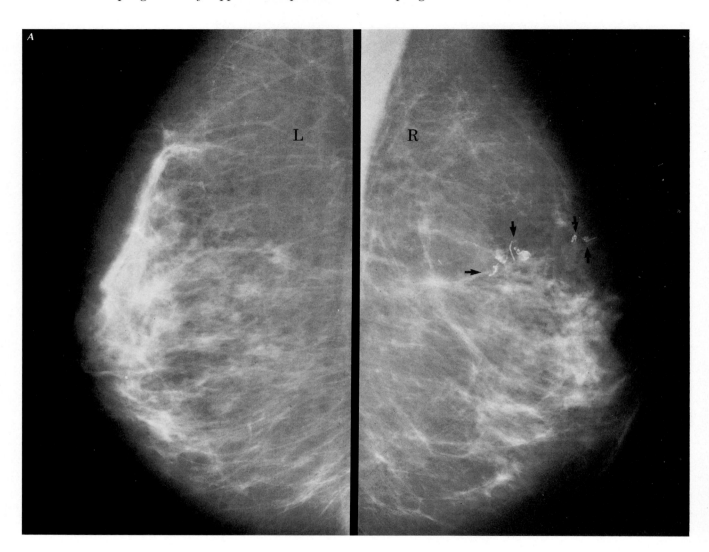

MAMMOGRAPHIC INTERPRETATION AND RECOMMENDATION

OBL views (*A*) show calcified sutures on the right side (*arrows*) from the radiation therapy. The left breast has no dominant mass or suspicious calcifications. All densities are unchanged from multiple previous mammograms (this patient was receiving annual mammography because of her personal history of breast cancer on the right side).

In view of the "normal" mammogram, there are three options. The first is to follow the area of skin dimpling clinically. The second would be to perform a biopsy under the area of skin dimpling on the chance of excising a nonpalpable carcinoma. The third option is to perform an ultrasound examination directed to the area of skin dimpling. This third option was recommended, and an ultrasound over the area of the skin dimpling was performed.

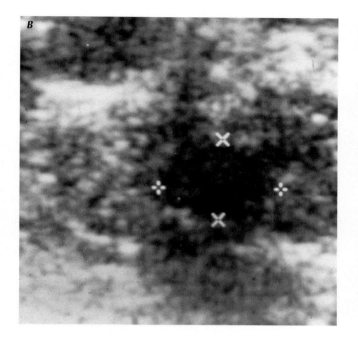

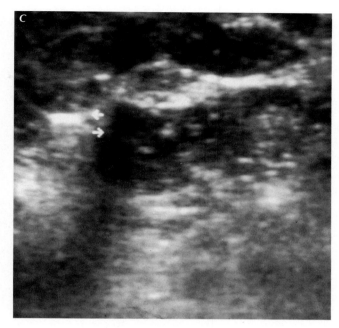

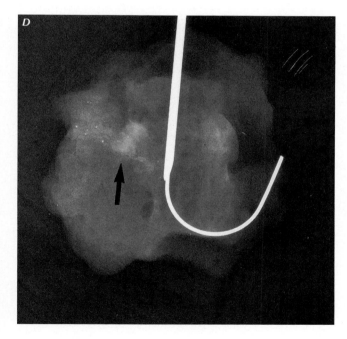

DISCUSSION

Ultrasound (*B*) revealed a hypoechoic mass under the area of skin dimpling. Needle localization was performed under ultrasound guidance. The upper arrow on the ultrasound localization film (*C*) is the needle tip, and the lower arrow points to the hypoechoic mass. Magnification specimen radiography (*D*) revealed that a stellate mass with microcalcifications was excised. Histology showed invasive ductal carcinoma. In selected cases, directed ultrasound can complement mammography in the search for occult carcinoma. Needle localization of a nonpalpable breast lesion can be successfully performed under ultrasound guidance.

Case 21

OK

OK

HISTORY

Routine screening mammogram was performed on a 67-year-old woman in 1984. Two years later another routine screening mammogram was performed.

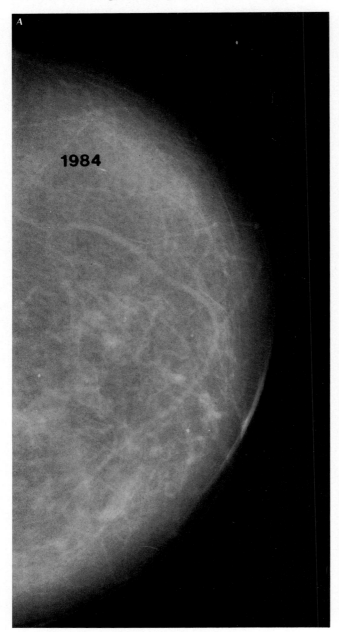

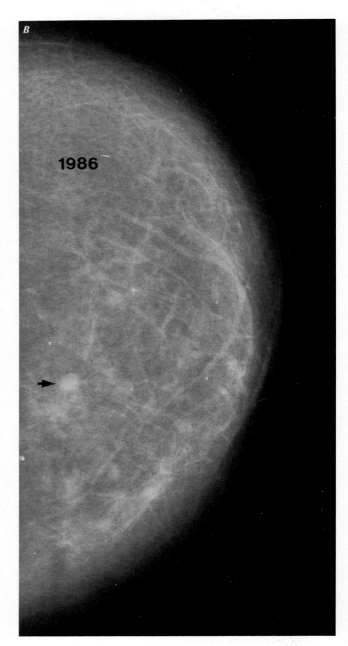

MAMMOGRAPHIC FINDINGS AND RECOMMENDATION

CC views (**A** and **B**) show that within this two-year interval a neodensity has developed (*arrow*).

Perform an ultrasound examination to rule out the possibility that this density represents a simple cyst. If the mass is solid, it should be excised. If nothing is identified by ultrasound, the neodensity should be excised after it is localized by needle. Ultrasound examination was performed and revealed neither cyst nor mass. The clinician ordered a repeat mammogram in six months.

256

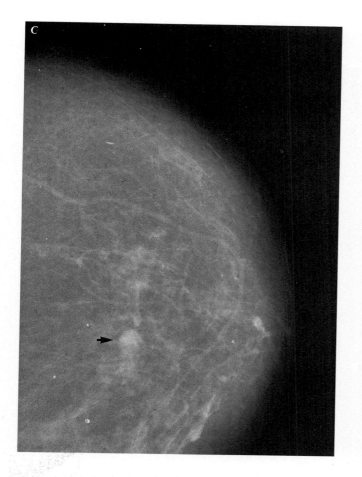

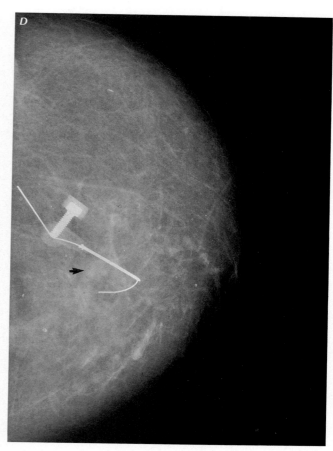

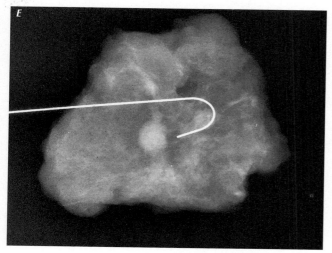

DISCUSSION

Within this six-month interval the mass has grown larger (*C*). The mass was still nonpalpable. Needle localization (*D*) and excision were performed. Specimen radiography (*E*) confirmed excision of the mass, and histology revealed an invasive ductal carcinoma. This case illustrates that when the ultrasound revealed neither cyst nor mass, this should have been understood as noninformation and biopsy should have been performed. Unless there is an ultrasound correlation for a definite mammographic abnormality, the ultrasound examination should not weigh into the decision of management.

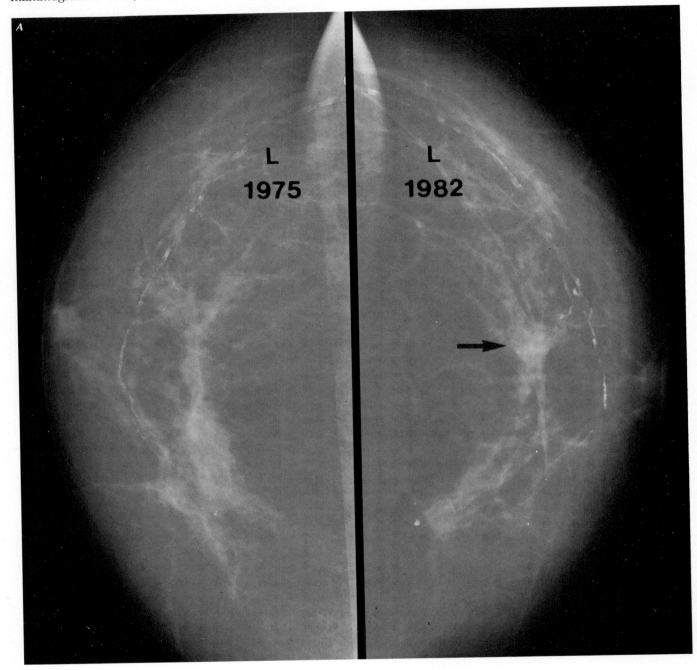

HISTORY

A 73-year-old woman underwent a routine screening mammogram in 1975, and another one 7 years later.

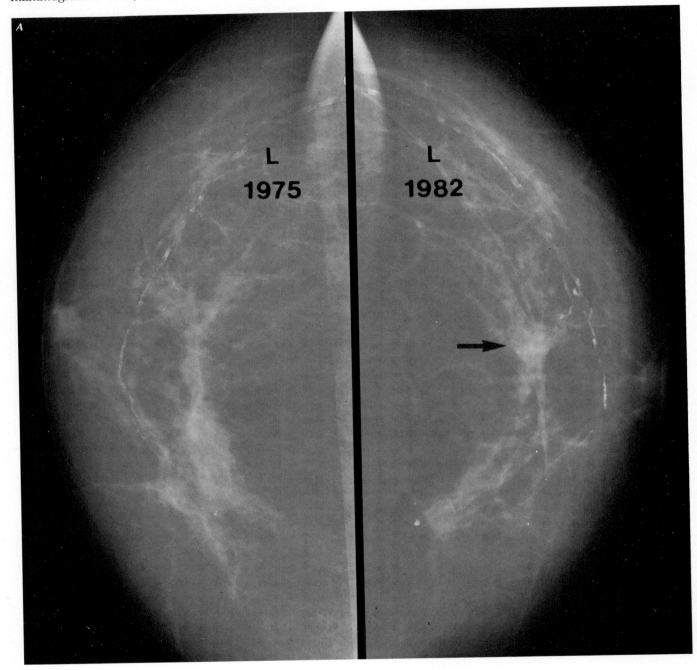

MAMMOGRAPHIC FINDINGS AND RECOMMENDATION

CC views (*A*) comparing the left breast in 1975 and 1982 show that a neodensity (*arrow*) has developed.

If the area remains nonpalpable on directed repalpation, it should undergo preoperative needle localization prior to excisional biopsy.

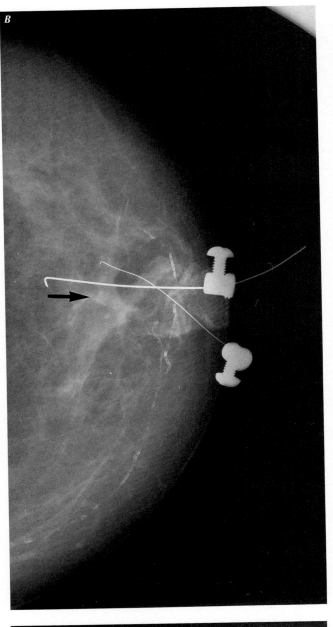

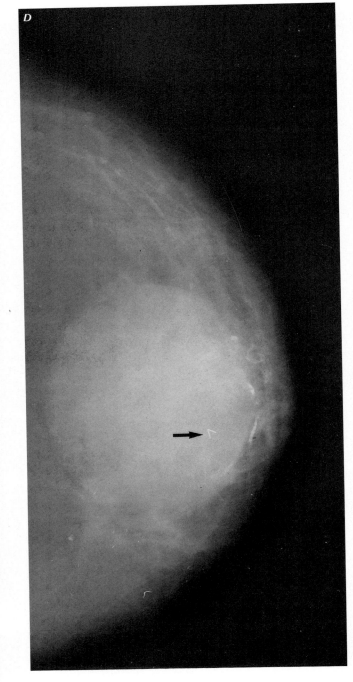

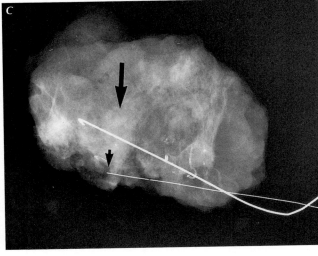

MAMMOGRAPHIC FINDINGS

Percutaneous localization was performed using needle-wire systems that could not be repositioned. Postlocalization CC view (**B**) shows that two wires were left in vivo. Specimen radiograph (**C**) confirms excision of the noncalcified mass (*large arrow*). It was firm to palpation, and histology revealed invasive ductal carcinoma. Notice that the hooked end of one of the wires (*small arrow*) is not contained on the specimen radiograph. Postoperative mammogram (**D**) reveals a large hematoma at the biopsy site. The hooked end of the wire is evident (*arrow*).

DISCUSSION

The patient did not want breast conservation therapy, and so a modified radical mastectomy was performed. There are two important points illustrated by this case. Transection of a localization wire is not negligent, but it is one of the potential complications of the needle localization procedure. If I were using a wire that could be transected, I would have this included as a potential complication in the consent form, which I have every patient sign prior to performing the localization procedure. Finally, when thin wires that can be transected are used for localization, the specimen radiograph should be evaluated to determine not only whether the nonpalpable lesion has been excised but *also* whether the entire distal end of the wire has been retrieved.

HISTORY ⎯⎯⎯⎯⎯⎯⎯⎯⎯

This 65-year-old woman presented for a routine screening mammogram. One year earlier she had undergone a needle localization and excision for what she said was a benign lesion. The postbiopsy skin changes beneath the nipple were visually apparent.

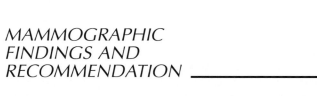

MAMMOGRAPHIC FINDINGS AND RECOMMENDATION ⎯⎯⎯⎯⎯⎯⎯

The LAT view (*A*) shows a stellate mass with associated skin thickening and retraction. These findings were confirmed on the CC view as well.

The mammograms from the previous needle localization must be obtained for review to determine what was removed and its relationship to the stellate mass seen on the current examination.

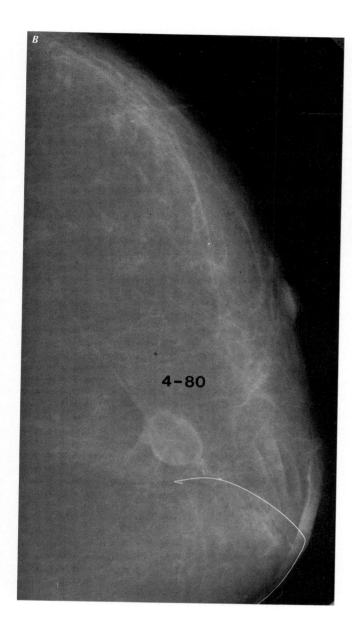

4-80

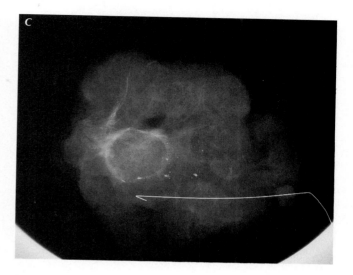

MAMMOGRAPHIC FINDINGS AND RECOMMENDATION

The mammogram from approximately one and a half years earlier was obtained (**B**), and it showed an unusual lesion containing a lucent center with irregular borders and associated microcalcifications. This film from the actual localization showed the precise path of the wire. An accompanying specimen radiograph (**C**) confirmed that the lesion was removed. The pathology report was also obtained, and the histology of the lesion was focal fibrosis with chronic inflammation and calcifications.

We now had proof that the localization and biopsy took place in the same area of the current mammographic changes. The lesion was completely excised and was benign. The stellate mass imaged on the current examination could represent a postoperative parenchymal scar. Since the breast palpation was also consistent with expected postbiopsy changes and did not identify a firm mass, the patient was placed into a follow-up protocol.

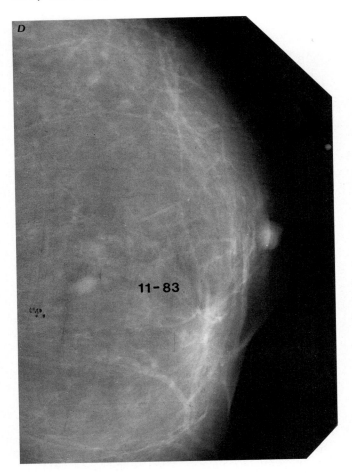

D

11-83

DISCUSSION

When postbiopsy changes are followed over time, they should either remain stable or regress. This LAT view (**D**) taken during the follow-up protocol shows definite regression of the stellate mass.

The radiologist always faces a difficult dilemma in trying to determine whether mammographic findings that would otherwise trigger a biopsy could be the result of postsurgical changes in a biopsied breast. No firm rules can be given but in general when the radiologist can obtain proof of where the actual biopsy took place, the needle path, and confirmation that the lesion was excised, at least follow-up becomes more of an option. Of course breast palpation findings always weigh into the decision. Finally the time elapsed between the biopsy and the current mammogram must be taken into consideration for there is no guarantee that during the interval, a cancer, totally unrelated to the excised benign lesion, has developed. The longer the time between the biopsy and the current mammogram, the greater the chance that an interval cancer could have developed.

HISTORY

Routine screening mammogram on a 38-year-old woman.

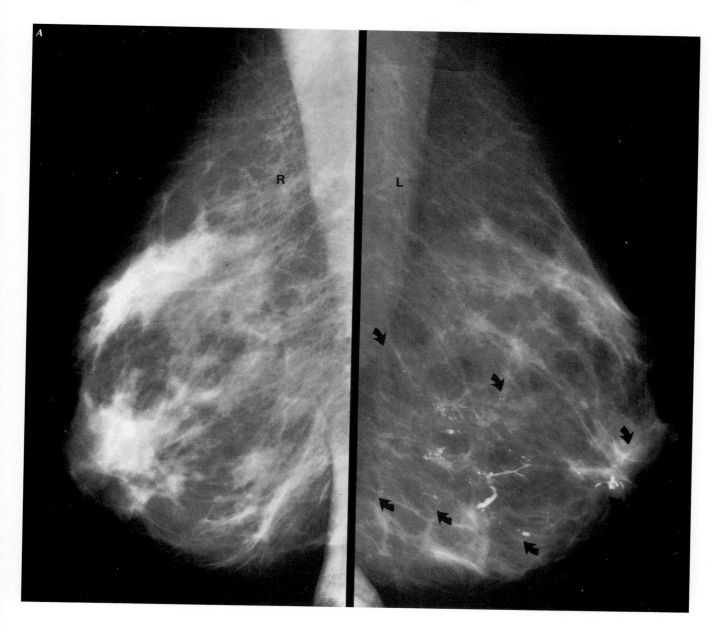

MAMMOGRAPHIC FINDINGS AND RECOMMENDATION

OBL views of both breasts (*A*) reveal a large geographic region of microcalcifications and macrocalcifications, including large ductal calcifications in the left breast. The microcalcifications are pleomorphic and too numerous to count. The process extends from the subareolar region to the chest wall. The right breast has no dominant mass or suspicious calcifications.

Perform an incisional biopsy of the left breast process. Needle localization is not necessary because of the extensive nature of the process. Specimen radiograph the excised tissue to document that some of the calcifications have been excised.

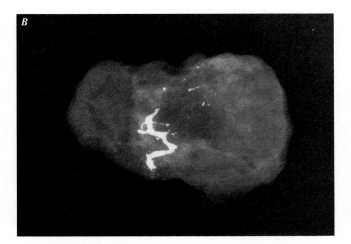

DISCUSSION

Specimen radiography (**B**) showed that the tissue contained calcifications. Histology revealed that all of the calcifications were contained within intraductal tumor. Since the process was so extensive, breast conservation therapy was not an option and a modified radical mastectomy was performed. Pathology revealed negative lymph nodes and no residual tumor in the mastectomy tissue. If indeed there was no residual tumor in the mastectomy specimen, then the tumor was really focal and breast conservation therapy could have been an option. I asked for the mastectomy tissue to be radiographed.

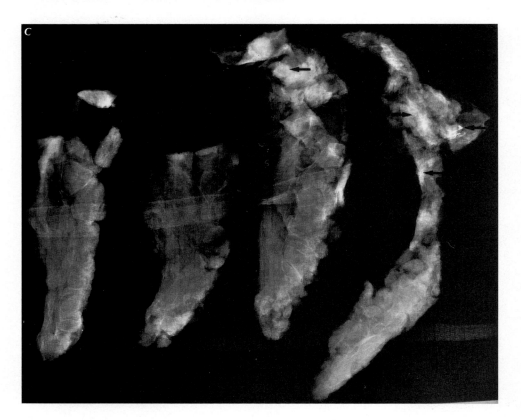

DISCUSSION

Radiography of the mastectomy sections (**C**) revealed numerous areas of calcifications (*arrows*). Histology of these areas revealed extensive intraductal carcinoma in every focus of calcification. This case dramatically illustrates that if microcalcifications are not isolated for the pathologist, there is no guarantee that they will end up on the slide for analysis. The radiologist must work with the pathologist to be certain that microcalcifications undergoing needle localization and excision are isolated for histologic review.

HISTORY

In 1985 a 34-year-old woman presented for evaluation of a palpable mass. It was excised and histology revealed invasive ductal carcinoma. She opted for breast conservation therapy. The cancer was excised with clear margins, and she underwent radiation therapy. In 1989 a new cluster of microcalcifications was detected on an annual screening mammogram.

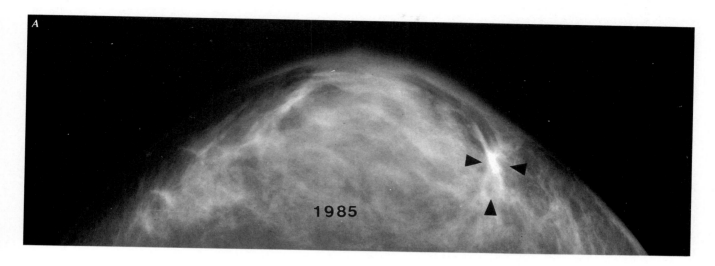

1985

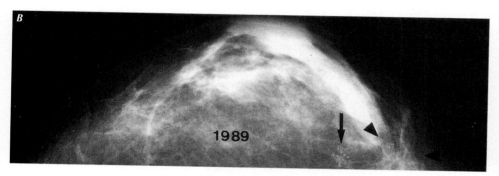

1989

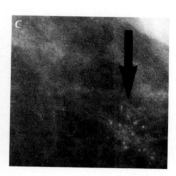

MAMMOGRAPHIC FINDINGS AND RECOMMENDATION

A CC view (*A*) in 1985 reveals the lumpectomy site (*arrowheads*). The generalized skin thickening is the result of the breast irradiation. In 1989 a CC view (*B*) shows that a cluster of microcalcifications (*arrow*) has appeared adjacent to the lumpectomy site (*arrowheads*). Closeup view (*C*) shows the new cluster to better advantage.

Needle localization and excision of the microcalcifications should be performed to evaluate the possibility of recurrent tumor at the lumpectomy site or the development of a new focus of breast carcinoma.

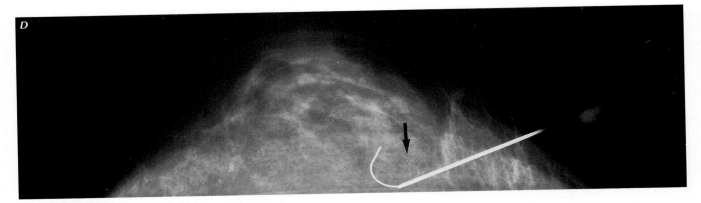

D

DISCUSSION ─────────────

Needle localization (**D**) was performed. Although an excisional biopsy was to be done, not all of the calcifications were contained in the specimen radiograph. Histology revealed a very dysplastic lesion with marked atypia. Although no definite areas of malignancy were present, the lesion looked so dysplastic that the pathologist said that more tissue should be excised to exclude the possibility of malignancy. The woman had to choose the option of another localization and biopsy versus a mastectomy. She was told that even if the lesion proved to be benign, her cosmesis after the repeat localization and biopsy would be poor. She opted for a mastectomy with eventual breast reconstruction. The pathologist reported that the mastectomy specimen revealed no residual tumor. I asked for the mastectomy specimen to be radiographed in order to locate the microcalcifications.

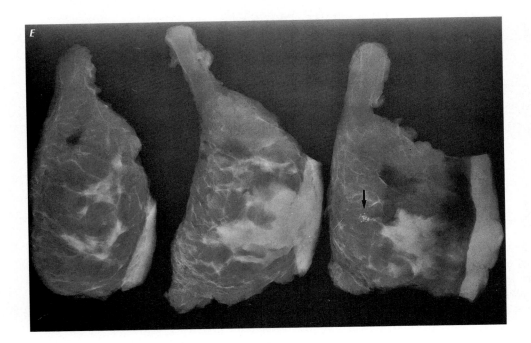

E

DISCUSSION ─────────────

Radiography of the mastectomy sections (**E**) identified the focus of microcalcifications (*arrow*). Histology revealed comedocarcinoma with areas of early invasion. This is another dramatic example of the questionable reliance that can be placed upon a pathology report stating "no evidence of tumor" if the mammographic calcifications have not been positively isolated for the pathologist to sample for histologic analysis.

HISTORY

Two different patients presented to be evaluated for breast conservation therapy. Patient #1 is a 37-year-old woman, and patient #2 is a 52-year-old woman.

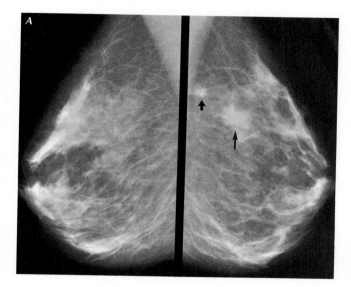

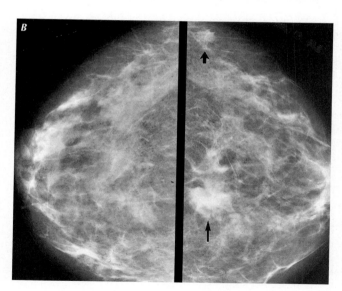

MAMMOGRAPHIC FINDINGS AND RECOMMENDATION

OBL views (**A**) and CC views (**B**) from patient #1 reveal the palpable proven carcinoma (*long arrow*). However a smaller irregular nonpalpable mass (*short arrow*) is also present.

LAT view (**C**) from patient #2 shows a large postoperative hematoma (*arrowheads*) at the site of excisional biopsy of a palpable carcinoma. There are two noncalcified masses present, one in the upper part of the breast (*thin arrow*) and another in the lower part of the breast (*thick arrow*). Ultrasound revealed that the small mass in patient #1 and the 2 masses in patient #2 were all solid.

Perform a needle localization of the small irregular mass in patient #1 and perform a simultaneous needle localization of both masses in patient #2.

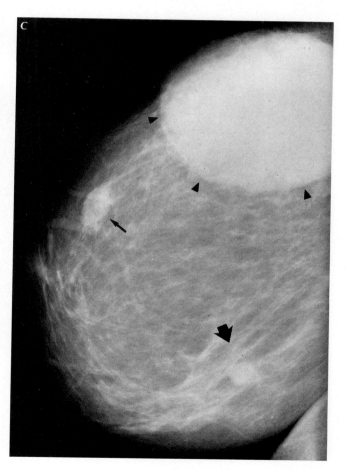

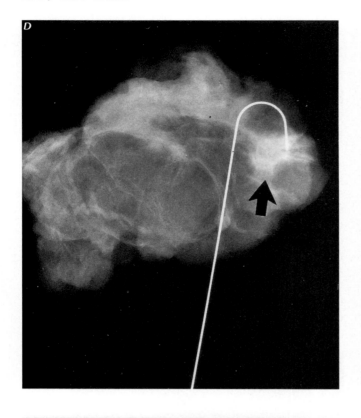

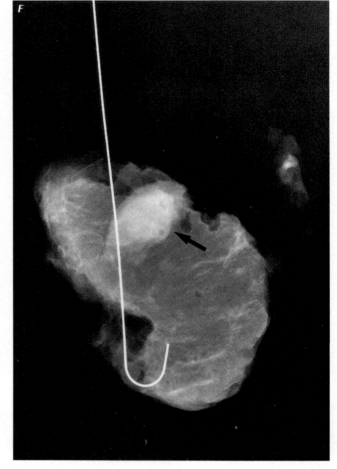

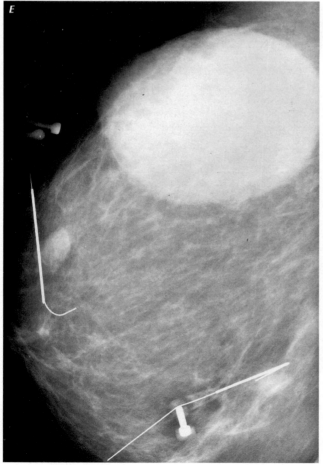

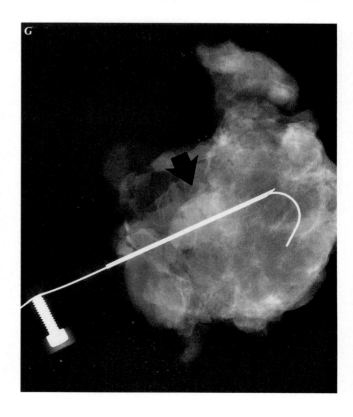

DISCUSSION

Specimen radiograph (**D**) confirms excision of the small mass in patient #1. Histology revealed invasive ductal carcinoma. LAT view (**E**) from patient #2 shows the bilateral simultaneous needle localization. Specimen radiograph (**F**) of the mass in the upper half of the breast in patient #2 confirms its excision, and histology revealed a benign fibroadenoma. Specimen radiograph (**G**) of the lower mass confirms its excision, and histology revealed invasive ductal carcinoma.

Since both patient #1 and patient #2 had distant foci of tumor, acceptable cosmesis could not be achieved so breast conservation was no longer an option. Both patients underwent modified radical mastectomies. These cases illustrate the important role of the radiologist in evaluating the patient with known breast carcinoma. The presence of occult disease totally changes management. Mammography prior to mastectomy and prior to breast conservation therapy should be an integral part of the evaluation of patients considering breast conservation therapy.

HISTORY

Routine screening mammogram was performed on a 63-year-old woman in 1987. Follow-up was suggested because of asymmetric densities. Another mammogram was performed in 1989. The patient was still asymptomatic and had a normal breast palpation.

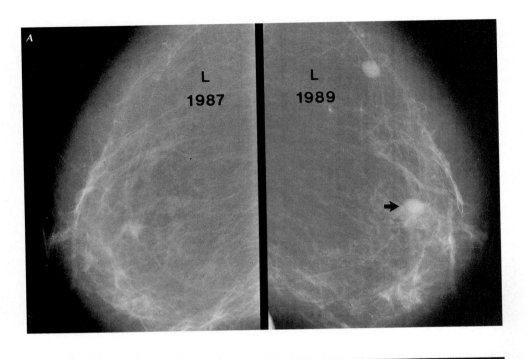

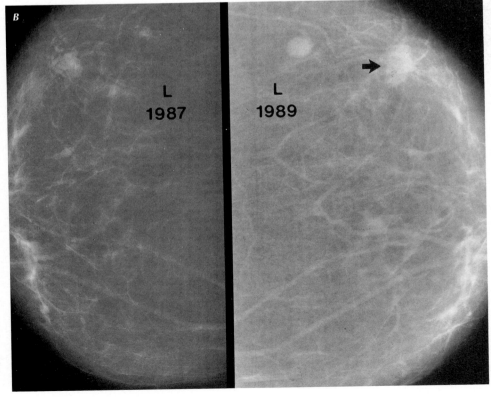

MAMMOGRAPHIC FINDINGS AND RECOMMENDATION

Within this two-year interval LAT views (**A**) and CC views (**B**) show that an ill-defined mass (*arrow*) in the left breast at the 3 o'clock position has grown larger, and a second mass with sharp margins in the left upper outer quadrant has also enlarged. The poorly defined mass was needle localized and excised. Histology revealed invasive ductal carcinoma. The patient was referred for management.

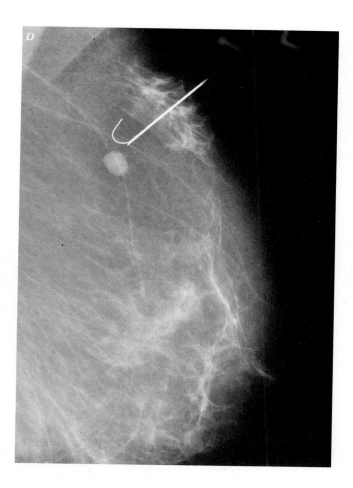

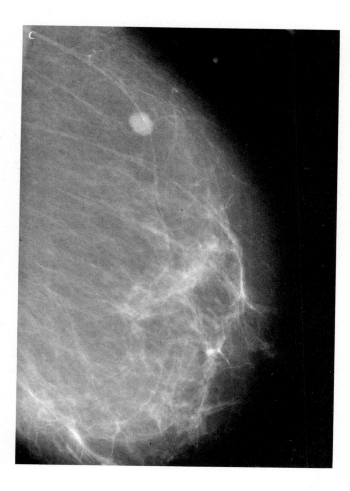

MAMMOGRAPHIC FINDINGS AND RECOMMENDATION

This single LAT view (**C**) of the left breast shows the postbiopsy changes at the site of the excised carcinoma, and the well-defined mass. Ultrasound showed that the mass was solid.

The well-defined mass could represent an enlarged lymph node involved with metastatic tumor. If management depends upon knowing whether the lymph node is involved with tumor, it can be needle localized and excised to establish its histology.

DISCUSSION

Needle localization (**D**) was performed, and specimen radiography confirmed excision of the mass. Histology revealed an intramammary lymph node replaced with tumor. An axillary dissection was then performed, and 13 of 13 lymph nodes were free of tumor.

The patient opted for breast conservation therapy. It was important to establish whether the sharply defined mass was involved with tumor because radiation therapy is less effective when bulk disease is left in the breast.

HISTORY

Fourteen years ago, at the age of 19, this woman had a palpable mass excised, which was an invasive ductal carcinoma. She opted for breast conservation therapy. Her tumor was excised with clear margins, and her breast was irradiated. She comes in for annual breast palpation and mammography.

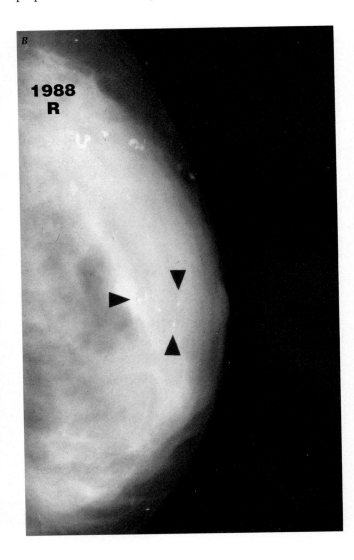

MAMMOGRAPHIC FINDINGS AND RECOMMENDATION

Film (**A**) is a LAT view taken when the patient was 32 years old. Calcified suture material (*arrows*) resulting from the breast irradiation is evident. Film (**B**) is a LAT view taken one year later. A new geographic focus of microcalcifications (*arrowheads*) has appeared in the subareolar area. A closeup view (**C**) shows the calcifications to better advantage.

Perform a subareolar biopsy to establish the histology of the microcalcifications. Needle localization is not necessary for the subareolar biopsy, but the specimen must be radiographed to confirm that the microcalcifications have been sampled.

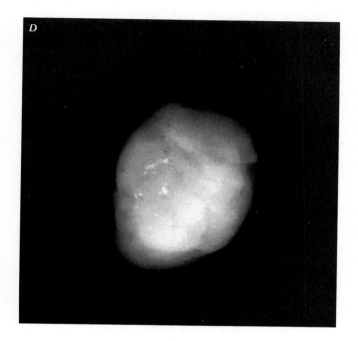

MAMMOGRAPHIC FINDINGS

The subareolar biopsy (**D**) contains some of the microcalcifications. Histology revealed invasive ductal carcinoma.

DISCUSSION

A patient with a personal history of breast cancer has the highest risk for developing either a recurrence from treatment failure or a new primary elsewhere either in the ipsilateral or contralateral breast. It was felt that in this case the malignancy represented a new primary appearing 14 years after the initial tumor. Since the breast irradiation was finished long ago, these new microcalcifications could not be attributed to postradiation calcium and so biopsy was immediately performed. After the malignant nature of the microcalcifications was established, the patient underwent a modified radical mastectomy.

HISTORY

Routine screening mammogram on a 46-year-old woman.

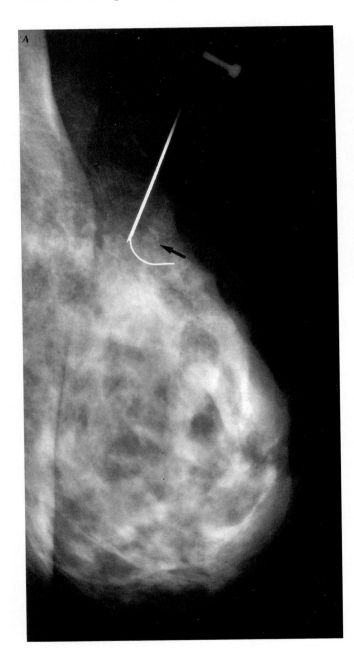

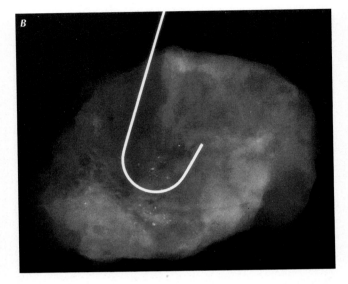

MAMMOGRAPHIC FINDINGS AND RECOMMENDATION

OBL view (*A*) of the left breast revealed a solitary geographic cluster of microcalcifications. Needle localization and excision were successfully performed. Specimen radiography (*B*) confirmed excision of the lesion. Histology revealed intraductal carcinoma with clear margins. The patient opted for breast conservation therapy, and no further treatment was given.

This patient with proven breast carcinoma should have annual mammography.

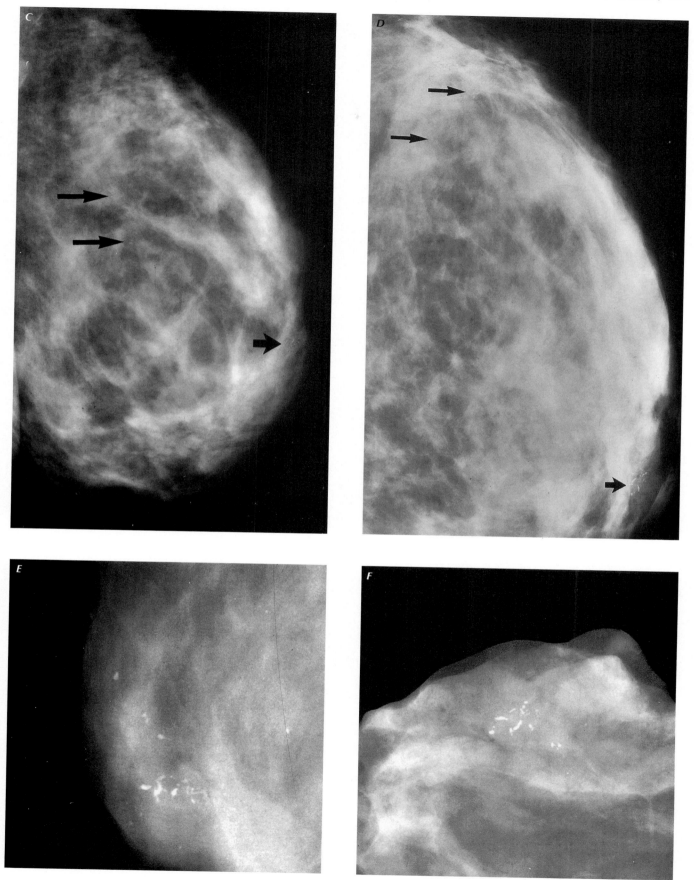

MAMMOGRAPHIC FINDINGS

The examination one year later (*C*) showed the development of new microcalcifications in the subareolar area (*one arrow*) as well as new microcalcifications at the lumpectomy site (*2 arrows*). Magnification view (*D*) shows these areas of calcifications to better advantage. The lumpectomy site was reexcised (*E*), and a subareolar biopsy was performed (*F*). Neither case required needle localization. Histology revealed both intraductal and invasive ductal carcinoma at both sites. The patient underwent a modified radical mastectomy.

DISCUSSION

This case dramatically illustrates how quickly new sites of tumor can appear and be detected by mammography. Tumor appeared both at the lumpectomy site as well as at a distant site. In patients undergoing breast conservation therapy, the radiologist's attention must not be limited to the treated region.

HISTORY

Routine screening mammogram on a 38-year-old woman.

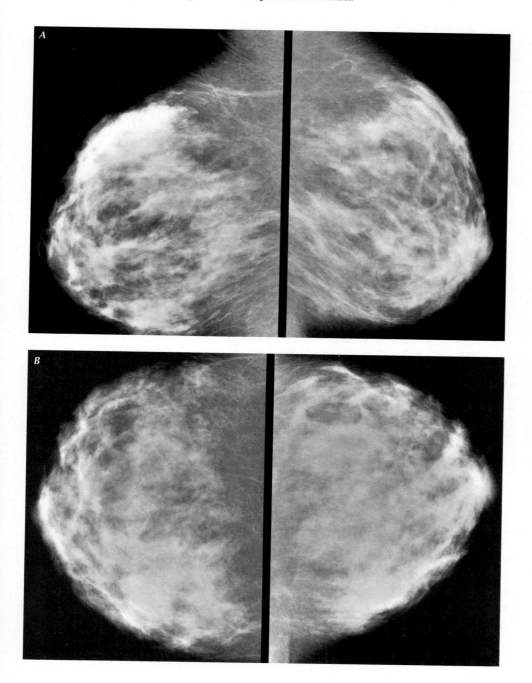

MAMMOGRAPHIC FINDINGS AND RECOMMENDATION

OBL (*A*) and CC (*B*) views reveal multiple bilateral asymmetric densities without a dominant mass. There are no suspicious microcalcifications in either breast. Place the patient into a follow-up protocol.

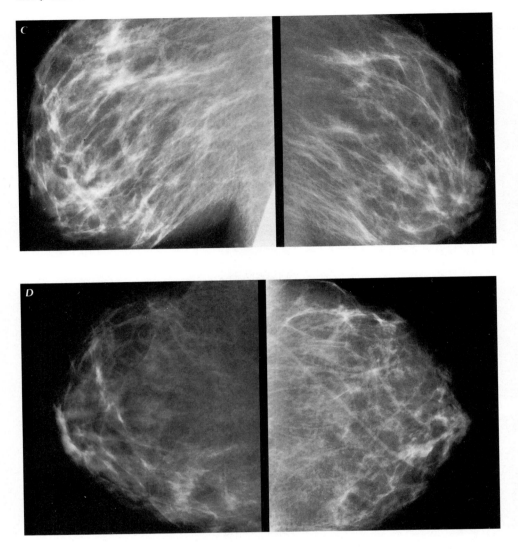

MAMMOGRAPHIC FINDINGS

There has been a dramatic change on this six-month examination. OBL (*C*) and CC (*D*) views reveal that the asymmetric densities have regressed. The examination now shows no dominant mass or suspicious calcifications.

DISCUSSION

A phone call to the referring clinician revealed that the patient was breast feeding at the time of the initial mammogram. It makes no sense to obtain a "baseline" mammogram when the baseline will change in the near future. Had we known the patient was breast feeding, the mammogram would not have been performed. We try not to perform routine mammography on women until at least three to six months after they have stopped breast feeding (and preferably longer). This case illustrates how the breast can return to normal within this time interval. Of course if the patient is symptomatic, the examination is not routine and will be performed even if the patient is still breast feeding. To avoid performing a routine mammogram on a woman who is breast feeding, letters can be sent out to referring clinicians advising them against this practice. But the foolproof way to eliminate this problem is to have the technologist question the patient about breast feeding at the time she takes her history and notify the radiologist if there is a problem.

HISTORY

A 33-year-old woman presented for evaluation of a palpable, soft, mobile mass at the 6 o'clock position in the left breast. It was aspirated and became nonpalpable. The fluid appeared "benign" and was not sent for cy-tological analysis. One month later the same mass became palpable again. Ultrasound was performed, the mass was aspirated, and the fluid was sent for cytological analysis. A postaspiration mammogram was performed. The mass became palpable again two weeks later.

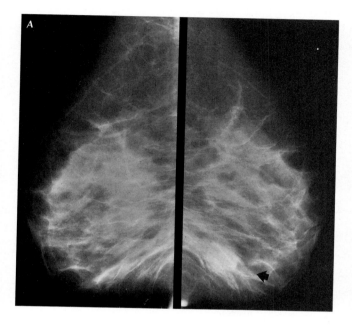

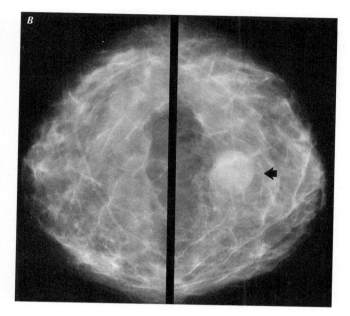

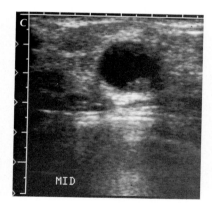

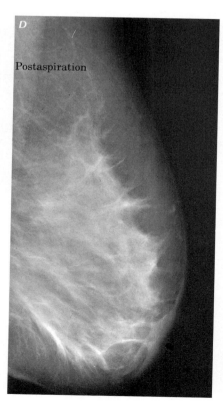

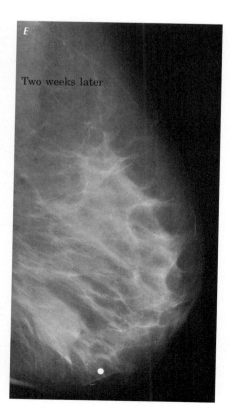

MAMMOGRAPHIC FINDINGS AND RECOMMENDATION

LAT (*A*) and CC views (*B*) performed prior to the ultrasound examination show that the mass is noncalcified and has moderately well-defined margins. There are no other masses in either breast. The ultrasound examination (*C*) revealed that the mass was partially cystic, with thick irregular walls, and had a small mass adherent to the posterior wall. A postaspiration mammogram (*D*) shows that the mass has totally disappeared. A single LAT view (*E*) obtained two weeks later, when the mass became palpable again, shows the recurrent lesion.

Based upon the ultrasound findings, biopsy was recommended with the preoperative diagnosis of intracystic carcinoma. The fluid sent for cytology contained malignant cells. Since the mass became palpable again, preoperative needle localization was not necessary. Histology revealed intracystic carcinoma with areas of invasion.

DISCUSSION

There were several indications for biopsy, including the abnormal ultrasound examination and the positive cytology. In addition, a solitary recurring cyst is a clinical indication for excisional biopsy. Although a pneumocystogram would have produced dramatic images, it would not have added anything to patient management. Finally, as illustrated in this patient, aspirated fluid is not always automatically sent for cytology. Many clinicians believe that given the high incidence of cysts, and the rarity of intracystic carcinoma, it is not reasonable to routinely send aspirated cyst fluid with a benign appearance for cytologic analysis.

HISTORY

This 43-year-old woman had a large mobile mass in the left upper outer quadrant measuring 8 cm in greatest diameter. It was judged to be a fibroadenoma on clinical grounds. It was not excised and had remained stable over many years. She presents at this time for the evaluation of an enlarged, painless left axillary lymph node. At the time the lymph node was excised, the large breast mass was also removed. The mass proved to be a benign fibroadenoma. No calcifications were present in any of the histologic sections. The lymph node contained poorly differentiated adenocarcinoma. Workup for an occult malignancy was unrevealing.

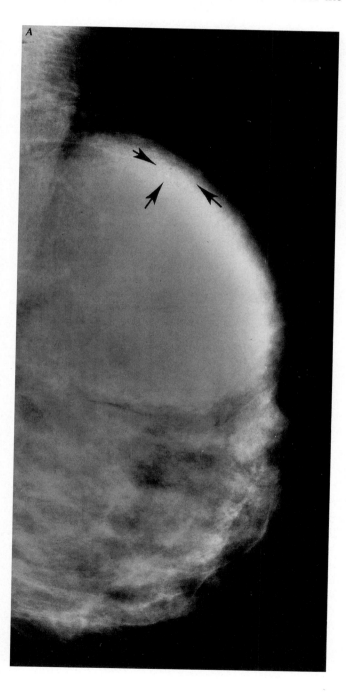

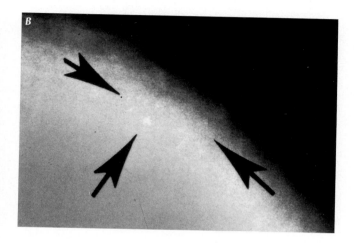

MAMMOGRAPHIC FINDINGS AND RECOMMENDATIONS

An OBL view (*A*) from the preoperative mammogram showed the large mass in the upper half of the left breast. A subtle cluster of microcalcifications was also present (*B*). The calcifications were geographic and unlike the usual calcifications seen in a fibroadenoma.

Repeat the mammogram. If the microcalcifications are still present, they should be needle localized and removed to establish their histology. If the mammogram shows that the microcalcifications are no longer present, the paraffin blocks must be radiographed to locate the microcalcifications so they can be evaluated histologically.

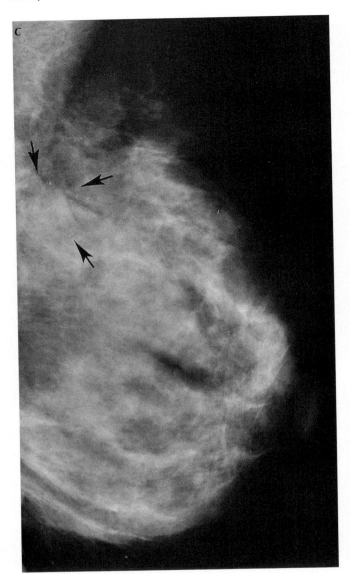

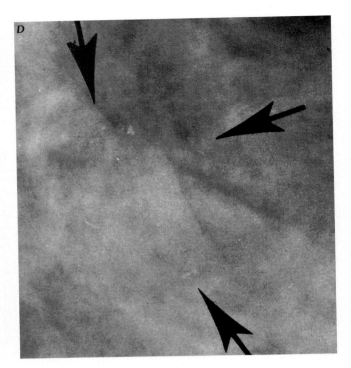

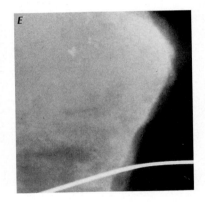

DISCUSSION

Repeat OBL mammogram (*C*) and close-up (*D*) shows that the microcalcifications were still present. They were localized and excised. Specimen radiograph (*E*) confirmed their excision, and histology revealed an invasive ductal carcinoma. A modified radical mastectomy was performed, and 2 of 11 lymph nodes contained tumor. There was no extracapsular extension.

Breast cancer manifesting itself as an enlarged lymph node is an uncommon but well-recognized presentation. Difficulty occurs if the lymph node is shown to contain adenocarcinoma when the breast palpation and mammograms are normal. This specific case illustrates that benign and malignant disease can coexist in close proximity to each other. As in all other areas of imaging, the radiologist must try to avoid concentrating only on the obvious abnormality. This case also shows that tumor size alone cannot predict its biologic activity. Finally, detecting the breast cancer permitted the correct aggressive therapy to begin. Mastectomy would not have been performed if the primary breast cancer remained undetected. (*Radiographs reprinted by permission of the publisher from Abrams RA, O'Connor T, May G, Homer MJ: Breast Cancer Presenting as an Axillary Mass: Case Report and Review. Breast Disease 3:39–46, 1990. Copyright © 1990 by Elsevier Science Publishing Co., Inc.*)

HISTORY

This 67-year-old woman had nipple eczema which did not resolve after appropriate therapy. It was biopsied, and histology revealed superficial Paget's carcinoma. The patient was referred for management. She wanted breast conservation therapy.

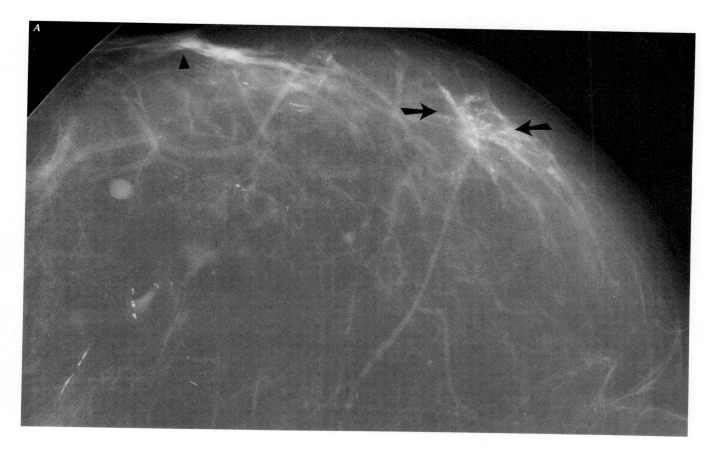

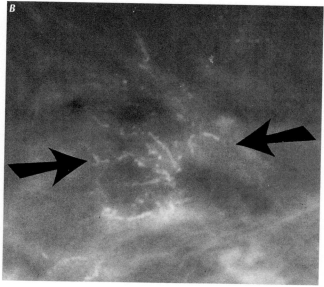

MAMMOGRAPHIC FINDINGS AND RECOMMENDATION

A CC view (**A**) shows the area of biopsy-proven Paget's carcinoma (*arrowhead*). In the outer portion of the same breast was a geographic area of irregular punctate and linear microcalcifications (*arrows*). Closeup view (**B**) shows the calcifications to better advantage. Further history revealed that in the past the patient had a previous biopsy in the area of the calcifications for what proved to be benign disease. On repalpation there was a firmness at the biopsy site, which the clinician believed corresponded to the location of the calcifications.

These calcifications did not have the appearance of dermal calcifications that might form in a scar. They have very "malignant" characteristics. The firm area should be excised and radiographed to be certain that it contains the microcalcifications.

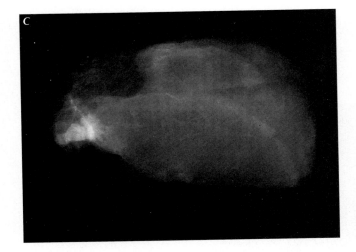

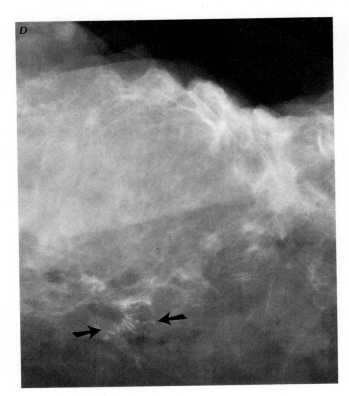

DISCUSSION

Specimen radiography (**C**) of the biopsy scar showed that it contained no microcalcifications. At this point, the patient changed her mind and wanted a modified radical mastectomy instead of breast conservation therapy. Mastectomy was performed (**D**). The area of microcalcifcations (*arrows*) was isolated in the mastectomy specimen and proved to be extensive invasive ductal carcinoma. There are two very important teaching points illustrated by this case. The mammographic abnormality of microcalcifications was not the palpable abnormality. Without the specimen radiograph, it might have been incorrectly assumed that the mammographic abnormality and the palpable abnormality were the same process. The second point is that superficial Paget's carcinoma is often associated with a deeper carcinoma, either intraductal or invasive. The presence of a deeper focus of tumor may eliminate any option other than mastectomy.

HISTORY

A mammogram was performed prior to excisional biopsy for a palpable mass in the upper half of the left breast in this 43-year-old woman.

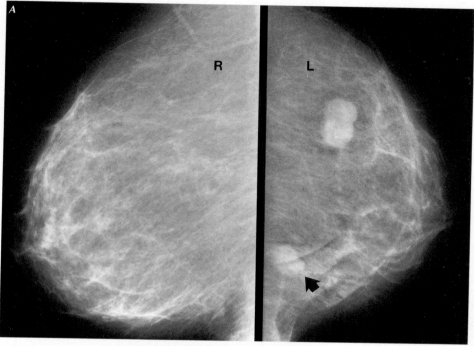

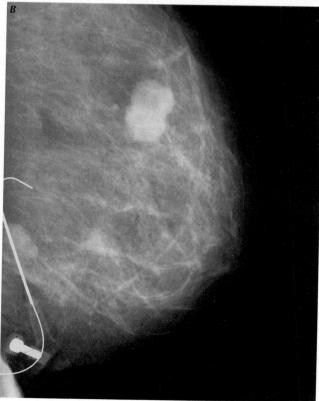

MAMMOGRAPHIC FINDINGS AND RECOMMENDATION

An OBL view of each breast (**A**) reveals no dominant mass or suspicious calcification in the right breast. The palpable mass in the upper half of the left breast has lobulated margins and contains microcalcifications. There is another noncalcified lobulated mass with some poorly defined borders in the lower half of the left breast (*arrow*).

Perform needle localization of the nonpalpable mass and excise both the palpable and nonpalpable masses at the same time.

Needle localization was performed (**B**). Both the palpable and nonpalpable masses were excised, and histology revealed fibrocystic disease of the breast with cyst formation, prominent apocrine metaplasia, and intraductal hyperplasia and papillomatosis with foci of moderate dysplasia.

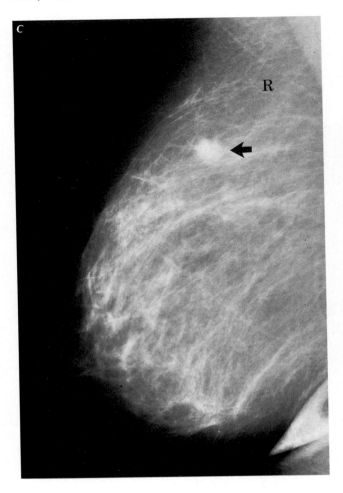

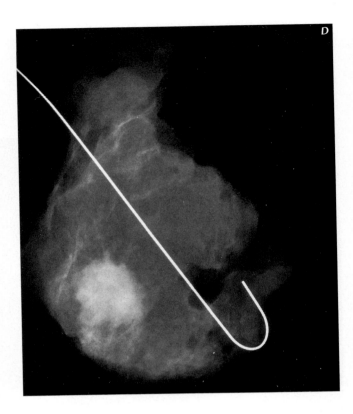

MAMMOGRAPHIC FINDINGS

Two years later on another routine screening mammogram an OBL view (*C*) of the right breast shows that a noncalcified poorly defined mass (*arrow*) has developed. It was needle localized and excised (*D*). Histology revealed a 1-cm invasive ductal carcinoma.

DISCUSSION

This case illustrates that each mammographic finding must be evaluated on its own basis. While the first two lesions were benign, the third proved to be malignant.

HISTORY

This 46-year-old woman felt a palpable mass in the upper *inner* quadrant of her right breast. It was excised and proved to be an invasive ductal carcinoma measuring less than 1 cm in greatest diameter. She presents to be evaluated for breast conservation therapy.

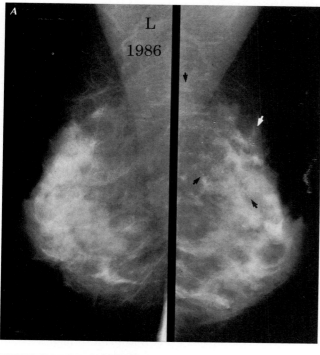

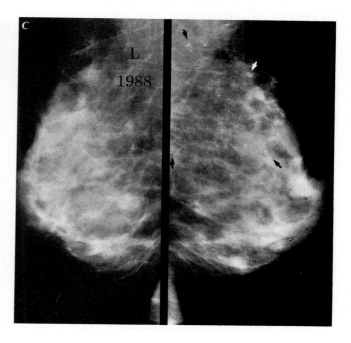

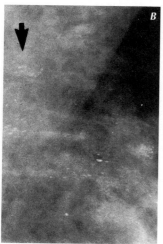

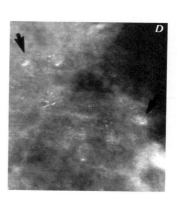

MAMMOGRAPHIC FINDINGS AND RECOMMENDATION

OBL (**A**) views and close-up (**B**) from 1986 show a solitary geographic area of microcalcifications in the right upper *outer* quadrant (*arrows*). The calcifications are primarily punctate with the suggestion of a few milk-of-calcium forms. Oblique views (**C**) from 1988 taken after excision of the palpable mass show that the calcifications remain geographic, and more calcifications, including milk-of-calcium forms, have developed in the interval. Close-up view (**D**) shows calcification to better advantage.

Since there is no palpable abnormality in the right upper outer quadrant, this area should be needle localized to obtain some tissue for histologic analysis.

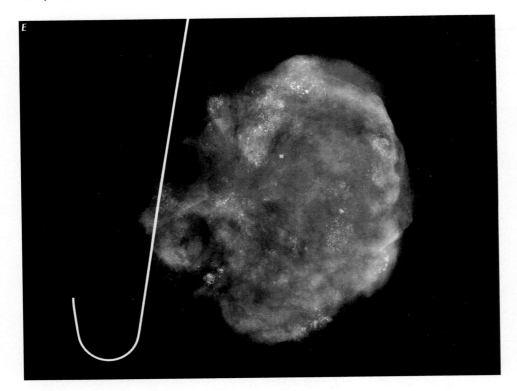

DISCUSSION

Magnification specimen radiograph from needle localization (*E*) shows that many of the calcifications have been excised. Histology revealed foci of intraductal, invasive ductal, in-situ lobular, and invasive lobular carcinomas. The patient was told that because of the extensive nature of the process and because it was in a different quadrant than her palpable carcinoma, breast conservation was not an option. She underwent a modified radical mastectomy.

There are many instructive points in this case. The first is that even an extensive carcinoma can remain nonpalpable over the years and evoke no other clues to its malignant nature such as skin thickening or skin retraction. The next point is that even though milk-of-calcium forms were present, this does not guarantee that the entire lesion is benign. The milk of calcium may reflect ducts obstructed by tumor. A mixed lesion (one containing *both* milk-of-calcium and nonmilk-of-calcium forms) must either be followed or excised. The films between 1986 and 1988 showed that the process was not stable, but was creating more calcium, and also that over this time period the process remained geographic. Both of these features indicated that biopsy was necessary.

HISTORY

Routine screening mammogram on a 47-year-old woman.

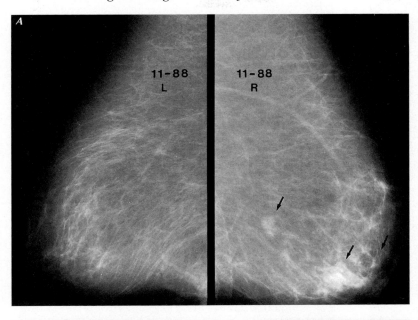

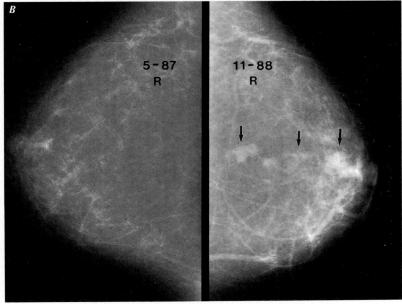

MAMMOGRAPHIC FINDINGS AND RECOMMENDATION

OBL views (*A*) reveal that there are several noncalcified densities extending from the right subareolar region to the mid-portion of the right breast (*arrows*). The left breast has no such pattern. CC views of the right breast (*B*) reveal that this process was not presented on a prior examination of 1987.

Perform a needle localization and excision to establish the nature of the process.

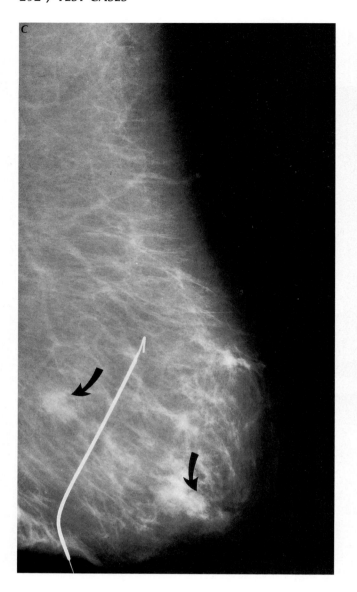

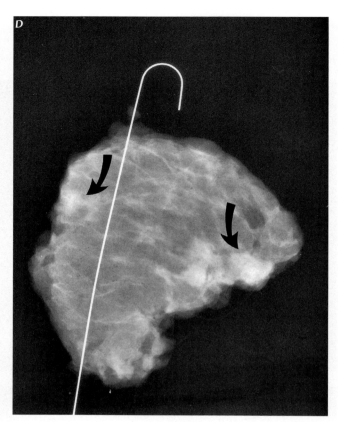

DISCUSSION _____

Using an inferior approach, the central portion of the process was localized (*C*). Specimen radiography (*D*) confirms excision of many of the densities. Histology revealed invasive ductal carcinoma. Since the process was so extensive, the patient underwent a modified radical mastectomy. There are several interesting points in this case. As is sometimes the case, this cancer is not making a single volumetric mass or microcalcification but is infiltrating in a fashion that can be mistaken for breast parenchyma. The obvious clues to its abnormality are its asymmetry as well as its change in appearance since the last examination. It is remarkable that such an extensive cancer can appear within 1 1/2 years in a fatty breast and still be nonpalpable.

HISTORY

Routine screening mammogram on a 64-year-old woman.

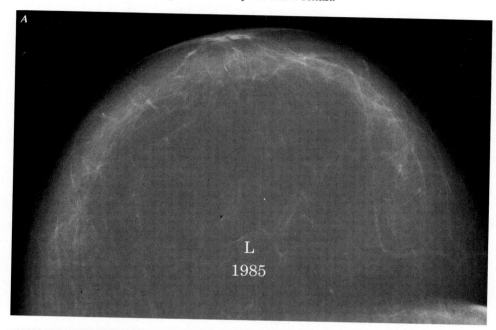

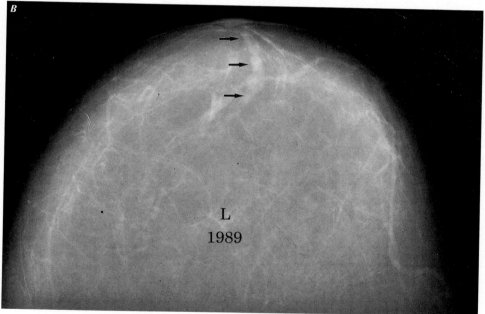

MAMMOGRAPHIC FINDINGS AND RECOMMENDATION

Film (*A*) is a CC view of the left breast showing a very fatty breast without any evidence of a dominant mass or suspicious calcifications. Film (*B*) is a CC view of the same left breast taken four years later, when the woman was age 64. In the interval, a solitary dilated duct measuring approximately 5 cm in length has developed. It contains no calcifications.

Excise the duct to determine the nature of its contents. A needle localization is not necessary because of its size and subareolar location.

DISCUSSION

Histology revealed ductal ectasia. The duct contained debris and mild focal epithelial hyperplasia. A solitary enlarged duct is one of the localizing signs of breast cancer. However, without any other finding such as nipple discharge, retraction, or eczema, the chance of it containing carcinoma is very low. In the asymptomatic patient, many radiologists either follow the solitary enlarged duct or consider it a manifestation of benign secretory disease and do not recall the patient for a follow-up. In this case, a more aggressive approach was taken because the solitary duct enlarged over time. However the underlying process still proved to be benign.

HISTORY

Routine screening mammogram on a 32-year-old woman.

Five years earlier she had acute mastitis on the left side treated successfully with antibiotics. A mammogram was performed at that time.

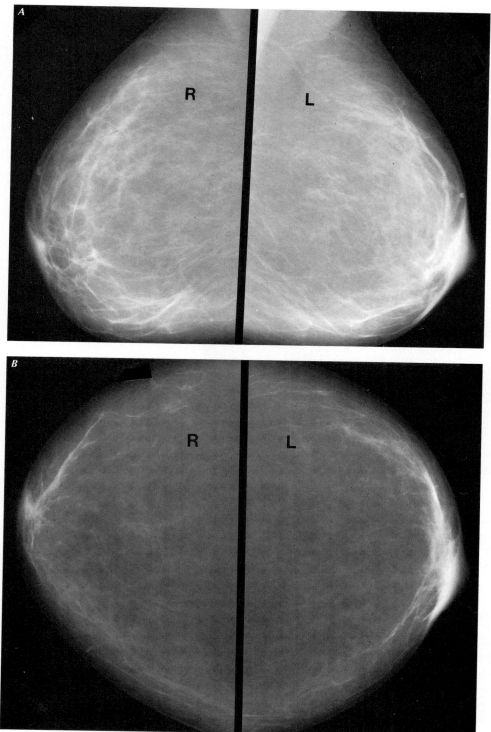

MAMMOGRAPHIC FINDINGS AND RECOMMENDATION _____

LAT (**A**) and CC (**B**) views demonstrate left periareolar skin thickening and increased left subareolar density.

Obtain old mammograms. Repalpate the left subareolar area carefully.

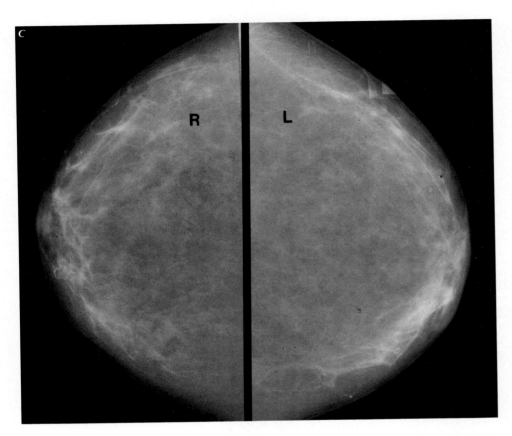

MAMMOGRAPHIC FINDINGS _____

CC views (**C**) taken during the episode of the acute mastitis showed increased left subareolar density.

DISCUSSION _____

The breast repalpation was normal. In view of the fact that the old mammograms confirmed that the area involved with mastitis was in the left subareolar region, two management options were reasonable. The left subareolar region could be biopsied, since there was no reason to believe that a cancer hadn't developed in the interval. However because the mammographic findings were consistent with the sequellae of an inflammatory process and because the breast repalpation was normal and there were no associated nipple abnormalities, placing the patient into a follow-up protocol was also an option. The patient was placed into a follow-up protocol. She has remained asymptomatic, and the mammographic findings remain stable. As in many cases, there is no one correct answer to the case but only a choice of reasonable management options.

HISTORY

Routine screening mammogram on a 61-year-old woman.

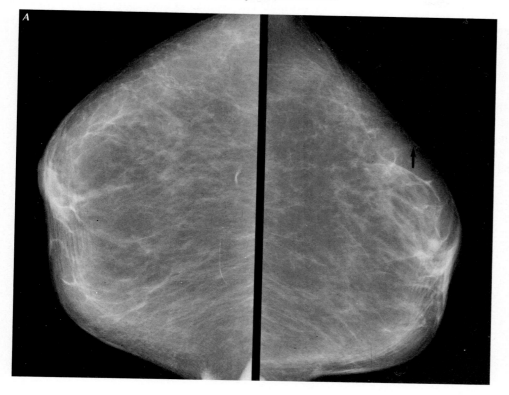

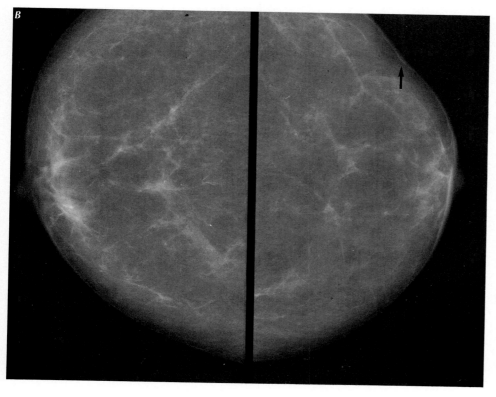

MAMMOGRAPHIC FINDINGS AND RECOMMENDATION

On the LAT (*A*) and CC (*B*) views there is a localized area of skin retraction and minimal thickening (*arrows*) in the left upper inner quadrant. There is no underlying parenchymal abnormality in these fatty replaced breasts.

Reexamine the woman with special attention to the left upper inner quadrant. If nothing is evident to explain the mammographic findings, ask her if anything ever happened to that part of the breast that didn't happen to any other part of that breast or the other breast.

DISCUSSION

Visual inspection and palpation of the area initially were normal. The woman stated that when she was a child, her mother accidentally spilled boiling water on that part of her breast and she had suffered a severe burn. When the woman held her breast in the appropriate position, a subtle dimpling was evident.

Compressing the breast is the mammographic equivalent of examining the breast with maneuvers designed to stretch Cooper's ligaments such as lifting the arms up or holding them close to the sides in upright position. This burn is obviously of no clinical significance, but it is important to know the etiology of the mammographic findings so that they can be dismissed as not significant. Mammography is so sensitive an examination that skin thickening or retraction may be identified before they are clinically evident. Asking the woman a simple question about the area of concern may be all that is required to explain the mammographic findings.

HISTORY

This 68-year-old woman presented for evaluation for new onset right nipple retraction. There was no associated discharge or nipple eczema.

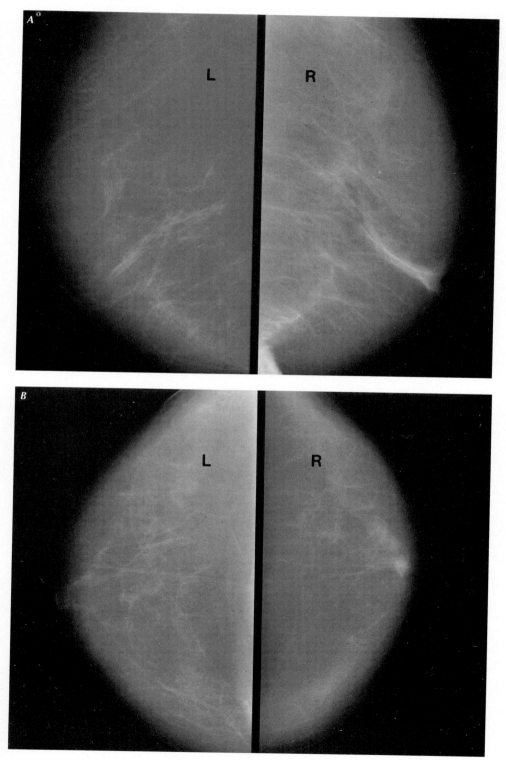

MAMMOGRAPHIC FINDINGS AND RECOMMENDATION

On the LAT (*A*) and CC (*B*) views there is an abnormality of the right nipple and subareolar region. There is nipple retraction and prominent density, which could represent pathologically dilated ducts.

Subareolar biopsy is mandatory to establish histology of the process. Needle localization is not required.

DISCUSSION

A subareolar biopsy was performed, and histology revealed dilated ducts with moderate periductal fibrosis. There was no evidence of malignancy. Unexplained new onset of nipple retraction almost always demands a subareolar biopsy even if the mammogram is unremarkable. In this case, the clinical finding associated with the mammographic abnormality made malignancy a prime possibility. This case illustrates that mammography is a sensitive but nonspecific examination and that every sign of malignancy can be caused by a benign process.

HISTORY

In 1984 a routine screening mammogram was performed on a 42-year-old woman. In 1985 a mammogram was performed because of the new clinical finding of right breast skin thickening.

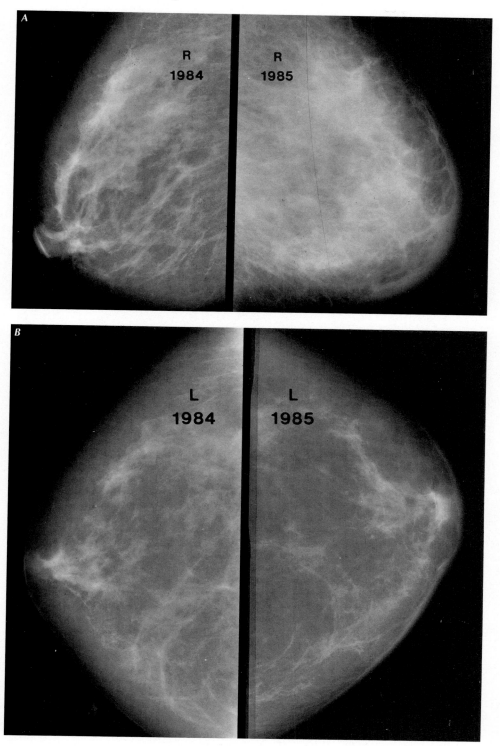

MAMMOGRAPHIC FINDINGS AND RECOMMENDATION

Between 1984 and 1985 generalized skin thickening has appeared in both the right (**A**) and left (**B**) breasts. Neither breast has a dominant mass or suspicious calcifications.

Differential diagnosis includes bilateral inflammatory breast carcinoma and lymphatic obstruction from other causes such as a primary pulmonary process. None of the other causes of generalized skin thickening such as acute mastitis, anasarca, radiation, etc. applied to this case. If the chest x-ray is normal, dermal punch biopsies of the breast may be performed to evaluate the possibility of inflammatory breast cancer.

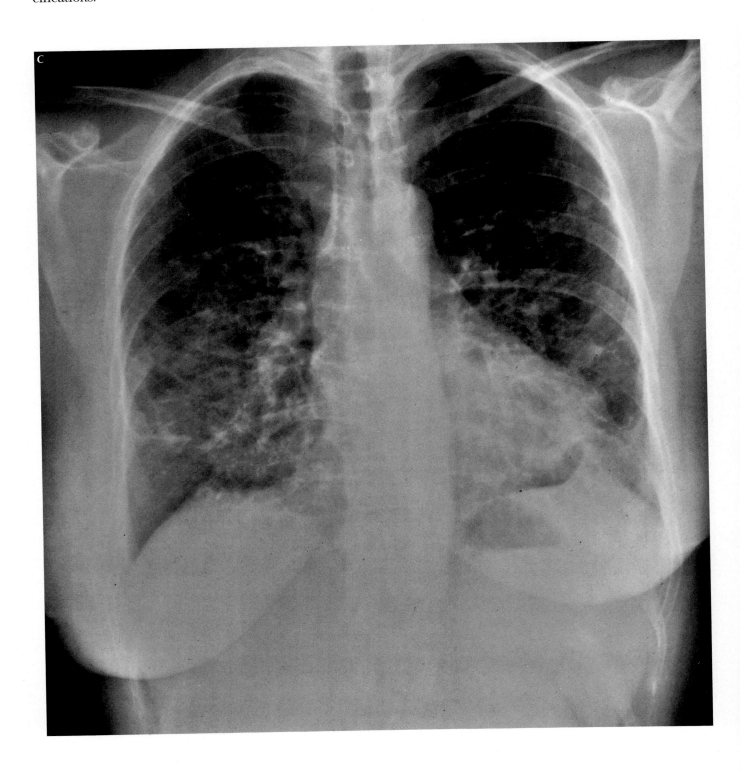

RADIOGRAPHIC FINDINGS

A chest radiograph (*C*) demonstrates a bilateral interstitial process involving both lungs consistent with lymphangitic spread of tumor.

DISCUSSION

Dermal biopsies from both breasts contained no tumor. Pleural and lung biopsies from the left lower lung zone revealed adenocarcinoma. The presumptive diagnosis was metastatic tumor from a distant primary, probably from the GI tract, spreading via lymphatics to the lungs and causing secondary obstruction of the draining lymphatics from the breast. When the mammogram shows generalized skin thickening, either unilateral or bilateral, a recent chest radiograph should be reviewed to be certain that the mammary findings do not reflect lymphatic blockage from a pulmonary process. One final point is that although the mammogram clearly demonstrated generalized skin thickening on the left side, the breast palpation was only abnormal on the right side. The mammogram is more sensitive to early skin thickening than is breast palpation.

HISTORY

A 68-year-old woman was admitted to the hospital for an abnormal chest x-ray. A diagnostic thoracentesis on the right was performed, and 200 mL of a bloody exu-date was obtained. It contained adenocarcinoma. A work-up for an occult primary was begun. On day #8 the mammogram requisition was submitted, and the history stated "Pre-discharge mammogram. Looking for an occult malignancy."

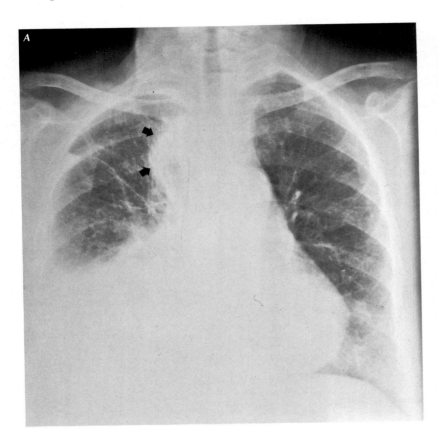

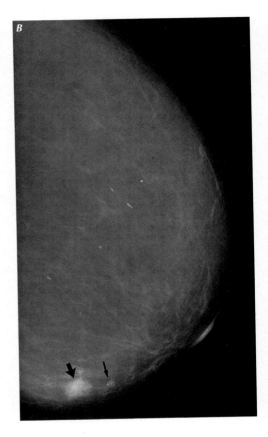

MAMMOGRAPHIC FINDINGS AND RECOMMENDATION

The admission chest radiograph (**A**) showed a unilateral right effusion and a pleural based mass (*arrows*). A LAT view of the right breast (**B**) revealed a very fatty breast, and within 1 cm from the surface was an irregular non-calcified 1.5-cm mass (*thick arrow*) with an adjacent solitary cluster of microcalcifications (*thin arrow*).

Repalpate the area of the breast containing the mass and microcalcifications. If something is palpable, it must be excised. If nothing is palpable, the area should be needle localized prior to excision.

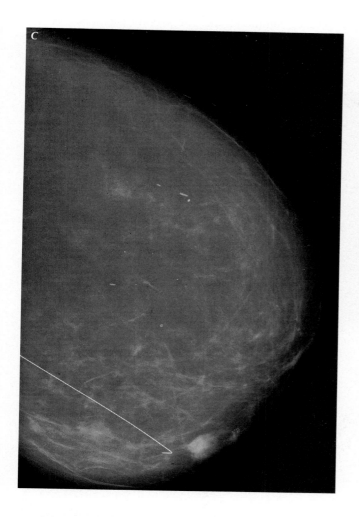

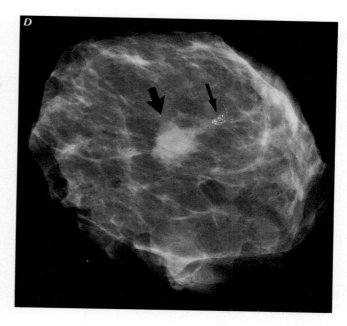

DISCUSSION

Nothing was palpable on repeat examination of the breast. Needle localization was performed (**C**). Specimen radiograph (**D**) confirms excision of both lesions. The mass was invasive ductal carcinoma, and the microcalcifications were a separate focus of intraductal carcinoma.

There are several interesting points to this case. Since two of the more common malignancies in the female are chest and breast, a chest radiograph *and* a mammogram should be among the initial diagnostic tests performed in the work-up for an occult malignancy in the female. Some clinicians still believe that while they may not be able to palpate a lesion in a firm breast, they have little problem in the fatty replaced breast. These two superficially located cancers remained nonpalpable on directed breast repalpation.

HISTORY

Two different patients who had undergone bilateral reduction mammoplasties presented for mammography.

The first was a 41-year-old woman who had a routine screening mammogram. The second was a 54-year-old woman who presented for evaluation of a palpable subareolar firm mass.

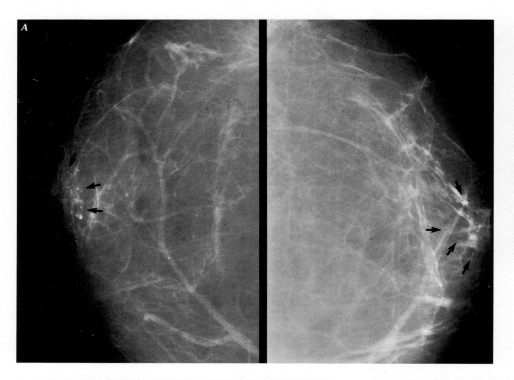

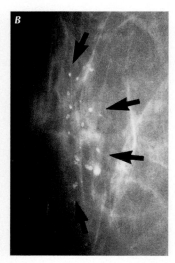

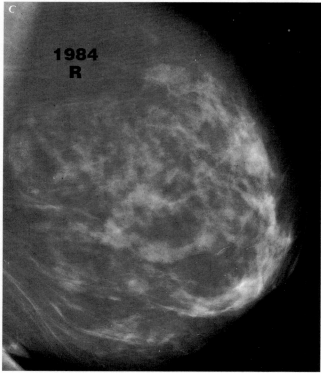

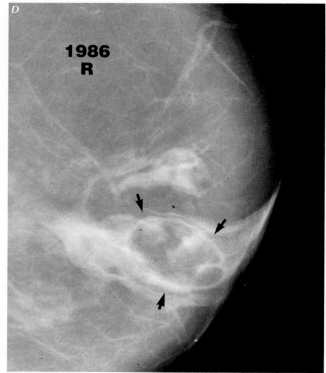

MAMMOGRAPHIC FINDINGS AND RECOMMENDATION

CC views (*A*) from a routine screening mammogram in patient #1 revealed bilateral periareolar microcalcifications (*arrows*). Some which were imaged in tangent were clearly dermal in location. The calcifications had a punctate appearance (*B*), but no lucent centers were present.

LAT view (*C*) of right breast is from a preoperative mammogram prior to the reduction mammoplasties in patient #2. LAT view two years later (*D*) shows the palpable subareolar mass (*arrows*). It has a lucent center and appears to be surrounded by a capsule. It is unassociated with microcalcifications.

The bilateral periareolar calcifications in patient #1 are dermal and are often seen after augmentation or reduction mammoplasties. Recommend future mammography as per usual clinical indications.

The subareolar mass seen in patient #2 is characteristic of posttraumatic fat necrosis surrounded by a fibrous capsule. Recommend future mammography as per usual clinical indications.

DISCUSSION

Since augmentation and reduction mammoplasties are increasing, radiologists must become familiar with expected mammographic findings in order to avoid unnecessary surgery in these patients where cosmesis is so important. At NEMCH plastic surgeons are encouraged to obtain premammoplasty mammograms on patients over age 30 to be certain that an occult malignancy is detected before the major surgery is performed. In patient #2 the subareolar mass was excised because it was firm and its presence bothered the patient. Histology revealed fat necrosis.

HISTORY

This 44-year-old woman had bilateral breast prostheses. She presents for evaluation of multiple firm masses in the right upper outer quadrant.

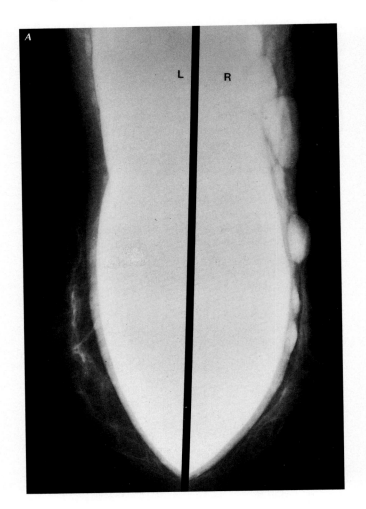

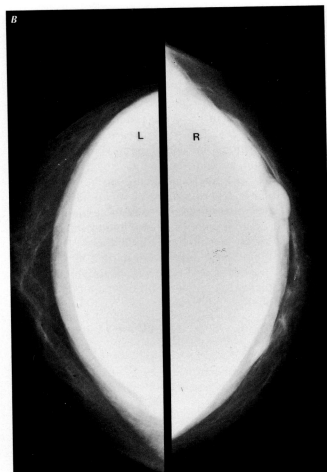

MAMMOGRAPHIC FINDINGS AND RECOMMENDATION

LAT (*A*) and CC (*B*) views show that the right breast prosthesis has ruptured, and its contents have leaked out into the breast tissue.

The numerous palpable masses represent leakage of the contents of the right breast prosthesis. Given the decreased sensitivity of mammography in breasts with implants, there is no dominant mass or suspicious calcifications.

DISCUSSION

Rupture of a breast prosthesis is one of the known complications of breast augmentation with prostheses. From a technical point of view, it is better if the implants are placed behind the pectoralis muscle rather than in front of it so that the prosthesis would obscure less breast tissue on the mammographic examination.

This examination was performed prior to the article (*Eklund GW, Busby RC, Miller SH, Job JS: Improved Imaging of the Augmented Breast. AJR 151:469–473, September 1988*) describing a modified technique for visualizing more breast tissue in patients with breast prostheses. This technique requires the technologist to push the prosthesis toward the chest wall and compress only breast tissue rather than including the implant in compression. Had this technique been used, more breast tissue would have probably been imaged. Radiologists and technologists performing mammography should be familiar with this technique.

HISTORY

These are two different patients presenting for routine screening mammograms. Both have had free silicone injected into their breasts for augmentation.

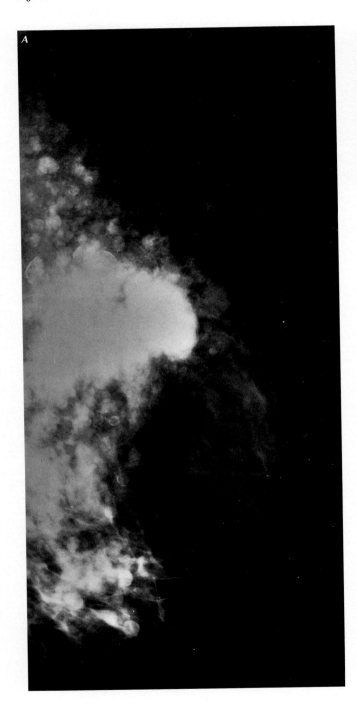

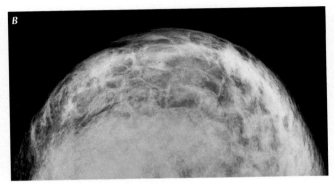

MAMMOGRAPHIC FINDINGS AND RECOMMENDATION

OBL view (*A*) from the first patient reveals masses of varying sizes, some with rim calcification. The masses are extremely dense. A CC view (*B*) from the second patient shows a diffuse increased density throughout the breast.

Both patients have findings seen when free silicone is injected into the breast. The silicone obscures normal breast parenchyma and can make a cancer manifesting itself either as a mass or microcalcifications impossible to detect. While there are no different guidelines for screening women who have undergone silicone injections, the referring physician and the patient should both realize that the false-negative rate of mammography is even higher in this situation.

DISCUSSION

It is now illegal in the United States to inject silicone into the breast for augmentation. The silicone can create granulomas with calcification as seen in the first patient. The technique for these mammograms is often poor because penetrating the dense silicone causes overpenetration of the normal breast tissue. In the second patient, the silicone has diffused throughout the breast, and instead of creating discrete masses, it created an overall increased density to the breast.

Routine screening mammogram in a 56-year-old woman.

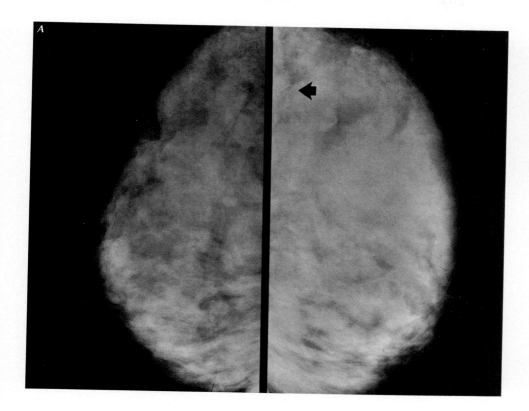

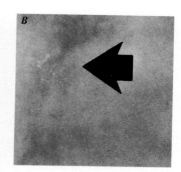

MAMMOGRAPHIC FINDINGS AND RECOMMENDATION

A LAT view of each breast (*A*) shows extremely dense breast tissue. In the upper portion of the right breast (*arrow*) is a solitary geographic cluster of microcalcifications (*B*). The contralateral left breast was just as dense but contained no microcalcifications.

Repalpate the breast with special attention to the area of microcalcifications. If nothing is palpable, the area can be needle localized prior to excision.

DISCUSSION

The patient was repalpated, and a mass was detected corresponding to the site of the microcalcifications. It was excised and was an invasive ductal carcinoma. This case demonstrates the value of directed breast repalpation. A needle localization was avoided. Even in retrospect, the palpable mass could not be detected on the mammogram. In a dense breast such as this, the false-negative rate of mammography is much higher than the usual 10 to 15 percent.

Even though the radiologist may feel frustrated in evaluating the dense breast, knowing full well that a large mass could be missed, it should always be remembered that these breasts are often firm to palpation and difficult to examine clinically as well. The dense breast provides a challenge to both palpation and mammography in breast cancer detection. However, since many cancers will eventually make microcalcifications, even though the tumor mass may remain hidden, a cancer can be detected by recognizing its microcalcifications.

HISTORY

In 1984, a 67-year-old woman had a routine screening mammogram. A 9-mm noncalcified mass present in the left upper outer quadrant was unchanged in appearance from numerous prior examinations. In July of 1986 the patient presented for evaluation of a palpable mass in the left upper outer quadrant.

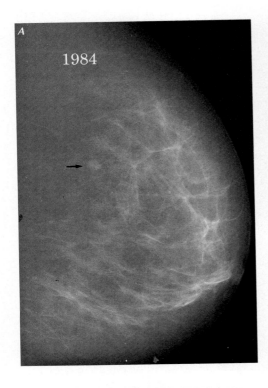

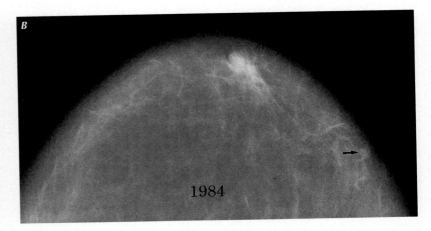

MAMMOGRAPHIC FINDINGS AND RECOMMENDATION

The 1984 screening mammogram shows the stable mass (*arrow*) in the LAT (*A*) and CC (*B*) views. The 1986 mammogram (*C, D*) reveals that this mass has enlarged and is the clinically palpable mass. It has sharp margins and a lucent center seen best on the LAT view.

The clinical decision was made to excise the palpable mass. Its mammographic appearance was consistent with a lymph node. Three weeks later, the mass was no longer palpable. A repeat mammogram was performed.

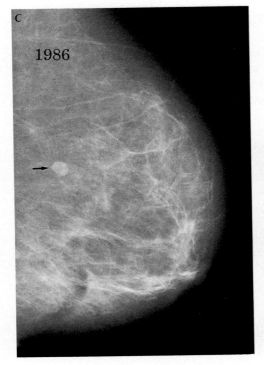

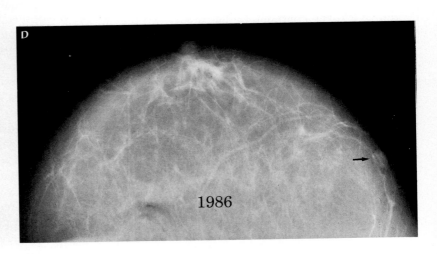

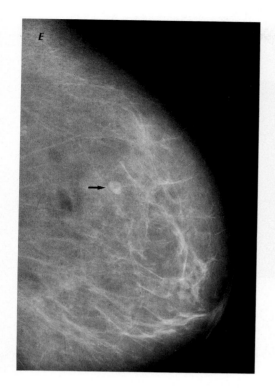

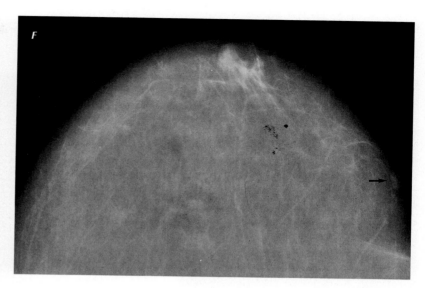

DISCUSSION

LAT (*E*) and CC (*F*) views show that the mass has decreased in volume. It still has sharp margins and a lucent center. Breast cancers do not spontaneously decrease in size so the biopsy was canceled. An aspiration was not performed so this couldn't have been an explanation for the decrease in size of the mass. The mass was probably an intramammary lymph node which was reacting to something. The patient never had an apparent infection, such as a dermatitis, to explain its enlargement. Although the cause for the enlargement was never ascertained, the biopsy was averted.

HISTORY

Routine screening mammogram on a 49-year-old woman.

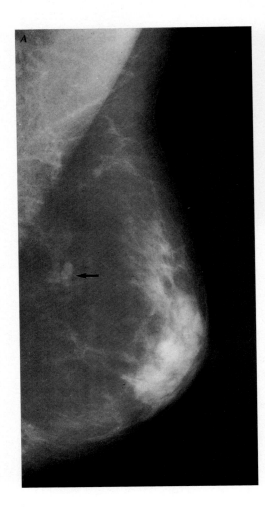

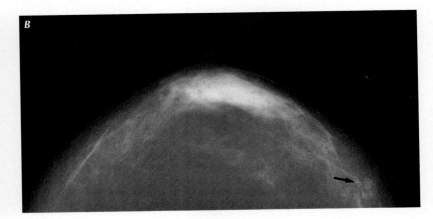

MAMMOGRAPHIC FINDINGS AND RECOMMENDATION

OBL (*A*) and CC (*B*) views of the right breast reveal several (approximately 4 to 5) small well-defined non-calcified masses in the upper outer quadrant (*arrow*). Despite their peripheral location on the CC view, they were nonpalpable.

While the appearance of these masses was quite unusual for multifocal carcinoma, that possibility could not be ruled out. None of the tiny masses had recognizable central fat or a central notch or hilus. The sharp margins of the masses weighed in favor of a benign process. While follow-up was clearly an option, needle localization and excision was favored to establish the histology of the process.

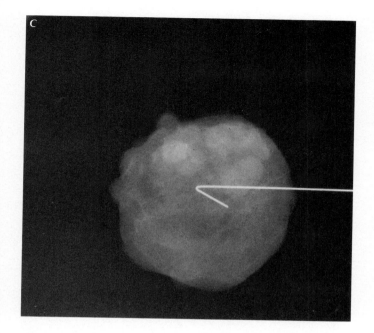

DISCUSSION

Specimen radiography (*C*) confirmed excision of the small masses. Histology revealed several normal intramammary lymph nodes. Now that both the common occurrence of normal intramammary lymph nodes and the fact that they can be multiple are well-known, in the future, follow-up rather than biopsy can be recommended.

Routine screening mammogram on a 74-year-old woman.

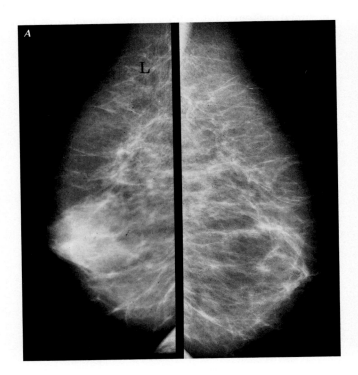

MAMMOGRAPHIC FINDINGS AND RECOMMENDATION

On the LAT views (*A*) and the CC views (*B*) there is increased left subareolar density, compared to the right side. There are no skin or nipple abnormalities. There are no suspicious microcalcifications in either breast.

The patient should be repalpated with special attention to the left subareolar region. If there is a palpable abnormality, its management should be based upon clinical grounds. If there is no palpable abnormality, then there are two options. A subareolar biopsy can be performed to obtain some tissue to establish the histology of the asymmetric density. Needle localization would not be required. Alternatively, the area can be evaluated by ultrasound, and if no mass or cyst is present, the patient can be placed into a follow-up protocol.

DISCUSSION

The chance of this rather large, superficially located asymmetric density representing a malignancy in an asymptomatic patient with a normal breast palpation is very low. Asymmetry in the subareolar region is a common mammographic observation. We would strongly encourage the woman to opt for the follow-up protocol. We have found ultrasound to be helpful in this situation because when it reveals that there is no subareolar pathology, this provides more reason to avoid a biopsy.

HISTORY

A mammogram was performed to evaluate a possible right retroareolar mass in this 67-year-old woman.

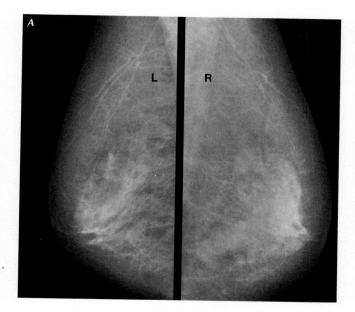

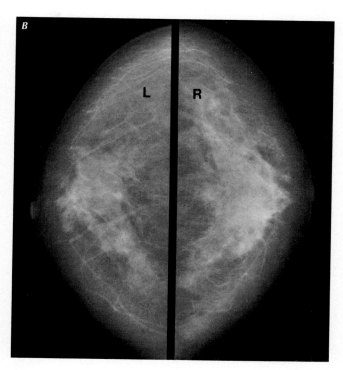

MAMMOGRAPHIC FINDINGS AND RECOMMENDATION

On OBL (*A*) and CC (*B*) views there is increased right retroareolar density, compared to the contralateral left side. There is no defined mass present, nor are there any microcalcifications present in the right retroareolar area. Excise the palpable area.

DISCUSSION

The palpable area was excised, and histology revealed invasive ductal carcinoma. This case is not really an example of asymmetric density but rather increased density on the right, compared to the left. The mammographic findings indicate that there is a right retroareolar process causing more tissue to form. Since the invasive carcinoma was not forming a defined mass, the clinician did not palpate a definite mass but recognized a difference in firmness between the right and left retroareolar regions. If a palpable abnormality is not present, the radiologist should still recognize the difference in density as a possible abnormality. A subareolar biopsy or follow-up should be considered if a repalpation of the area remains unremarkable. In this case, ultrasound may prove helpful in determining whether a right retroareolar mass is present.

HISTORY

Routine chest x-rays were performed on two different female patients.

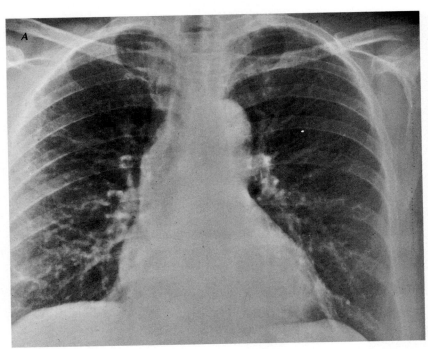

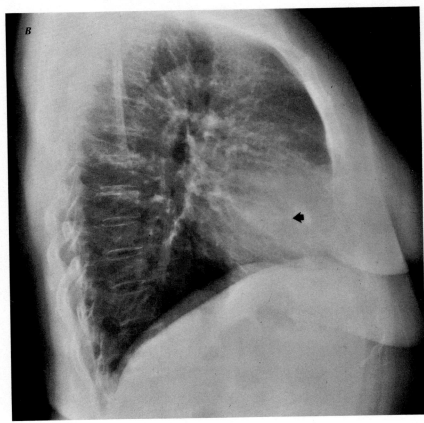

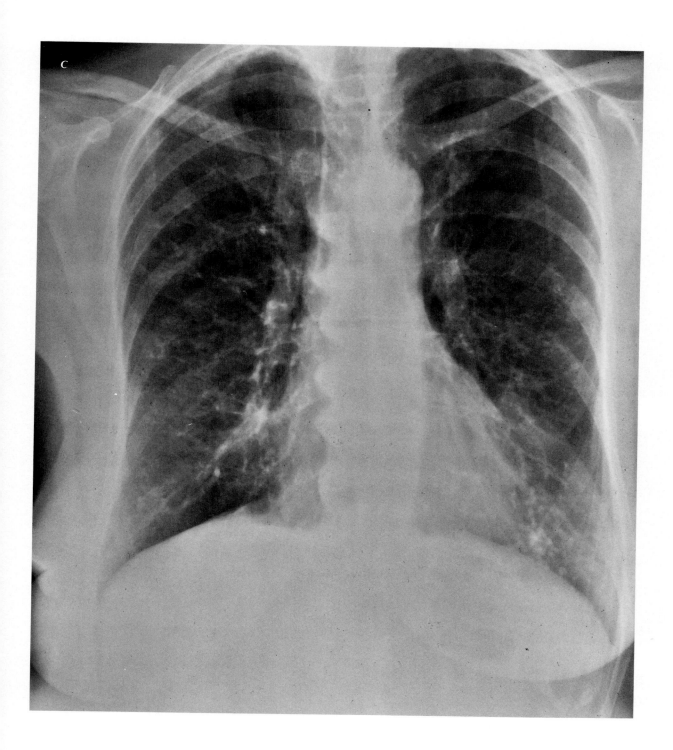

MAMMOGRAPHIC FINDINGS AND RECOMMENDATION

The PA chest radiograph (**A**) from patient #1 was normal. The lateral view (**B**) showed a 3-cm mass (*arrow*) overlying the cardiac shadow. Only a PA chest radiograph was obtained in patient #2 (**C**). It showed cal-

cifications in the left lower lung zone. Both patients had no prior history of pulmonary disease.

Before assuming that the mass or califications are in the lung, we should be certain that there is no breast pathology to explain the findings. This can be accomplished by visual inspection of the breasts or by mammography.

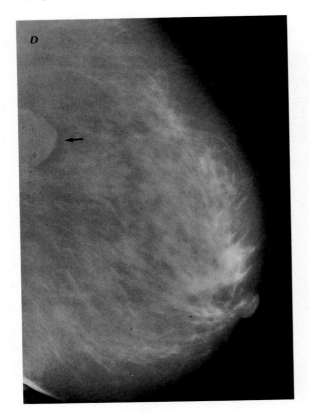

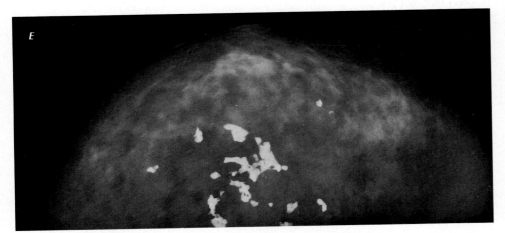

MAMMOGRAPHIC FINDINGS

LAT mammogram from patient #1 (**D**) shows a large lipoma, and CC view (**E**) from patient #2 shows large benign macrocalcifications.

DISCUSSION

Entities in or on the breast can masquerade as pulmonary disease on the chest radiograph, since breast tissue is positioned in front of the lower lung zones. The apparent mass in patient #1 was a skin lesion (lipoma) on the right breast, and the apparent pulmonary calcifications in patient #2 represented benign macrocalcifications within the left breast. The radiologist must always consider the possibility of a breast process appearing as an intrinsic pulmonary process.

HISTORY

Routine screening mammogram on a 70-year-old woman.

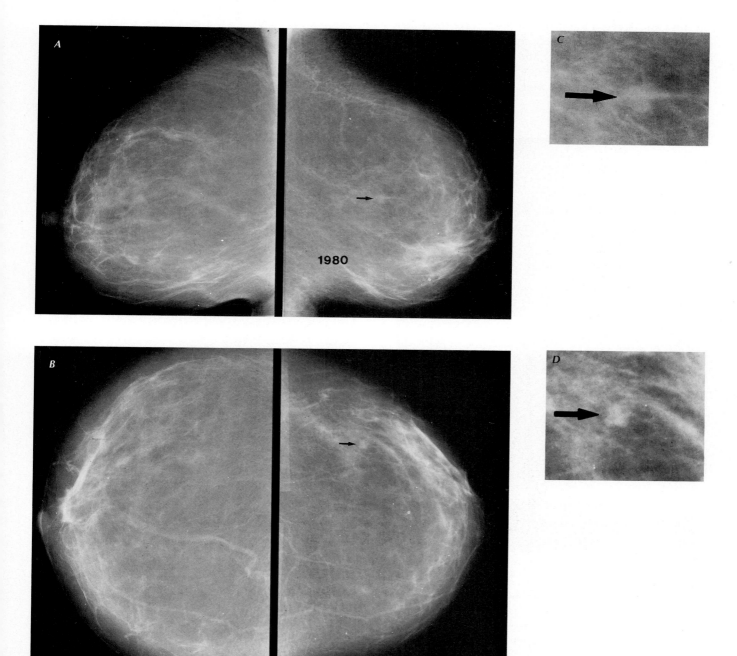

1980

MAMMOGRAPHIC FINDINGS AND RECOMMENDATION

On the OBL view (*A*) and the CC view (*B*) there is a subtle 5-mm mass in the left upper outer quadrant. Close-up views of OBL (*C*) and CC (*D*) projections show that the small mass is not calcified, and though its borders are moderately well-defined, they are not entirely sharp.

This finding was overlooked in the context of this routine screening study. The mass does not fulfill the criteria for a *sharply* marginated noncalcified mass less than 1.5 cm in greatest diameter, for which a follow-up is recommended. A magnification view probably would have demonstrated the irregular margins of this mass much more clearly. If the mass had been detected, the recommendation for management would have been excision to establish the histology of the lesion.

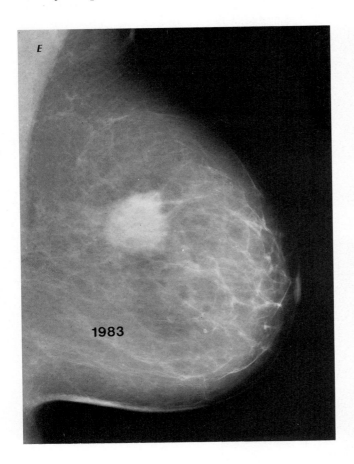

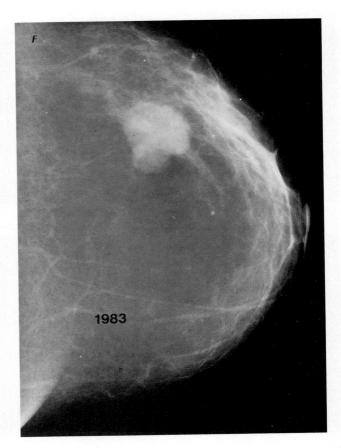

DISCUSSION

Three years later, in 1983, the woman presented with a palpable mass in the left upper outer quadrant. The OBL view (*E*) and the CC (*F*) view show that the 5-mm cancer has grown dramatically in the interval. This case illustrates how the exquisite sensitivity of mammography can detect early occult disease.

HISTORY

This is a baseline routine screening mammogram performed on a 39-year-old woman.

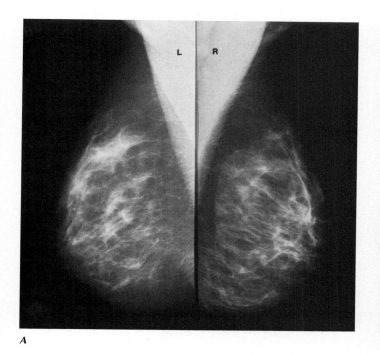

A

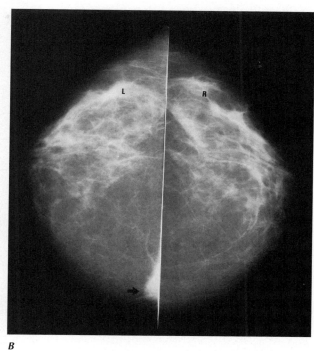

B

MAMMOGRAPHIC FINDINGS AND RECOMMENDATION

Present only on the left CC (**B**) view far medially is a noncalcified density measuring 1.5 cm in greatest diameter (*arrow*). By its appearance and location, the density is consistent with the sternal insertion of the pectoral muscle. The patient should be carefully palpated in this area to be certain that there is no palpable abnormality. Since there was no palpable abnormality, the patient was recalled for a diagnostic mammogram. An exaggerated CC view of the medial aspect of left breast and a repeat CC view of the right breast, with the technologist attempting to pull the breast out as much as possible from the chest wall, were obtained.

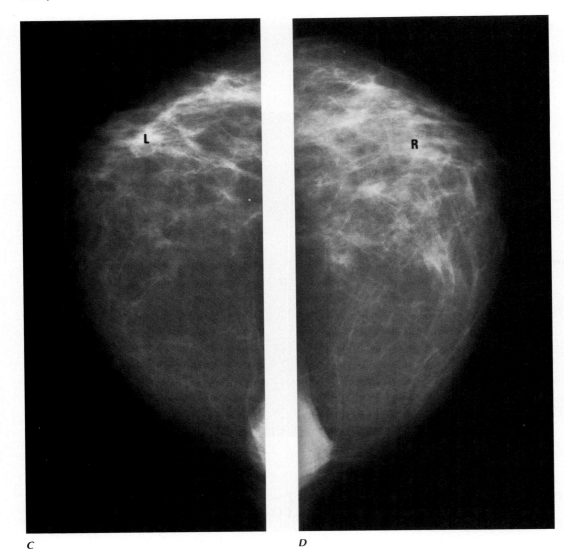

C

D

MAMMOGRAPHIC FINDINGS AND RECOMMENDATION ⎯⎯⎯⎯⎯⎯

The medial exaggerated CC view of the left breast (*C*) shows that the density is still present but has a changed contour and extends over a longer length of the breast at the chest wall. The repeat CC view of the right breast (*D*) shows that a rather similar symmetrical density is able to be produced. The diagnosis of normal sternal insertion of the pectoral muscle was made.

DISCUSSION

The possibility of sternal insertion of the pectoral muscle should always be considered when there is a density present far medially on the CC view. The base of the muscle abuts the film edge and the sides gradually slope towards the apex of the density. This normal anatomic structure is often produced in patients where the pectoral muscle is especially prominent and this is commonly the case in muscular patients. This muscle insertion will be visualized more often as our technologists learn to vigorously pull out the breast as much as possible before applying compression. If there is still uncertainty of the diagnosis, an ultrasound or even a CT scan can be performed to document the absence of a medial mass. A left CC view (*E*) of another patient (*below*) illustrates the edge of the medial pectoral muscle along a greater length of the chest wall.

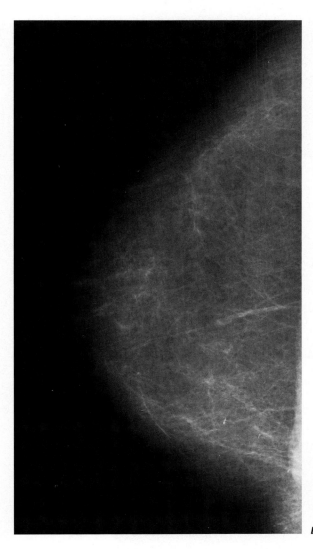

E

HISTORY

This is a screening mammogram on a 50-year-old woman.

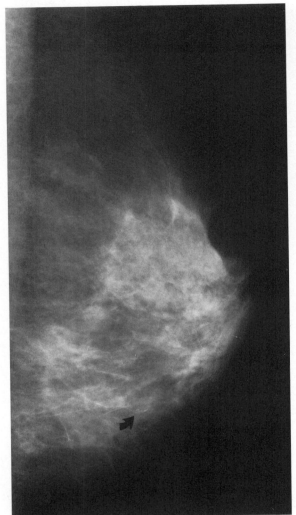

A

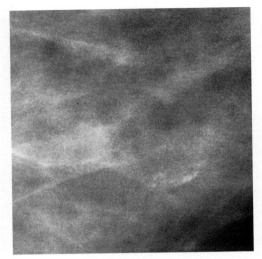

B

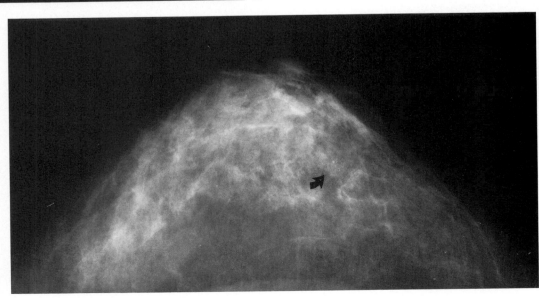

C

326

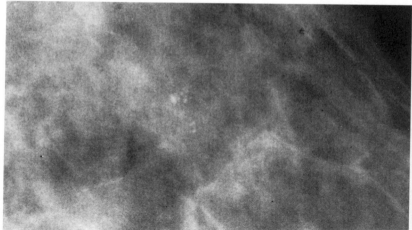

D

MAMMOGRAPHIC FINDINGS AND RECOMMENDATION

On the OBL view (*A*) and close-up view (*B*) as well as the CC view (*C*) and close-up view (*D*) there is a dominant cluster of microcalcifications located in the left lower inner quadrant. The calcifications are quite subtle but number more than five and are of varying sizes and shapes. This was confirmed by magnification views (not shown). Review of a prior mammogram showed that the cluster is new. The recommendation is for needle localization to establish histology.

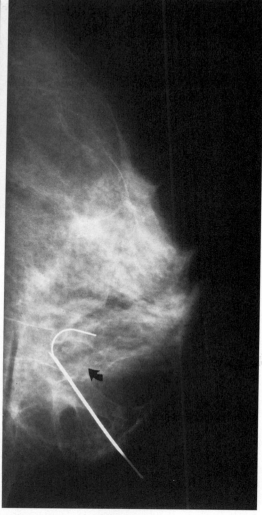

E

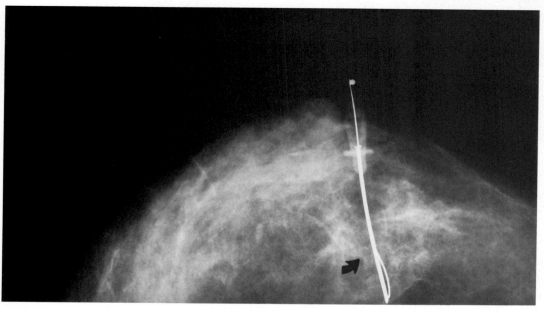

F

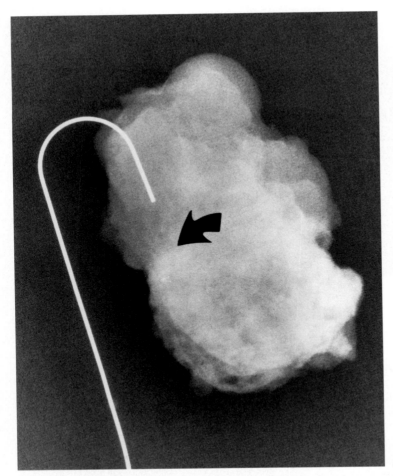

G

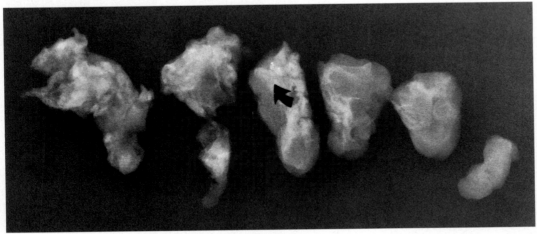

H

MAMMOGRAPHIC FINDINGS AND RECOMMENDATION

A needle localization was performed. The LAT view (**E**) and the CC view (**F**) show that the cluster is within 5 mm of the distal end of the needle. Specimen radiography (**G**) confirms that the cluster was excised. The specimen was sliced and the precise location of the microcalcifications (**H**) was marked for the pathol-ogist. The pathology report stated "Mild fibrocystic change. No microcalcifications were found." It is clear from this report that the pathologist had not identified the mammographic target. The first recommendation was to review the slides using polarizing light since the mammographic calcifications might have been calcium oxalate crystals which may be invisible using regular light. However, even with the use of polarizing light, no calcifications were identified. The next recommenda-tion was to radiograph the paraffin blocks.

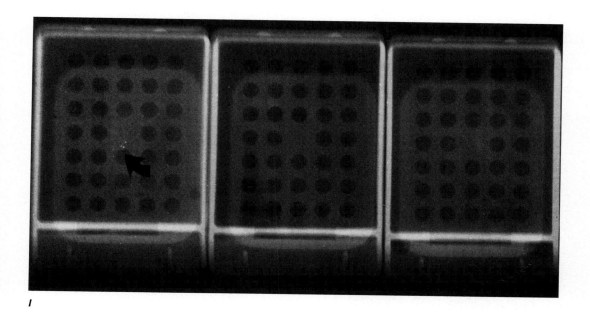

I

DISCUSSION

Radiography of the paraffin blocks identified the location of the microcalcifications. Additional slices from this block revealed that the calcifications were contained within dilated microcystic terminal ductules. This case demonstrates the close interaction required for a needle localization to be successful. The localization is successful when the mammographic lesion has been removed or sampled, and the pathologist evaluates the histology of the mammographic target. Even though there was a successful needle localization and excision, the procedure would not have been considered successful since the calcifications were not identified by the pathologist. This pitfall was avoided because the pathologist and radiologist, working together, recognized that the mammographic calcifications were not identified and took appropriate actions. As illustrated in this case, when microcalcifications are unequivocally excised but not identified by the pathologist, the first possibility to consider is that the calcifications are calcium oxalate crystals and the slides should be reexamined using polarizing light. If this fails to identify the calcifications, the paraffin blocks should be radiographed with the assumption that the calcifications are contained within a block but the pathologist did not section the block deeply enough to reach the level containing the calcifications.

HISTORY ———————

This is the first baseline screening mammogram on a
51-year-old woman.

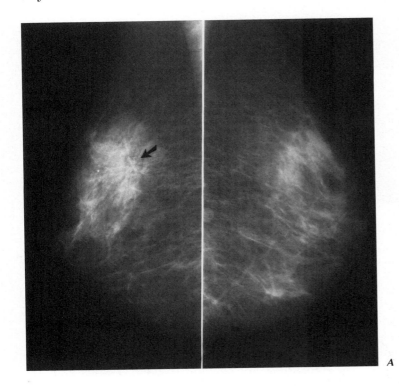

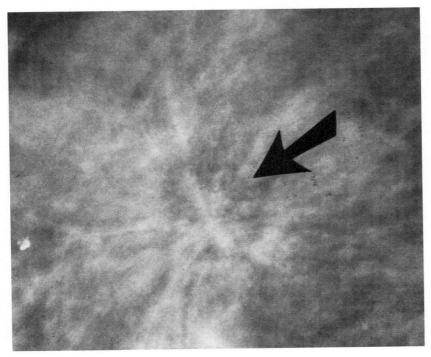

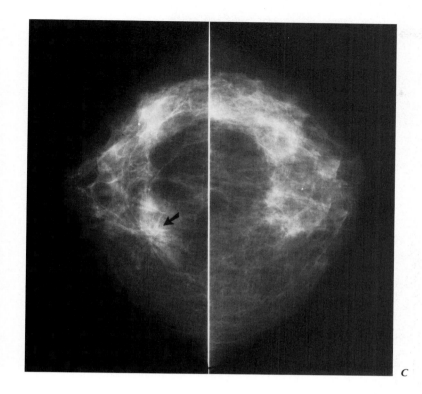

C

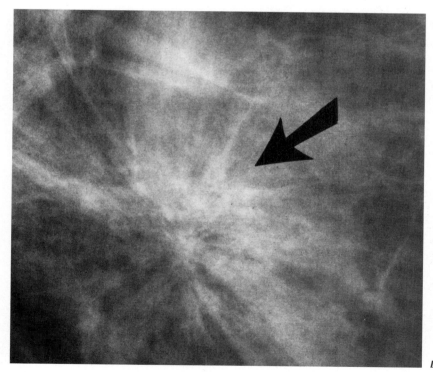

D

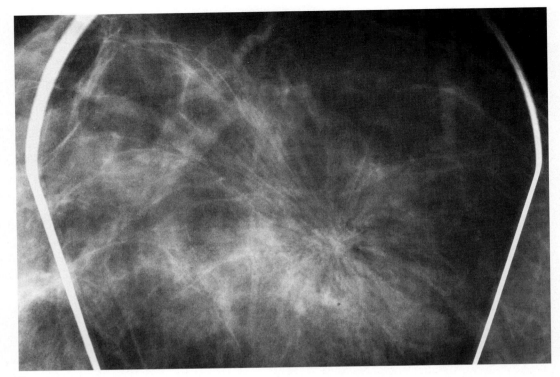

E

MAMMOGRAPHIC FINDINGS AND RECOMMENDATION

On the OBL view (**A**) and close-up (**B**), and on the CC view (**C**) and close-up (**D**), there is an area of archi-tectural distortion. A compression magnification view (**E**) confirms these findings and shows that there are no associated microcalcifications. Since there was nothing palpable on directed breast repalpation, a nee-dle localization was recommended to establish histology.

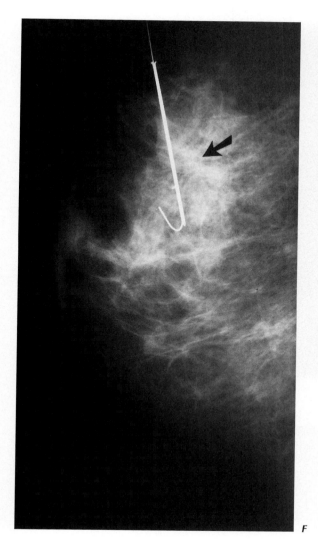

F

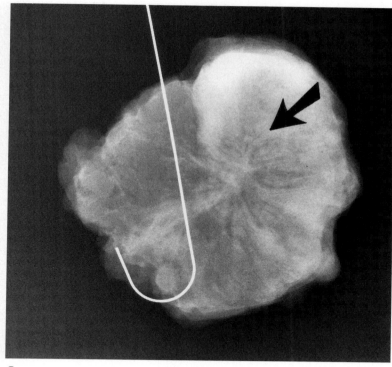

G

DISCUSSION

Needle localization was performed and a LAT view (**F**) shows that the needle is adjacent to the area of architectural distortion. Specimen radiography (**G**) confirms that the area of architectural distortion has been excised. Histology revealed a radial scar. Mammography cannot reliably differentiate between a radial scar and a ductal carcinoma. This radial scar had no central mass. Below (**H**) is an example of a radial scar that has a central mass of elastosis and a different example of a tubular carcinoma (**I**) that has no central mass.

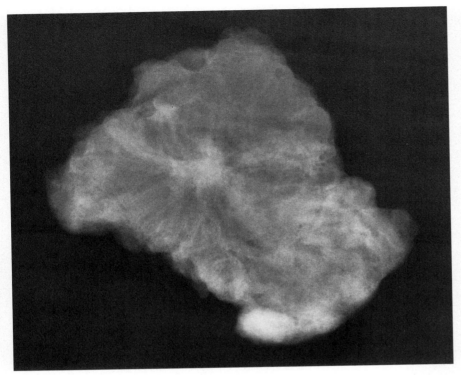

H

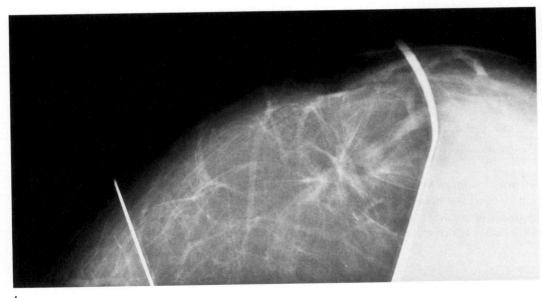

I

HISTORY

This 39-year-old woman underwent needle localization for a dominant solid noncalcified 1-cm mass with irregular margins.

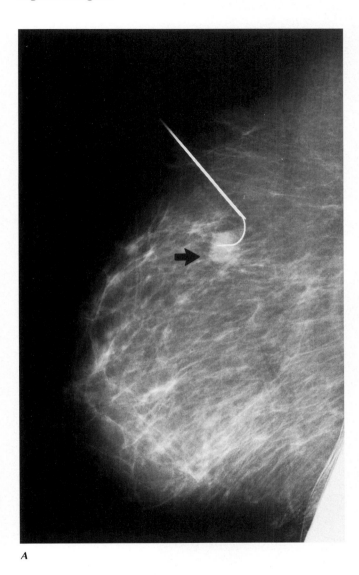

A

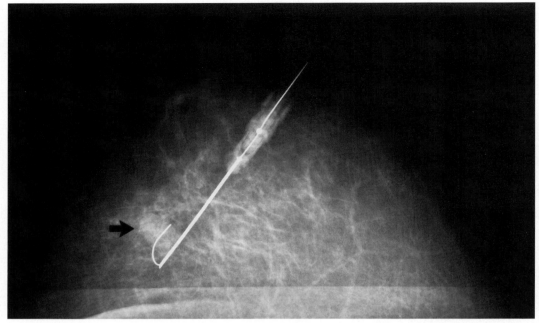

B

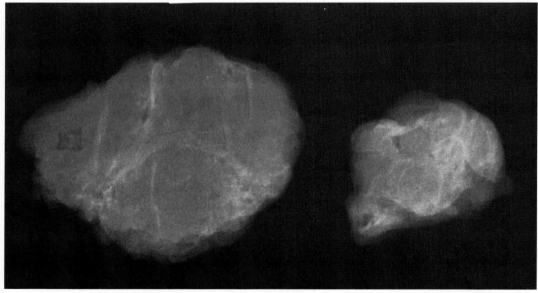

C

MAMMOGRAPHIC FINDINGS AND RECOMMENDATION

LAT (**A**) and CC (**B**) views from the needle localization show that the mass is at the tip of the needle and is skewered by the end of the "J" wire. Specimen radiography (**C**) does not confirm excision of the mass.

The surgery was terminated and the patient was told that the radiologist could not confirm that the mass was excised. The patient was told she might need a postoperative mammogram and possibly a repeat needle localization after review of histology of the breast tissue removed. Histology revealed no evidence of malignancy.

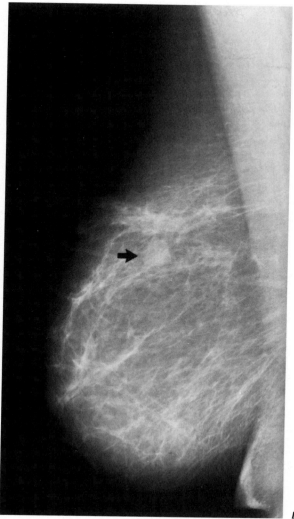

D

MAMMOGRAPHIC FINDINGS AND RECOMMENDATION

The postoperative mammograms (**D, E**) show that the mass is clearly present. There is some postoperative edema at the surgical site. The recommendation was to perform a repeat needle localization.

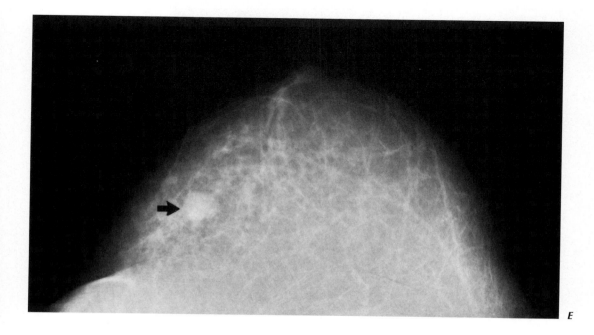

E

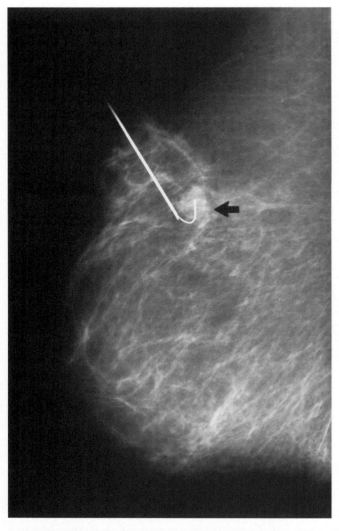

F

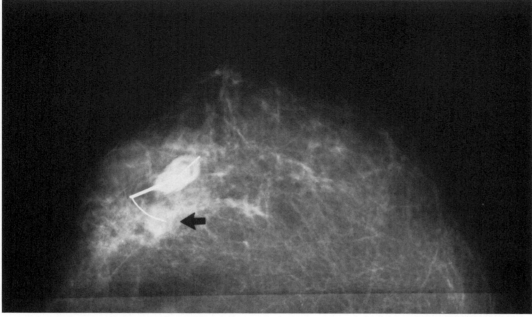

G

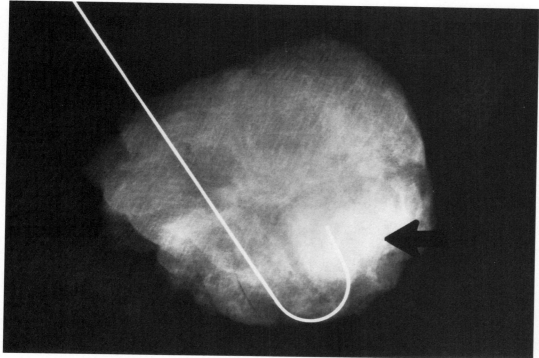

H

DISCUSSION

A repeat needle localization was performed. The mass is again at the distal end of the needle and is skewered by the "J" wire (*F, G*). Specimen radiography (*H*) confirmed removal of the mass and histology revealed sclerosing adenosis. Failure to excise a nonpalpable mass undergoing needle localization is not below standard of care as long as the case is subsequently managed appropriately. We have a failure-to-excise rate of 2 percent and the patient is informed of this during the consent procedure. We await review of the histology before recommending another needle localization since, sometimes, even though the mammographic mass is not excised, the diagnosis of malignancy is still made by the pathologist because of the presence of histologic malignancy which is not evident by mammography.

The repeat postoperative mammogram is difficult for the technologist to perform because optimal compression often cannot be obtained on the recently biopsied breast. In addition, interpretation may be difficult because postbiopsy edema or hemorrhage can obscure the location of the mammographic lesion making it impossible for the radiologist to determine whether or not it is still present. Nevertheless, when the mammogram is performed, one of three possibilities will become evident. Either it will be clear that the mammographic lesion still remains in the breast (as in this case), or that the mammographic lesion is no longer present (such as when a complex cyst undergoing needle localization has been inadvertently ruptured during excision), or that the location of the mammographic lesion is so obscured by postoperative density that it cannot be evaluated. In this last situation, follow-up mammography, after the postoperative density regresses, may allow the radiologist to determine whether the mammographic lesion is still present.

HISTORY

This is the first baseline screening mammogram on a
64-year-old woman.

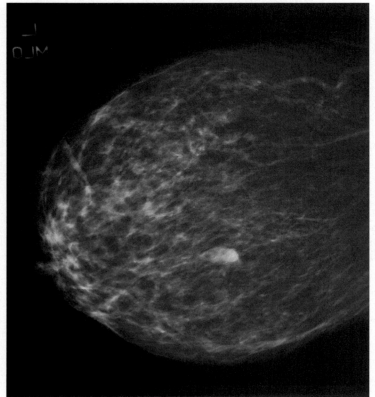

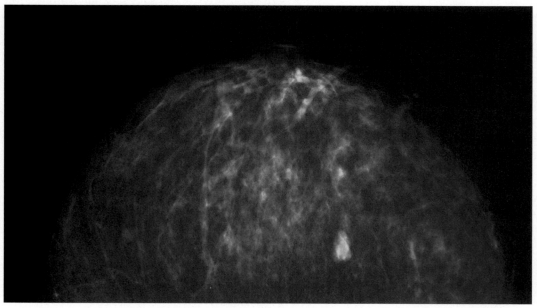

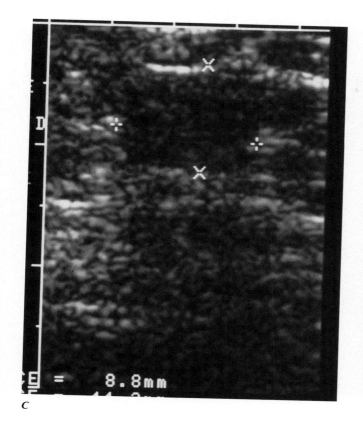

C

D

MAMMOGRAPHIC FINDINGS AND RECOMMENDATION _____

On the OBL (**A**) and CC (**B**) views a 2-cm noncalcified lobulated mass with poorly defined margins was identified in the breast approximately 10 cm deep to the left nipple. Ultrasound (**C**) showed that it was solid. Needle localization under ultrasound guidance was performed (**D**). The recommendation was to obtain a mammogram prior to surgery.

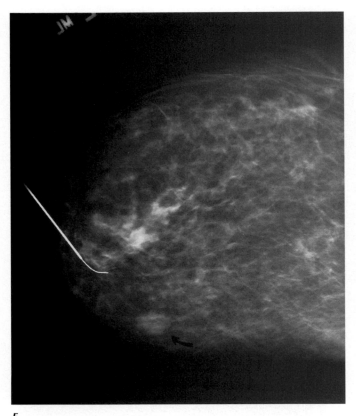

E

MAMMOGRAPHIC FINDINGS AND RECOMMENDATION _____

The preoperative LAT (*E*) and CC (*F*) views showed that the localizing needle was not near the mammographic abnormality (*curved arrow*). Under mammographic guidance (see below) another needle was placed next to the mammographic mass. The CC (*G*) and LAT (*H*) views show that the mass is adjacent to the needle shaft. Specimen radiography (*I*) confirmed excision of the mammographic mass. A second biopsy was performed at the distal end of the needle placed under ultrasound guidance. Histology of the mammographic mass revealed a fibroadenoma, and histology of the second breast biopsy revealed an area of focal fibrosis.

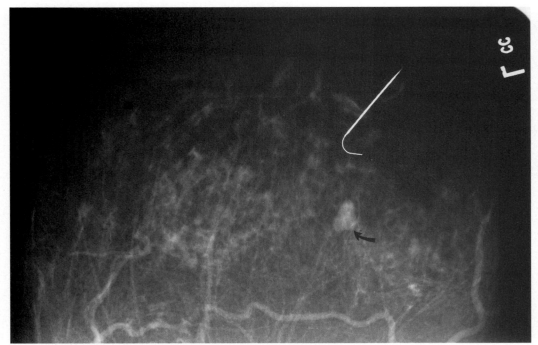

F

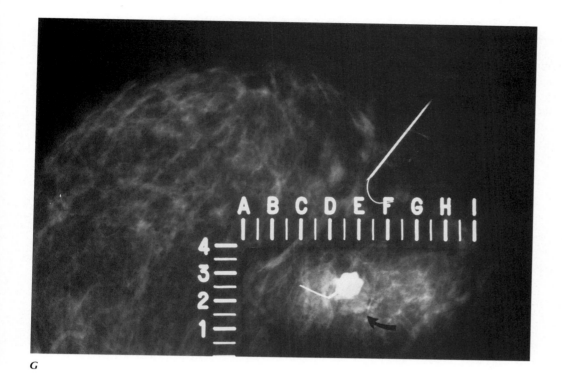

G

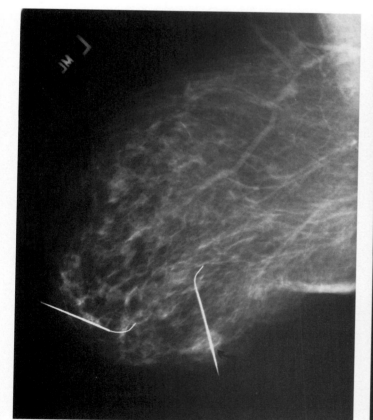

H

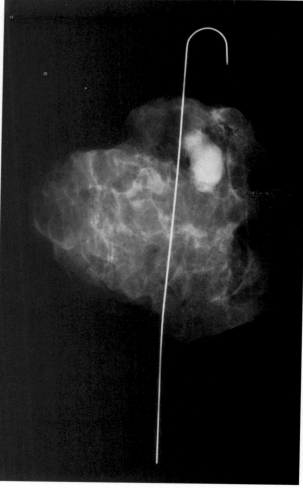

I

DISCUSSION

In every case when ultrasound is performed to evaluate a nonpalpable mammographic mass, the question must be asked whether the ultrasound mass is the mammographic mass. In this case, the mammographic mass was not the ultrasound mass. In one study, it was determined that in 10 percent of cases, the mass identified by ultrasound was not the mammographic mass. (*Conway WF, Hayes CW, Brewer WH. Occult breast masses: use of a mammographic localizing grid for US evaluation. Radiology **181**:141–146, 1991.*)

HISTORY

This 63-year-old woman presented with large, symmetrical, hard, palpable masses located in the 12 o'clock position of each breast. The preoperative diagnosis was bilateral breast cancer and the plan was to perform bilateral mastectomies after confirmation of the diagnosis by either fine needle aspiration or core biopsy. A preoperative mammogram was performed.

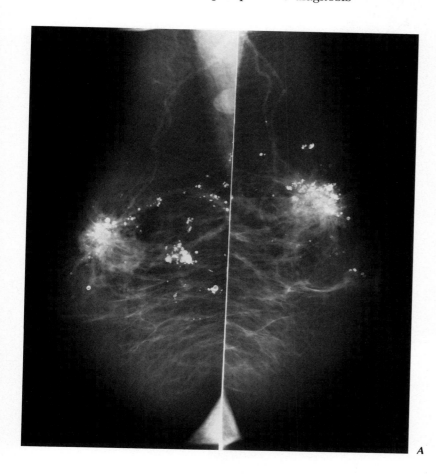

A

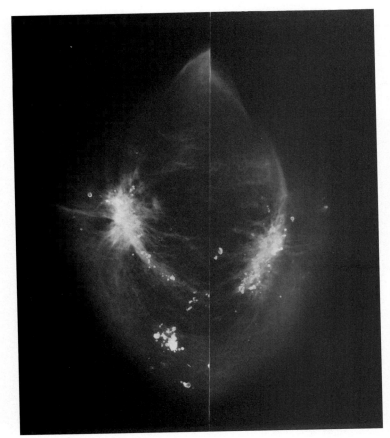

B

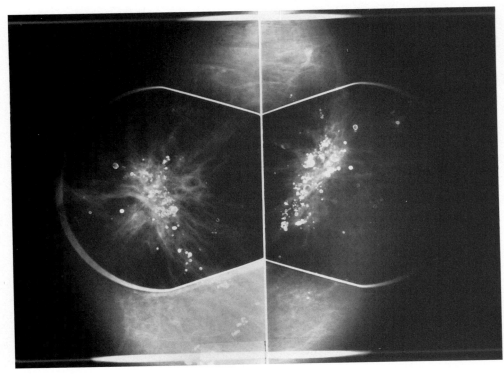

C

MAMMOGRAPHIC FINDINGS AND RECOMMENDATION

OBL (*A*), CC (*B*), and coned-compression magnification (*C*) views performed in CC projection reveal symmetrical masses containing benign macrocalcifications and rim calcifications surrounding areas of lucency consistent with lipid cysts. The possibility of extensive fat necrosis was raised. The symmetrical appearance also suggested the possibility of direct injection of a foreign substance into the breast. The patient was Asian and could not speak English so her daughter acted as the translator. The patient denied any trauma to the area or injections into the breast. Nevertheless, because the mammographic findings were not those of malignancy, the surgery was temporarily deferred.

DISCUSSION

The patient returned several days later with another family member acting as a translator. She finally admitted that many years earlier she had a substance injected into both breasts to make them firmer. She did not know what substance was injected. She said that she did not want to admit this in front of her daughter. Patient denial is not uncommon with breast problems. The usual case is the patient who has a lump but does not tell her primary care physician or the radiologist because she believes that if they cannot find anything on their own, the lump cannot be breast cancer.

HISTORY

This 67-year-old woman was referred to New England Medical Center after failure to excise a cluster of microcalcifications. A repeat needle localization was performed.

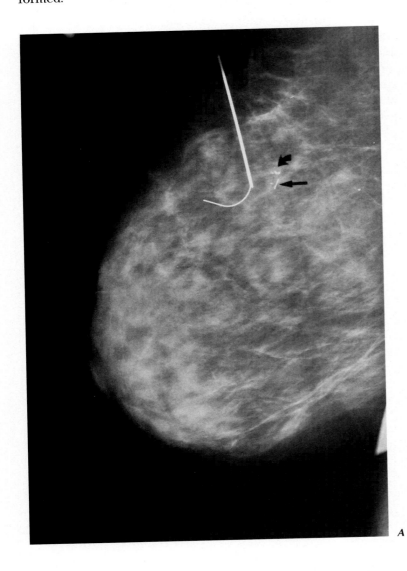

A

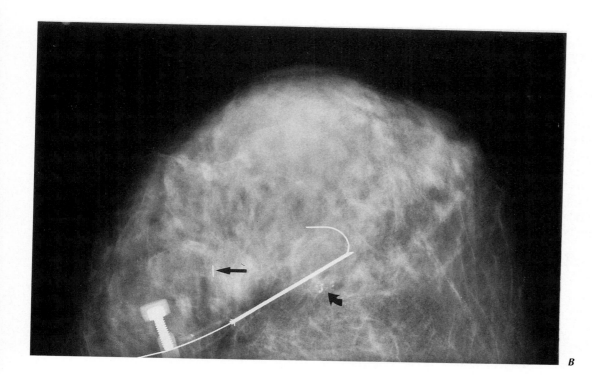

B

C

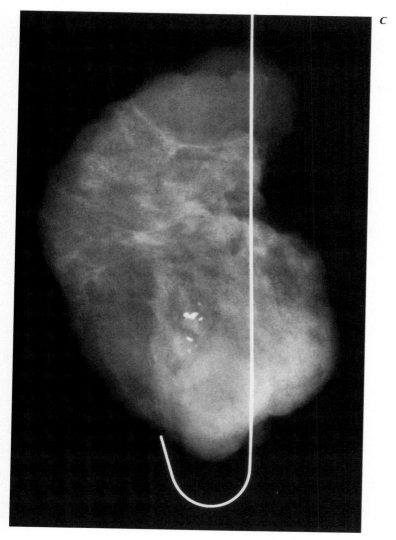

MAMMOGRAPHIC FINDINGS AND RECOMMENDATION

The LAT (*A*) and CC (*B*) postlocalization mammograms show that the cluster of microcalcifications (*curved arrow*) is within millimeters of the distal end of the localizing needle and "J" wire. The localization wire from the prior surgery, performed using a different localization device, had been transected and a fragment (*straight arrow*) remains within the breast. Specimen radiography (*C*) confirmed excision of the cluster of microcalcifications. Histology revealed that the calcifications were vascular.

DISCUSSION

At times, it is impossible for the radiologist to differentiate between parenchymal calcifications and early calcification of an artery. There was no clue from the morphology of the calcifications to have suggested their vascular nature. As discussed in Chap. 15, migration of transected wire fragments has been reported to occur to extramammary locations. There is no way to predict which wire fragments are destined to migrate.

HISTORY

This 53-year-old woman had a routine screening mammogram in 1996. She had known stable benign-appearing solid masses in the right breast which were thought most likely to represent intramammary lymph nodes.

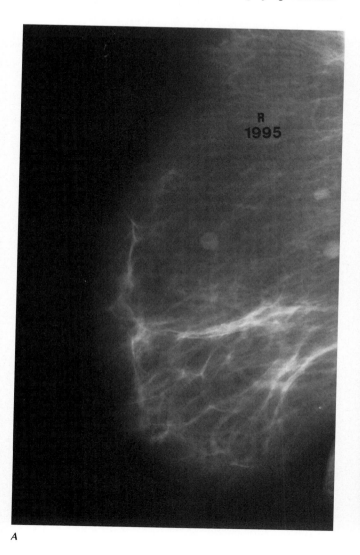

A

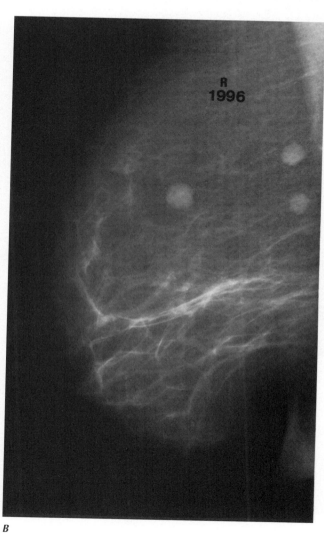

B

MAMMOGRAPHIC FINDINGS AND RECOMMENDATION

These LAT views show that, between 1995 (*A*) and 1996 (*B*), the three masses became larger. They maintained their sharp margins and remained noncalcified.

The possibility of reactive nodes was considered. A careful inspection of the skin revealed that the patient had recently developed a severe dermatitis beneath her right breast and she had just begun treatment. It was recommended that a repeat mammogram of the right breast be performed when the dermatitis resolved.

351

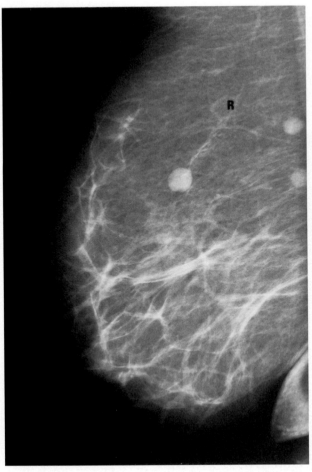

C

DISCUSSION

This LAT view obtained 2 months later (*C*) shows that the masses are decreasing in size. The differential diagnosis of reactive lymph nodes includes both benign and malignant etiologies. Regarding malignant etiologies, the concern was that the findings might be caused by an occult breast cancer spreading to adjacent intramammary lymph nodes. Although certainly a possibility, this was considered less likely because the breasts were almost completely replaced by fat, making the sensitivity of the mammographic examination in detecting occult cancer high. When the technologist is inspecting the breast prior to the performance of the mammogram, she should be trained to carefully inspect all surfaces of the breast, including the skin medially and inferiorly. In large-breasted women, visualization of these surfaces often requires the technologist to lift up the breasts to inspect the undersurfaces, and spread the breasts apart to inspect the medial surfaces.

HISTORY

This first baseline screening mammogram on a 62-year-old woman showed a well-defined, noncalcified 2-cm mass in the 12 o'clock position of the left breast. Ultrasound revealed a complex cyst. A needle localization was performed.

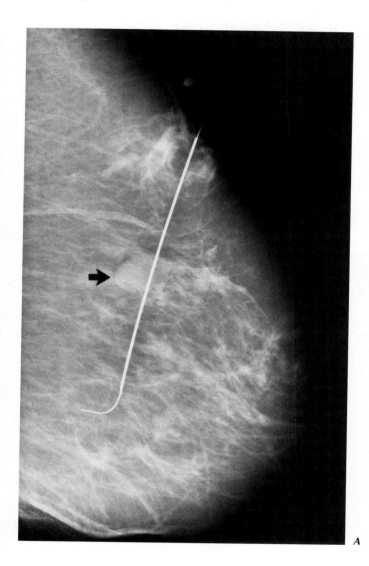

A

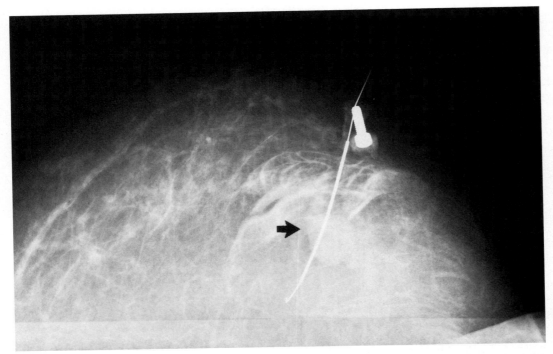

B

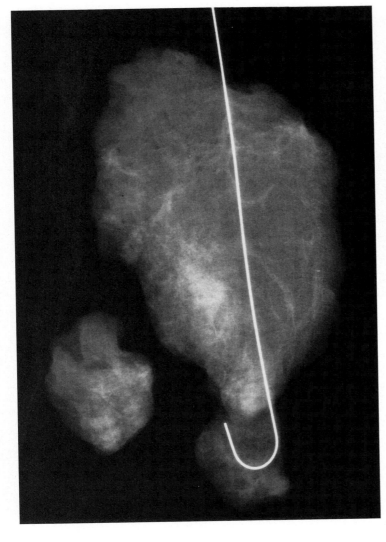

C

MAMMOGRAPHIC FINDINGS AND RECOMMENDATION

LAT (**A**) and CC (**B**) postlocalization films show that the mass (*arrow*) is skewered by the localization needle. A specimen radiograph (**C**) does not show the mass. The surgeon reported that during his dissection, he ruptured a cyst. Histology of the excised tissue revealed no evidence of malignancy. The recommendation was for a postoperative mammogram to be performed within the month.

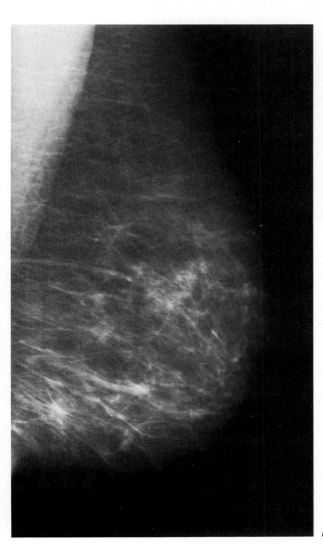

D

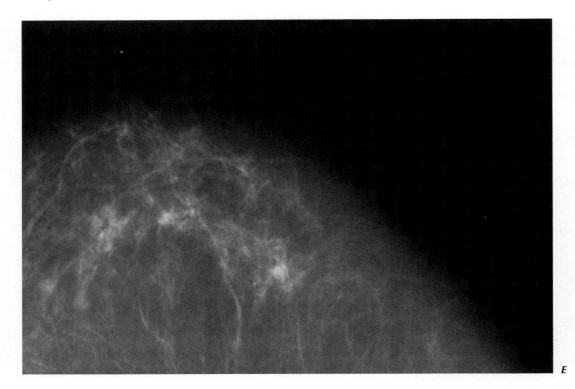

E

DISCUSSION

The LAT (*D*) and CC (*E*) views of the postoperative mammogram show no evidence of the mass. It is my policy that there must be unequivocal documentation that the nonpalpable lesion has been successfully ex-cised or sampled. While it is reasonable to assume that the cyst ruptured at surgery was the mammographic cyst, this assumption is not proof. When a patient undergoes an interventional procedure, it is prudent to document its outcome.

HISTORY

This mammogram and sonogram were performed on a 51-year-old woman who complained of recent onset of bilateral breast tenderness.

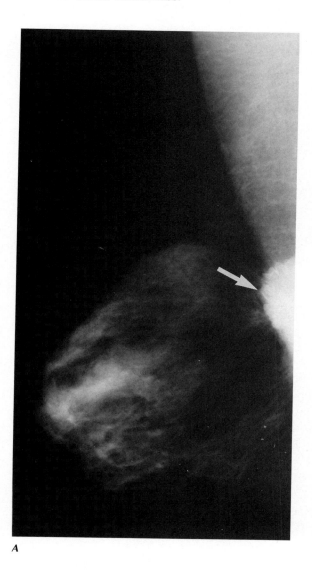

A

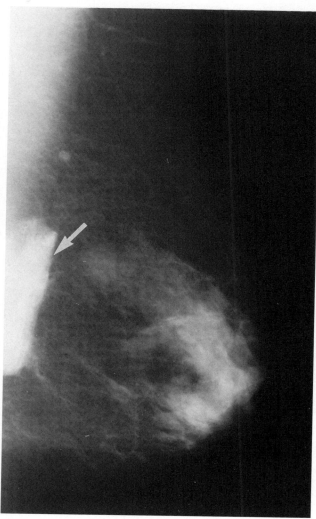

B

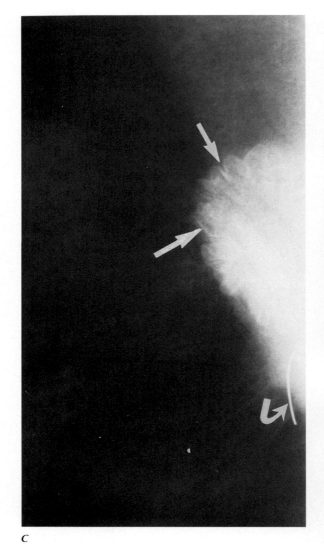

C

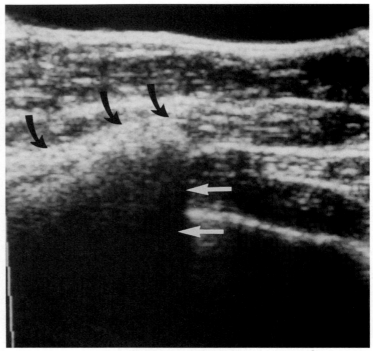

D

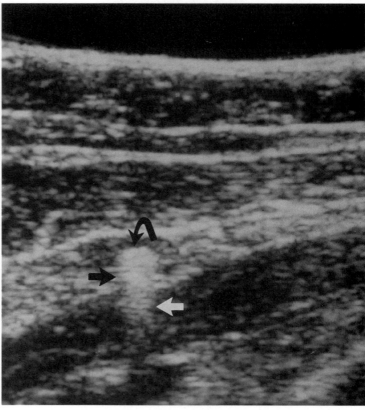

E

MAMMOGRAPHIC AND SONOGRAPHIC FINDINGS AND RECOMMENDATION

OBL views of the right (*A*) and left (*B*) breasts show bilateral high-density oval-shaped masses with lobulated borders (*arrows*). On the CC views (not shown) the masses were also visible and were located posteriorly and centrally. A close-up view of the right breast mass (*C*) revealed fine curvilinear calcifications (*straight arrows*) within the lobulated border. A cutaneous wire marks a surgical scar (*curved arrow*). Similar calcifications were associated with the left breast mass.

Ultrasound (*D*) revealed bilateral well-defined horizontally oriented echogenic areas (*curved black arrows*) with posterior acoustic shadowing and loss of detail posteriorly (*straight white arrows*). The pectoral muscle was obliterated in the area of acoustic shadowing. Ultrasound of the left axilla (*E*) revealed a small highly echogenic area (*curved black arrow*) with a well-defined anterior margin and propagation of echogenic sound posteriorly (*short white and black arrows*).

Additional history from the patient revealed that in 1980 she had saline implants which were replaced by prepectoral silicone implants in 1985. In 1989 the silicone implants were removed. The recommendation was to perform future mammography as per usual clinical indications.

DISCUSSION

At the time of surgical explantation, the silicone implants were removed through the capsulotomy incisions and the fibrous capsules were left in place. The mammographic masses represented the collapsed fibrous capsules which had developed capsular calcifications. The hyperechoic areas with acoustic shadowing demonstrated by sonography represented the collapsed fibrous capsules which may have contained some free silicone. The highly echogenic focus in the axilla represented silicone within a lymph node. Since no residual seromas or hematomas were identified, and since the small amount of silicone in the left axilla was causing the patient no problems, no further imaging studies were indicated.

HISTORY

This 46-year-old woman presented for evaluation of painful thickening associated with a hard mass in the left upper outer quadrant. There was a history of prior trauma.

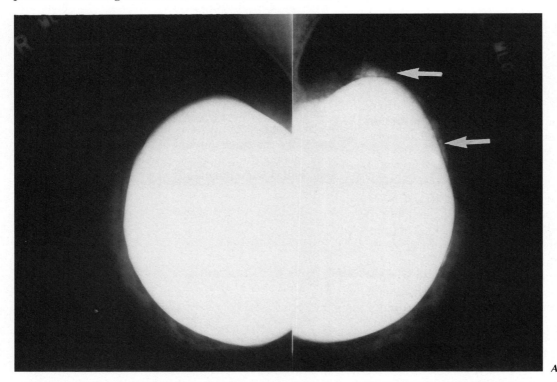

A

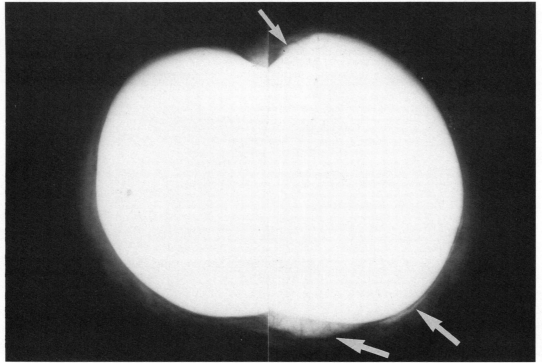

B

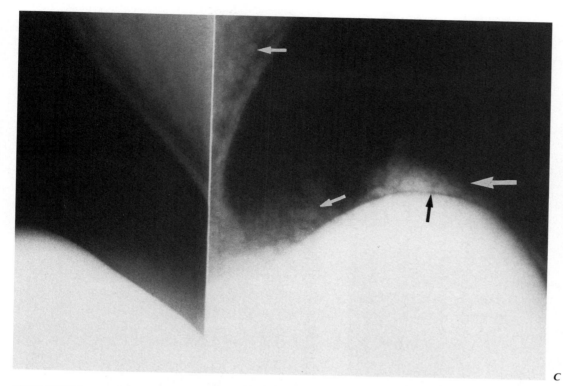

C

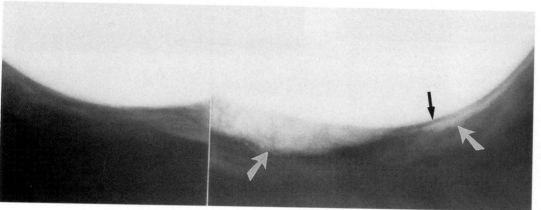

D

MAMMOGRAPHIC FINDINGS AND RECOMMENDATION

Side-by-side MLO (**A**) and CC (**B**) views revealed bilateral prepectoral silicone implants. Confluent collections of silicone are adjacent to the left implant (*arrows*). A close-up MLO view (**C**) of the left breast shows to better advantage the confluent collection of silicone (*long white arrow*) and smaller silicone globules (*short white arrows*) extending into the axilla. A close-up CC view of the medial aspect of the left breast implant (**D**) also demonstrates confluent collections of silicone (*white arrows*) in adjacent breast tissue.

A line of demarcation (*black arrows*) in panels **C** and **D** is evident between the more radiopaque silicone implant and the adjacent, less opaque free silicone. Implant rupture was diagnosed. An ultrasound was recommended to better evaluate the extent of spread of the free silicone and to rule out a concomitant breast lesion as the cause of the palpable mass. The contralateral right breast was also evaluated by ultrasound to rule out the possibility of an unsuspected asymptomatic rupture.

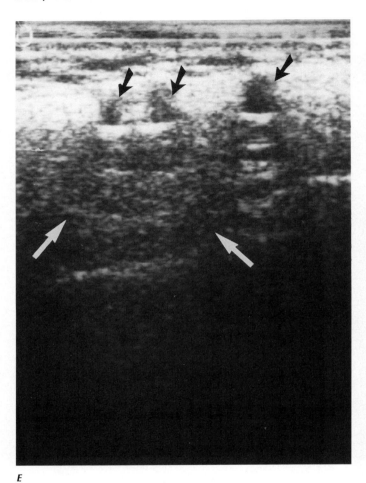

E

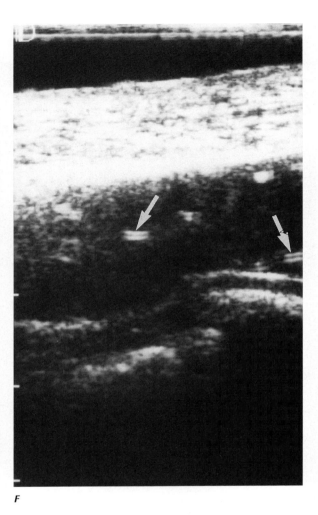

F

SONOGRAPHIC FINDINGS AND RECOMMENDATIONS

Ultrasound of the right breast revealed no evidence of implant rupture. Ultrasound of the left breast revealed no solid or cystic parenchymal lesions. Sonography of the palpable mass (*E*) revealed a highly echogenic area (*white arrows*) with loss of all detail posteriorly. Within the echogenic area are three hypoechoic areas with posterior enhancement (*black arrows*). Ultrasound of the implant (*F*) demonstrated short parallel horizontal lines (*arrows*) and low level echoes throughout. The recommendation was for the patient to be referred to a plastic surgeon.

DISCUSSION

Silicone granulomas associated with implant rupture can present clinically as hard painful masses or areas of thickening in the breast, axilla, or chest wall.

Evaluation by mammography and sonography of the palpable masses can differentiate true breast lesions from implant rupture. Sonography can better evaluate the extent of spread of free silicone. In this case, mammography confirmed the presence of free silicone beyond the confines of the implant. Sonography also demonstrated the presence of extracapsular silicone by the characteristic echogenic "snowstorm" pattern which represents silicone microglobules (oil) mixed within the tissues (water). This corresponded to the palpable mass. The small hypoechoic masses within the echogenic area in panel *E* represent larger confluent globules of silicone which act sonographically like "miniature implants." The short horizontal parallel lines in panel *F* represent the collapsed elastomer shell called "doublets" or the "stepladder sign" which are analogous to the linguine sign seen with MRI. Although initially the clinically palpable mass was quite worrisome for breast carcinoma, the mammographic and sonographic findings demonstrated that the palpable area represented a foreign body granulomatous reaction to the free silicone resulting from an extracapsular implant rupture.

HISTORY

This 54-year-old woman had a prior history of right breast cancer treated by mastectomy followed by a TRAM flap reconstruction. She presented for evaluation of two palpable masses in the right breast reconstruction.

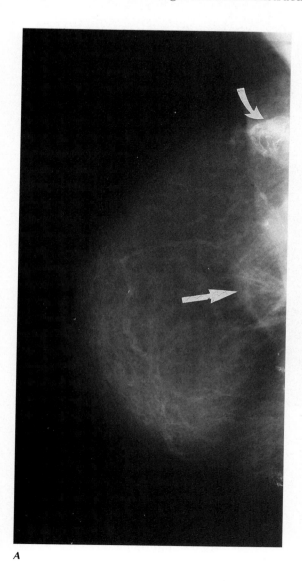

A

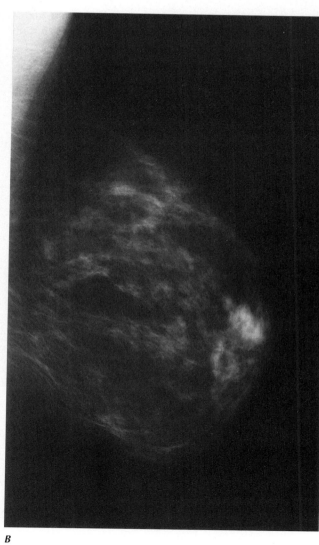

B

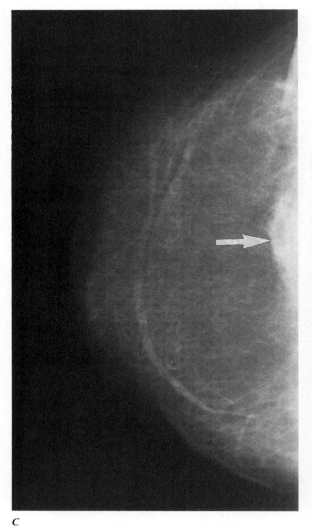

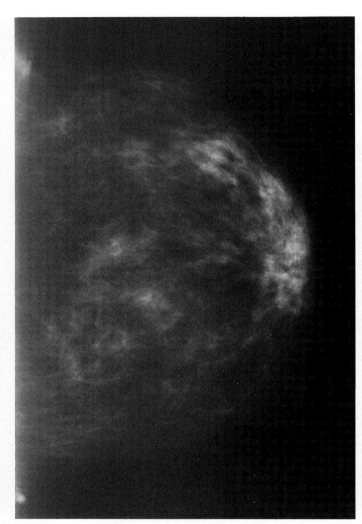

C

D

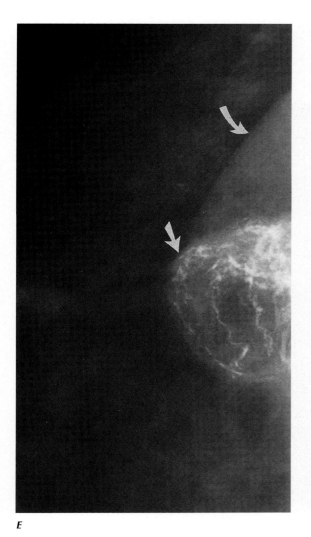

E

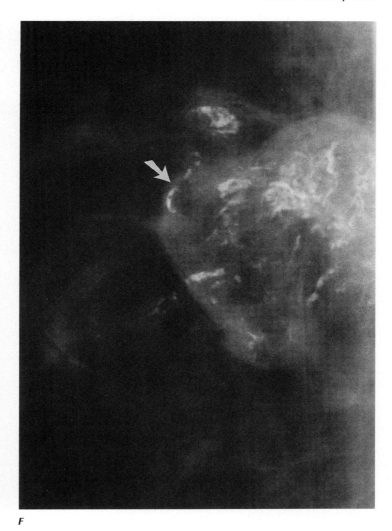

F

MAMMOGRAPHIC FINDINGS AND RECOMMENDATION —————————

The left breast is unremarkable in appearance on the MLO (**B**) and CC (**D**) views. As expected, the right breast mound on the MLO (**A**) and CC (**C**) views is devoid of ductal and glandular tissue and is composed primarily of adipose tissue. On both views there is an oval-shaped, posterior density with a well-defined margin (*straight arrows*). In addition on the right MLO view (**A**) there is a mass containing calcifications (*curved arrow*) which corresponded to one of the palpable masses. Magnification views of each palpable mass (**E, F**) showed the calcifications (*straight arrows*) to overlie the posterior, well-defined marginated density. Ultrasound of the two palpable masses revealed them to be solid and using a metal marker the palpable masses were proved to correspond to the sites of calcification seen mammographically. The patient and her physician were told that the palpable masses were benign and the recommendation was to continue annual mammography of the left breast only in this mastectomy patient.

DISCUSSION —————————

The posterior density with the well-defined margin represented the rectus abdominus muscle. This muscle and its blood supply, as well as the overlying adipose tissue and skin, constitute the breast mound. In asymptomatic patients who have had autologous tissue reconstruction, routine mammography or ultrasound of the reconstructed breast are not indicated. However, in this patient, an imaging work-up was requested because of the presence of palpable masses which were thought to represent recurrent carcinoma.

Although the intact arterial supply is transplanted along with the muscular pedicle, areas of ischemia and fat necrosis can occur with musculocutaneous TRAM flap breast reconstruction. In this patient, an inflammatory reaction to the ischemic tissue presented as palpable masses. Dystrophic calcifications which developed within the necrotic tissue and radiolucent oil cysts had the characteristic mammographic appearance of benign fat necrosis.

Case 65

Case 65

HISTORY

This asymptomatic woman presented for a routine screening mammogram.

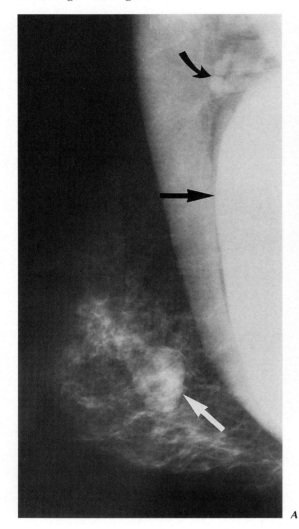

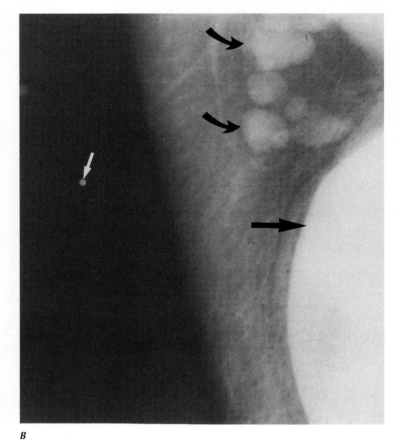

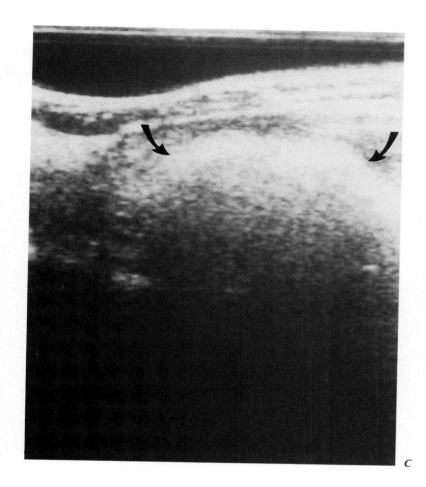

C

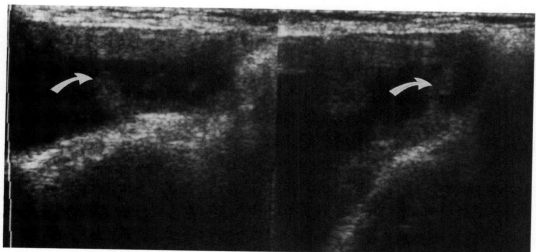

D

MAMMOGRAPHIC AND SONOGRAPHIC FINDINGS AND RECOMMENDATION

The MLO view (*A*) of the right breast revealed a well-circumscribed, oval, high-density mass in the mid-breast (*white arrow*). There is a retropectoral silicone implant (*straight black arrow*) and several slightly prominent axillary lymph nodes (*curved black arrow*). A coned view (*B*) shows that the lymph nodes (*curved arrows*) are less radiopaque than the adjacent silicone implant (*straight arrow*). A metal marker (*white arrow*) had been placed on the skin over an area of echogenicity in the axilla which was identified by sonography.

Ultrasound showed that the right breast mass was a simple cyst. Ultrasound of the axilla (*C*) serendipitously detected the echogenic "snowstorm" pattern of free silicone (*arrows*). Ultrasound of the implant (*D*) revealed bizarre internal echoes with bands crossing the entire implant (*arrows*) in the side-by-side transverse and sagittal images. The recommendation was to perform MRI of the breast.

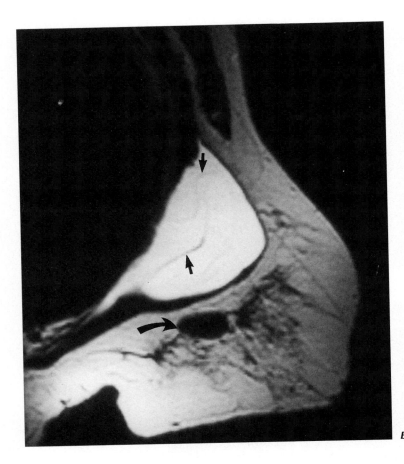

E

MRI FINDINGS AND RECOMMENDATION

The MRI (*E*) revealed the "linguine" sign (*straight black arrows*) compatible with an intracapsular leak. The breast cyst (*curved arrow*) was noted as a dark area on the fast spin echo with water suppression technique. The recommendation was for the patient to be referred to a plastic surgeon.

DISCUSSION

Ultrasound is highly sensitive in detecting small quantities of silicone mixed within the tissues because of the "snowstorm" pattern. In this case, ultrasound detected silicone within the axillary lymph nodes indicating extracapsular leakage and also suggested an intracapsular rupture. The "linguine" sign demonstrated in this patient, is an MRI sign of implant rupture. It represents the collapsed implant shell floating in silicone gel.

INDEX

Page numbers followed by "*f*" indicate figures; page numbers followed by "*t*" indicate tables.

ISBN 0-07-029720-7